Breast Cancer

CANCER SURVEYS

Advances and Prospects in Clinical, Epidemiological and Laboratory Oncology

Published for the

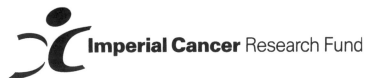

Imperial Cancer Research Fund

Breast Cancer

Guest Editors
I S Fentiman
J Taylor-Papadimitriou

COLD SPRING HARBOR LABORATORY PRESS 1993

CANCER SURVEYS
Breast Cancer
Volume 18

Copyright 1993 by Imperial Cancer Research Fund
Published by Cold Spring Harbor Laboratory Press
Printed in the United States of America
ISBN 0-87969-394-0
ISSN 0261-2429

Cover and book design by Leon Bolognese & Associates, Inc.

All Cold Spring Harbor Laboratory Press publications may be ordered directly from Cold Spring Harbor Laboratory Press, 10 Skyline Drive, Plainview, New York 11803-9729. Phone: Continental US & Canada 1-800-843-4388; all other locations (516) 349-1930. FAX: (516) 349-1946.

Contents

Breast Cancer

Introduction

J TAYLOR-PAPADIMITRIOU[1] • **I S FENTIMAN[2]**

[1]*Imperial Cancer Research Fund, 44 Lincoln's Inn Fields, London, WC2A 3PX;*
[2]*ICRF Clinical Oncology Unit, Guy's Hospital, London SE1 9RT*

Recent years have seen a remarkable convergence of experimental laboratory results and clinical research in breast cancer. At last, there is a new understanding of the biological basis of the disease, and this has led to exciting ideas for innovative therapies. This volume brings together work from both basic and clinical scientists that is likely to have a major impact on the outlook for women with breast cancer.

Cultured cells provide an important experimental system for analysing differences between normal and malignant cells. The well characterized system described by Stampfer and Yaswen for culturing normal human mammary epithelial cells has allowed the authors to investigate the responses of these cells to growth factors and how these responses can change when the cells are immortalized or transformed. They show that the signals generated by activated epidermal growth factor receptor (EGFR) are necessary for the growth of both the cell strains and immortalized cells. However, the inhibition of growth seen in these cells when they are treated with transforming growth factor beta is not seen in transformed cells. Demonstrably malignant cells are difficult to grow from primary breast cancers, so their dependence on epidermal growth factor generated signals has not been directly proven. However, breast cancer cell lines derived from metastatic lesions, mainly pleural effusions, are widely available, and studies with these cell lines, reported by Callahan and Salomon, suggest that EGFR as well as the p185 c-erbB2 receptor may be a suitable target for breast cancer therapy. These authors discuss in detail the various growth factors (including oestrogen) involved in the stimulation or inhibition of growth of breast cancer cells and give an idea of the complex interactions between the factors that may be occurring in vivo.

Recent years have also seen an increase in the efforts of many investigators to identify and understand the genetic alterations associated with the malignant change in breast cancer, and these efforts are beginning to yield exciting results. The importance of this area of activity is reflected in the fact that four of the chapters in this volume deal with aspects of genetic change in breast cancer.

Callahan and Salomon summarize the changes that have been recorded, particularly those causing loss of heterozygosity. The most frequent genetic change seen in breast cancers is in the *TP53* gene, the "guardian of the genome" (Lane, 1992), and a full account of what is known about the function of the molecule and the various types of mutations seen in breast cancers is given by Eeles and colleagues. Although a mutation in *TP53* does not seem to be an early event in breast cancer, the presence of such a mutation in tumours appears to be an important prognostic indicator. Since cells with non-functional TP53 are prone to genetic alterations, it is easy to see why defects in this protein might accelerate the progression of the disease. Since patients can show immune responses to TP53, the suggestion that an immunotherapy based on TP53 may be a viable proposition, made by Callahan and Salomon, should be taken seriously. In those Li-Fraumeni families that have germline mutations in *TP53,* some form of gene therapy may also be possible.

The amplification of a group of genes on chromosome 11, discussed by Fantl and colleagues, was originally identified via the *FGF3/int2* gene, the mouse homologue of which is expressed in a fraction of mammary tumours induced by mouse mammary tumour virus. Although this gene appears not to be expressed in breast cancers, its chromosomal location has identified an amplicon encompassing other oncogenes that are expressed and that might have a role in tumorigenesis. The association of amplification of this region of chromosome 11 with oestrogen receptor positivity is intriguing.

In addition to *TP53*, two other genes are associated with an inherited susceptibility to breast cancer in women, namely the *BRCA1* gene on chromosome 17 (17q21) and the ataxia telangiectasia (*AT*) gene on chromosome 11 (11q21–22). The relative risks and proportions of breast cancers attributable to these genes are outlined by Easton and colleagues. Mutated *TP53* accounts for only 1% of breast cancers, whereas *BRCA1* and *AT* are estimated to account for 2% and 7%, respectively. The cloning of the *BRCA1* gene, which appears imminent, will allow the identification of young women at risk who can then be kept under close surveillance and be given counselling and possible preventive therapy. An understanding of the functioning of the gene product should also give insights into the mechanisms underlying the malignant change in sporadic breast cancers.

Histopathology has always provided a bridge between clinical and laboratory research, and this is even more obvious now that so many molecular markers for nucleic acids and proteins are becoming available. Holt and colleagues discuss how these may be used in diagnosis and to define prognosis, in particular in relation to non-invasive ductal carcinoma in situ. The use of differential screening of cDNA libraries to identify genes expressed at different levels in normal breast tissue and tumours could lead to the identification of other markers and may further our understanding of the phenotype of the malignant or potentially malignant cells.

In the past 10 years or so, great advances have been made in understanding some of the mechanisms involved in antigen presentation to and recognition by cells of the immune system. These advances, together with the identification of specific tumour associated antigens, give new hope for using the host defence mechanisms to reject tumours. The possibility of applying immunotherapy to breast cancer is discussed by Burchell and colleagues, with particular reference to the use of antigens based on the products of the *MUC1* gene. The product of this gene, polymorphic epithelial mucin (PEM), is expressed by normal epithelial cells but is overexpressed and aberrantly glycosylated in tumours. There are good reasons to expect that effective immunogens based on PEM will be found, since cellular and humoral responses to PEM have been detected in both breast and ovarian cancer patients, and the cytotoxic T cells recognizing this antigen are not dependent on presentation by HLA class I molecules. Clearly, antigen presentation is of crucial importance, since tumours have not been rejected in cancer patients even though the cancer cells express not only PEM, but also mutated oncogenes such as *TP53* or proto-oncogenes such as c-*erbB2*. This emphasizes the importance of preclinical studies with mouse models for evaluation of vaccine formulations, including the possible use of co-stimulatory molecules, such as B7, and DNA based vaccines. Preclinical studies in a syngeneic mouse model are encouraging, and a transgenic mouse expressing the human *MUC1* gene will provide an even more appropriate model.

Optimization of existing therapies is still perhaps the most important consideration for clinicians and for patients presenting now with breast cancer. Recent research from Guy's Hospital on the timing of surgery in premenopausal women and its effect on prognosis is described by Fentiman and Gregory. Of patients who underwent tumour excision at the time of unopposed oestrogen (days 3–12), the 10 year survival was 54%, compared with 84% for those undergoing surgery at other times of the menstrual cycle. This effect was mostly confined to patients with axillary node involvement, and the data are consistent with tumours being less cohesive under conditions of unopposed oestrogen. Further support has emerged from measurement of plasma progesterone in women with known and unknown last menstrual period. Node positive patients undergoing surgery during the luteal phase (days 14–28) had a significantly better prognosis. There has been controversy concerning this finding, and an overview has been conducted which showed that overall no significant effect was demonstrated but that the heterogeneity of the results suggests that the positive findings are not the chance result of a normal distribution.

Being able to predict response to therapy is clearly desirable to avoid the considerable side effects of some drugs if they are likely to be ineffective. Klijn and colleagues comprehensively review the data on prognostic factors and response to both endocrine and cytotoxic therapy. High levels of oestrogen receptor, progesterone receptor, androgen receptor and PS2 in tumours predict for response to endocrine therapy, whereas elevated levels of EGFR, c-erbB2, urokinase and glutathione S-transferase (pi) suggest a poor response. However, valuable prognostic factors may be worthless in determining response to therapy, and poor prognostic factors may predict response. For example, those tumours expressing c-erbB2 are more likely to respond to chemotherapy, unlike those displaying multidrug resistance. In premenopausal women, the primary tumour and metastatic disease may differ in response as a result of the endocrine effects of adjuvant chemotherapy. These biological markers may eventually serve as targets for new biological therapies.

Advanced breast cancer is not curable, and yet the long natural history of the disease means that it is a very common problem, which is discussed by Rubens. Optimal management takes into account not only duration, but also quality of survival. As more patients receive systemic adjuvant therapy, so the frequency of recurrent disease may be reduced. Bone metastases are a common problem and these can be successfully palliated with both bisphosphonates and beta-emitting radioisotopes, with response being monitored biochemically as well as by imaging.

With breast cancer, our aim is not just to diagnose the disease at an earlier stage and treat optimally with a multidisciplinary approach, but also to identify women at risk so that preventive strategies may be used. Morrow and Jordan review this timely topic, focusing on the use of tamoxifen, in the context of the National Surgical Adjuvant Breast Project trial which is now running in the USA. They conclude that although tamoxifen is likely to prove both safe and effective, there are some unanswered questions with regard to long term toxicity, and this must be determined by a prospective randomized trial.

In considering the body of breast cancer related work produced by scientists and clinicians, a survey of which is presented here, it becomes very clear that interaction between the laboratory and the clinic continues to be vital to progress in the development of diagnostic procedures and therapies. Although the clinical relevance of some laboratory research is still a distant prospect, much of this research has reached the stage where its "potential" needs to be tested in clinical practice. Dialogue between laboratory and clinic is of fundamental importance, but it is not the only factor that can limit the transition to the clinic, although it is probably the one with which we can easily cope. Other obstacles difficult to overcome are, firstly, the nature of the disease, which means that a long time is needed for evaluation of new therapies, and, secondly, the supply of funds. These factors are of course related, since the pharmaceutical industry must provide the money necessary for large scale clinical trials that in turn require lengthy follow up. The problem is now acute because there are many possible therapies based on the abundant new knowledge and techniques of molecular biology that need to be evaluated. Although these problems are not easy to solve because by and large they cannot be solved by the scientific community acting in isolation, they can at least be formulated, discussed and aired among as wide a range of individuals as possible. One obvious need that can perhaps be met is the development of adequate models for preclinical evaluation and comparison of different therapeutic approaches. The science has advanced tremendously; the challenge remains to make the exciting results coming from the laboratory into a practical benefit for the large number of women who are going to be confronted with the disease. It is our hope that this volume of *Cancer Surveys* takes a small step in the direction of achieving that aim.

References

Lane DP (1992) p53, guardian of the genome. *Nature* **358** 15–16

Culture Systems for Study of Human Mammary Epithelial Cell Proliferation, Differentiation and Transformation

MARTHA R STAMPFER • PAUL YASWEN

Life Sciences Division, Lawrence Berkeley Laboratory, University of California, Berkeley, California 94720

Introduction
Mammary gland differentiation
Growth and characterization of HMEC types in culture
Effects of EGF/TGFA on normal and transformed HMEC
Effects of TGFB on normal and transformed HMEC
Isolation and characterization of the NB1 gene/calmodulin like protein
Discussion and future directions
Summary

INTRODUCTION

The long term goal of our laboratory has been to develop a cell culture system using human epithelial cells to study the normal mechanisms controlling proliferation and differentiation in human cells and to understand how these normal processes may become altered as a result of immortal and malignant transformation. Underlying these goals are four assumptions. Firstly, prior knowledge of normal cell behaviour is necessary to determine what constitutes abnormal and deranged processes. Secondly, the aberrations that occur during epithelial cell carcinogenesis involve changes in the normal pathways of proliferation and differentiation. Thirdly, the understanding of normal and aberrant human epithelial cell growth control and differentiation will ultimately require examination of human epithelial cells. Non-human and non-epithelial cell studies may provide valuable information and suggest areas of research. However, the many differences that exist between these cell types in vitro as well as in vivo indicate that only examination of the cells in question will give an accurate picture of those cells' behaviour. Finally, in a situation where whole animal experiments are not possible (ie with human cells), and thus the contribution of whole body or whole organ factors cannot be systematically examined, the next best option is to develop culture systems that can as accurately as possible approximate to the in vivo state. Since normal and aberrant cellular processes in vivo involve complex interactions within three dimensional organ systems, culture systems need to be developed that can mimic in vivo cell-cell and cell-matrix interactions.

Guiding our work in developing a human mammary epithelial cell (HMEC) culture system has been the desire to facilitate widespread use of human epithelial cells for molecular and cellular biology studies. Therefore, we have tried to develop a system that is relatively easy to use, can provide large quantities of uniform cell populations and is relatively well defined. At the same time, there has been the need to balance the goals of making the system as amenable as possible to widespread use with the goal of trying to optimize the ability of the system to reflect in vivo biology. In considering possible use of this HMEC system, we first broadly formulated the questions that we would want to be able to address with it. The direction of system development has been influenced by the following general questions. Firstly, what are the differences in growth control between cells that are actively cycling and those that have ceased cycling through senescence? Secondly, what are the differences between cells that are cycling but have a finite lifespan and those that are capable of indefinite lifespan (ie transformed to immortality)? Thirdly, what are the differences between cells that require a specific growth factor, or are sensitive to specific growth inhibitors, and those whose growth is no longer responsive to these factors? Fourthly, what conditions influence expression of differentiated properties, and how does expression of differentiation interface with the controls on proliferation? Finally, what is the interface between differentiation and carcinogenesis, for example how does the differentiated state of a cell influence its capacity to become malignantly transformed, and how might superimposition of differentiated properties upon transformed cells influence their malignant behaviour?

We focused on the mammary gland as a model of human epithelial cell biology because it is the origin of the commonest cancer in women in Western countries, and it has the particular advantage that abundant quantities of normal epithelial cells from reduction mammoplasties and lactation fluids are readily available. Also, abnormal tissues can be obtained from mastectomies and metastatic effusions. In order to facilitate widespread use of this human epithelial cell system, our initial work concentrated on obtaining pure epithelial cell cultures, maximizing the number of cells available for experimentation and developing a serum free medium. We then sought to define the system more carefully in terms of the growth capacity of cells from individual donors, the phenotypes of HMEC in culture and the response of HMEC to chemical carcinogens and oncogenes, including the capacity to transform in culture. More recently, we have focused on positive and negative growth regulators of cell cycle progression. Although some of our studies have addressed the questions concerning the interface between carcinogenesis and differentiation, we believe that further improvements in the cell culture system will be necessary for the elucidation of these questions.

MAMMARY GLAND DIFFERENTIATION

A relationship between transformation and differentiation is suggested by the fact that many cancer cells reflect specific stages in the differentiation pathway of the organ system from which they arise and that loss of response to differentiation inducing agents is one of the earliest observed growth control aberrations in epithelial cell transformation. The human mammary gland, unlike most other organ systems, is not always in a functionally differentiated state even in adults, namely in pregnancy, lactation or involution. Other than cells obtained from lactational fluids, human mammary tissues are not readily available from pregnant or lactating glands. Consequently, analysis of human mammary gland functional differentiation in culture is very difficult. However, the absence of functionally differentiated cells in culture does not necessarily limit the usefulness of cultured HMEC for studies of carcinogenesis, since mammary carcinoma cells themselves are not functionally differentiated.

Although cultured HMEC may be difficult to study for properties associated with functional differentiation, they can be readily examined for the pathway of differentiation we have termed "maturation". This refers to the developmental history of a cell from a proliferative stem cell population to a cell with diminished reproductive capacity to a "terminally differentiated" cell no longer capable of division. The maturation lineage of human mammary epithelial cells in vivo has not been fully defined. The mammary gland consists of pseudo-stratified epithelium, with a basal layer resting upon a basement membrane and an apical layer facing the lumen of the ducts and alveoli. The basal layer of cells does not contact the lumen, whereas the apical layer may contact the basement membrane as well as the lumen. Apical cells display a polarized morphology, with microvilli at the luminal side. The myoepithelial cells, which contain muscle like myofilaments and contract on appropriate hormonal stimuli to cause expulsion of milk, lie in the basal layer. The factors that influence the maturation state of the mammary gland are of particular interest in the study of carcinogenesis because the phenotype of the cancer cells found in vivo, as well as that of most breast tumour cell lines in vitro, closely resembles the phenotype of the normal mature apical cell in vivo.

Examination of keratin expression and other marker antigens suggests that a stem cell population capable of differentiating into both myoepithelial cells and apical glandular epithelial cells resides in the basal cell layer of the rodent mammary gland (Dulbecco et al, 1986). In normal human mammary tissues, basal cells express keratins 5 and 14 and α-actin (Taylor-Papadimitriou et al, 1989). Some reports have indicated that a subpopulation expresses the common mesenchymal intermediate filament, vimentin (Guelstein et al, 1988; Rudland and Hughes, 1989). Luminal cells uniformly express keratins 8 and 18, and a subpopulation expresses keratin 19. Specific epitopes of the large polymorphic epithelial mucins (PEM) are also present. In culture, cells displaying keratin 19 and PEM have reduced proliferative potential, suggesting that they may represent the least proliferative, or most mature, luminal cell type in vivo (Chang and Taylor-Papadimitriou, 1983; Bartek et al, 1985a,b).

Only a small proportion of normal mammary epithelial cells in vivo are oestrogen receptor positive, and this positive population is preferentially localized in the non-basal layer (Petersen *et al*, 1987; Ricketts *et al*, 1991). Cells from breast tumour tissues and tumour cell lines display phenotypes similar to those found in the mature luminal cell population. They rarely express keratins 5 and 14 and nearly uniformly express keratins 8, 18, and 19 and specific PEM epitopes (Taylor-Papadimitriou *et al*, 1986, 1989). About 70% of breast tumour tissues also display high levels of the oestrogen receptor. Vimentin is not present in most tumour cells but is expressed in a subset of oestrogen receptor negative breast tumour cell lines and tissues (Sommers *et al*, 1989). These data indicate that breast tumour cells in vivo and in vitro display a phenotype that in normal HMEC is associated with low proliferative potential in vitro. The question remains whether this association is due to some requirement for maintenance of the tumour state following transformation or to a requirement for a certain maturation state to exist for a cell to be susceptible to transformation.

Another form of growth control displayed by cells of finite lifespan in culture is senescence. Normal human fibroblasts and epithelial cells in culture cease to grow after a fixed number of population doublings, which varies with cell type and culture conditions. These non-dividing senescent cells may remain viable for months in culture, and thus cellular senescence differs from the states that lead to cell death or apoptosis. The biological pathway to senescence (ie the controls that limit the number of times a given cell completes the cell cycle) may also be distinct from the pathways leading to maturation, or to non-dividing and ultimately non-viable terminal differentiated cells, since a cell can become senescent in culture without ever exhibiting the phenotype of the most mature or functionally differentiated cell type in its lineage. Human cells in culture differ significantly from the commonly used rodent model systems, in that escape from senescence (immortal transformation) is common in cultured rodent cells. Spontaneous transformation to immortality is an extremely rare event in cultured cells derived from normal human tissues. In most of the few reported cases of "spontaneous" transformation of human epithelial cells, the tissue source was not fully normal (Briand *et al*, 1987; Boukamp *et al*, 1988; Soule *et al*, 1990). Human tumour tissues frequently give rise to cells with indefinite lifespan, indicative of a fundamental change in growth control correlated with malignant transformation.

GROWTH AND CHARACTERIZATION OF HMEC TYPES IN CULTURE

Unlike most other human organ systems, large quantities of breast tissues with normal epithelial cell content can easily be obtained from healthy subjects. Early studies developed methods to process the discarded material from reduction mammoplasty operations in order to isolate pure epithelial clumps (organoids) free from stroma (Stampfer *et al*, 1980). The epithelial and stromal cells could be stored frozen in multiple ampoules, allowing experiments to be repeated with cells from the same individual. The initial medium developed for growing HMEC, designated MM, contains a variety of growth factors, including insulin, hydrocortisone, epidermal growth factor and cholera toxin, as well as 0.5% fresh fetal bovine serum and 30% conditioned media from other human epithelial cell lines (Stampfer, 1982). In MM, there is active epithelial cell division for between three and five passages at 1:10 dilutions. The cultures show a mixed morphology, with larger, flatter non-dividing cells eventually outnumbering the smaller dividing cells with a cobblestone morphology.

Subsequent studies defined an optimized growth factor supplemented serum free medium, designated MCDB 170, that contains 70 µg/ml bovine pituitary extract as its only undefined element (Hammond *et al,* 1984). In MCDB 170, there is initial active cell division for two or three passages of "cobblestone" cells. These cells gradually change morphology, becoming larger, flatter and striated with irregular edges and reduced proliferative capacity. As these larger cells cease growth and die, a small number of cells with the cobblestone morphology maintain proliferative capacity and soon dominate the culture. We have referred to this process, whereby only a small proportion of the cells grown in MCDB 170 display long term growth potential, as self selection. The postselection cells maintain growth for 7–24 passages (~45–100 population doublings in total), depending on the individual reduction mammoplasty specimen. At senescence, they appear flatter and more vacuolated while retaining the cobblestone epithelial morphology. Self selection can also be observed in primary cultures that are subjected to repeated partial trypsinization, a process wherein approximately 50% of the cells are removed and the remaining cells are allowed to regrow. After about ten partial trypsinizations, most of the cells remaining in the dish display the flat, striated morphology and cease division. However, nearly every organoid patch also gives rise to areas of the growing "cobblestone" cells, indicating a widespread distribution of the cell type with long term growth potential.

Most of the studies described below on normal HMEC biology use these postselection cells, which display long term growth in MCDB 170. These cells are particularly useful in molecular and biochemical studies because large batches can be stored frozen, permitting repetition of experiments with cells from the same frozen batch, as well as from the same individual. Furthermore, these postselection cells grow rapidly (doubling times of 18–24 hr) and will grow clonally with 15–50% colony forming efficiency. The active proliferative capacity displayed by these cells has meant that a virtually unlimited supply of uniform batches of normal human epithelial cells is available for experimentation. However, since the cells with long term growth potential represent a selected subpopulation of the mammary epithelial cells placed in culture, it was essential to try to characterize and compare the cell types grown in vitro with cell types grown in vivo. We, along with other collaborators, have examined the cultured HMEC for expression of potential markers of mammary epithelial cell maturation and differentiation, including intermediate filaments (keratins and vimentin), PEM, oestrogen receptor and milk products (caseins and α-lactalbumin).

Histochemical and northern blot analyses of our HMEC cultures (Taylor-Papadimitriou *et al*, 1989; Stampfer and Yaswen, 1992) have shown that normal primary HMEC grown in MCDB 170 and early passage cultures grown in MM are heterogeneous. Some cells have the basal pheno-type—keratins 5/14 and vimentin positive, PEM negative, α-actin positive. Other cells show the luminal phenotype—keratins 5/14 negative, keratins 8/18/19 positive, PEM positive. The cells that initially proliferate in MCDB 170 have the basal phenotype. However, postselection cells begin to express some properties associated with the luminal cell type, that is, keratins 8 and 18 and some PEM epitopes. Expression of these luminal properties increases with continued passage in culture, such that the senescent cells uniformly ex-press these markers. Senescent cells continue to express the basal keratins 5/14 and vimentin and remain viable. Neither keratin 19 nor oestrogen recep-tor is detected. All reduction mammoplasty derived HMEC thus far examined have shown a normal karyotype (Wolman *et al*, 1985; Walen and Stampfer, 1989), although we have not examined HMEC at or near senescence.

These results have led us to propose that the cells that display long term growth in MCDB 170 are derived from a multipotent cell population initially present in the basal layer of the gland, which is distinct from the myoepithelial cells in the basal layer. With increasing time in culture, these cells are capable of a partial differentiation towards the luminal phenotype. However, the ab-sence of keratin 19 and the presence of vimentin in the senescent cell popula-tion suggest that these cells have not acquired the fully mature luminal phenotype.

Since one of our objectives has been to understand the differences be-tween actively cycling and senescing cells, we have carefully characterized the growth of each cell batch in MCDB 170 until senescence so that the remain-ing reproductive potential of a given cell batch is known. Figure 1 illustrates some of these data from three of our most commonly used reduction mam-moplasty specimens. These observations have shown that cells from a given batch show a consistent population doubling capacity, independent of the number of times they have been frozen and replaced in culture. Cells from a given individual also show consistency in population doubling potential, al-though we have noticed occasional individual cell batches with increased reproductive capacity (eg batch 184SK in Fig. 1). We have grown cells from reduction mammoplasty tissues from 12 individuals aged 16–66 years (mean 26) and from non-tumour mastectomy tissues from six individuals aged 35–80 years (mean 42). We have not observed any significant correlation between the age of the specimen donor and the doubling capacity of the cells in culture. This result differs from some reports that doubling capacity in human fibroblast cells is correlated with donor age (Finch and Hayflick, 1976). This difference might be due to the fact that the HMEC displaying long term growth represent a selected subpopulation of the original cell population.

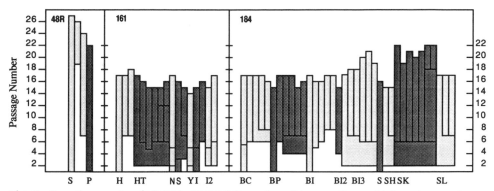

Fig. 1. Growth capacity of HMEC in MCDB 170 medium. Primary cultures obtained from reduction mammoplasties of three individuals were initiated and subcultured as described with about eightfold amplification per passage. The bottom horizontal lines indicate the passage level of initiation of frozen ampoules. The top horizontal lines indicate the passage level of no net increase in cell number. Internal horizontal lines indicate that cultures were frozen and reinitiated at that passage level. The changes in shading indicate cells derived from the different "selections". The letters indicate the designated names for each selection "batch"

These well characterized cell populations represent excellent substrates for studies on human cellular senescence.

To compare growth properties of normal finite lifespan HMEC with those of immortally or malignantly transformed HMEC, we attempted to induce in vitro transformation of normal HMEC. Our aim was to generate a series of cells, from the same individual, that might represent different stages in malignant progression. Primary cultures of normal HMEC from specimen 184 growing in MM were exposed to the chemical carcinogen benzo(a)pyrene (BaP) (Stampfer and Bartley, 1985). Previous studies had indicated that HMEC, but not fibroblastic cells from the same breast tissue, were capable of rapidly metabolizing the procarcinogen BaP to its active form (Stampfer *et al,* 1981a; Bartley *et al,* 1982) Selection for transformed cells was based on the ability of the BaP treated cells to continue growing past the time that the control cells senesced. Treated cultures typically contained cells with an extended lifespan compared with controls. These extended life cultures were very heterogeneous with respect to morphology and growth potential. Often, they represented the outgrowths of individual patches or colonies. However, almost all eventually ceased growth. In only two instances have we observed escape from senescence, leading to cell lines with indefinite lifespan. These two cell lines, 184A1 and 184B5, each show specific clonal karyotypic aberrations, indicating their independent origins from single cells (Walen and Stampfer, 1989). Some of the karyotypic abnormalities found in 184B5, for example 1q22 breaks and tetrasomy for 1q, are also frequently observed in cells obtained from breast tumours (Dutrillaux *et al,* 1990). Upon continued passage in culture, these two lines show some genetic drift, but very much less than is seen in most human breast tumour cell lines. Thus, the vast majority of the cells would be expected to remain karyotypically stable when studied over the course of a few passages in culture, but the presence of some genetic drift could give rise to rare variants in the cell population. Although 184A1 and 184B5 are immortally transformed, they do not have properties associated with malignant transformation. They do not form tumours in nude mice and they show very little or no capacity for anchorage independent growth (AIG) (Stampfer and Bartley, 1985).

We next tried to induce malignant transformation of these cell lines by exposing them to the carcinogen N-nitrosoethylurea (ENU). Selection in these experiments was based on the ability of the ENU treated cells to sustain growth in growth factor deficient media that did not support the growth of untreated 184A1 or 184B5 cell lines (Stampfer and Yaswen, 1992). We were able to induce growth factor independent variants by this method, for example the lines designated A1ZNEB, which does not require either epidermal growth factor (EGF) or the bovine pituitary extract, and B5ZNEI, which does not require EGF or insulin. These variants may represent a further step in malignant progression. However, none of the variants showed AIG, nor did they form tumours in nude mice. Thus, we have not been able to derive cells that showed tumorigenic properties following the use of chemical carcinogens alone. Malignant derivatives of 184A1 and 184B5 have been obtained following transfection or infection with specific oncogenes or oncogenic viruses. 184B5 was rendered malignant by the introduction of the mutated Ki-*ras* or mutated *erbB2* oncogenes (Stampfer and Bartley, 1988; Pierce *et al*, 1991; Zhai *et al*, 1993). A variant of 184A1 was made malignant by the combination of the SV40-T and the mutated Ha-*ras* oncogenes (Clark *et al*, 1988).

Examination of the immortalized cell lines 184A1 and 184B5 for markers of maturation has shown that they express keratins 5 and 14 but at a decreased level relative to normal 184 HMEC, whereas expression of keratin 18 mRNA is increased (Stampfer and Yaswen, 1992). These lines have barely detectable levels of vimentin mRNA and no detectable oestrogen receptor protein. 184B5 strongly expresses the luminal PEM antigens. Keratin 19 mRNA is not detected in these lines when grown in MCDB 170 on plastic. These results suggest that the transformed cells, particularly 184B5, have a more mature phenotype than that seen in the normal postselection HMEC. However, 184B5 still does not express the phenotype of the most mature luminal cells (which is also the phenotype displayed by breast tumour cells).

The cell lines have also been examined for expression of extracellular matrix associated protein and for markers of functional differentiation. In normal HMEC, fibronectin is one of the major secreted proteins (Stampfer *et al*, 1981b). Transformed cells from many different tissue types have been reported to have greatly reduced levels of fibronectin mRNA and protein synthesis. Consistent with this pattern, 184B5, and to a much greater extent 184A1, shows reduced fibronectin synthesis (Stampfer and Yaswen, 1992; Stampfer *et al*, 1993b). Other extracellular matrix associated genes, such as laminin and collagen type IV, are not reduced in these cell lines. We have not been able to detect markers of functional differentiation, that is, caseins and α-lactalbumin, in either the normal or transformed HMEC grown in MCDB 170 on plastic.

EFFECTS OF EGF/TGFA ON NORMAL AND TRANSFORMED HMEC

One of the general aims in the development of the HMEC system was to ask questions about growth control mechanisms such as those controlling expression of finite lifespan, senescence, escape from senescence (immortality) and the role of specific growth factors in normal and transformed cells. This information seemed to be essential for understanding the growth control aberrations that occur during carcinogenesis. We have assumed that control of these processes would be connected to control of the cell cycle and that in order to examine the cell cycle, it would be necessary to obtain synchronized cell populations. Therefore, we began studies several years ago to define a method of obtaining efficient cell cycle synchrony in normal HMEC. In particular, we wanted a method that would not involve use of metabolic inhibitors or general starvation and thus not be cytotoxic or stress inducing.

Early studies on the effects of EGF and transforming growth factor alpha (TGFA) on growth of normal HMEC indicated a stringent requirement for this class of growth factor for clonal growth (Stampfer and Bartley, 1988; Stampfer and Yaswen, 1992), although growth in mass culture proceeded without addition of exogenous EGF. Further study demonstrated that HMEC were able to grow in mass culture without addition of EGF, because of the presence of an autocrine loop resulting from endogenous production of EGF like ligands such as TGFA (Valverius et al, 1989; Bates et al, 1990) and amphiregulin (VanBerkum and Means, 1991). If EGF receptor (EGFR) signal transduction was blocked by use of a blocking antibody to the EGFR, growth of HMEC in mass culture was prevented (Bates et al, 1990).

These results suggested that blockage of EGFR signal transduction might provide a method of arresting these HMEC and possibly of achieving synchronous entry into the cell cycle following release from growth arrest. We therefore examined growth inhibition in detail and measured DNA and protein synthesis and expression of specific mRNA species, when normal HMEC were exposed to monoclonal antibody (mAb) 225 to the EGFR (Stampfer et al, 1993a). Normal HMEC exposed to EGF deficient medium containing mAb 225 acquire a less refractile morphology with increased cell-cell contact. Almost no mitoses are visible after 48 hours. If these cells are refed with medium containing EGF and no antibody, the typical cobblestone epithelial morphology and many mitoses are visible 24 hours later. We were able to maintain cultures for up to 18 days in EGF deficient medium plus mAb 225 before the small amount of continued growth led to confluence. At all times up to 18 days, the cells were able to regain a normal cobblestone appearance, with mitotic activity, after being refed with medium plus EGF and

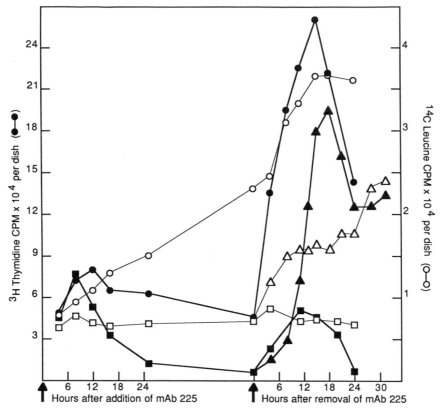

Fig. 2. Effects of blockage of EGF receptor signal transduction on DNA and protein synthesis by normal HMEC. Cells from specimen 184 were grown in 35 mm dishes in complete MCDB 170 until midconfluence. Treated cultures were then exposed to EGF deficient MCDB 170 plus 8 µg/ml mAb 225 for 49 hr; control cultures received complete MCDB 170. After 49 hr, all dishes were washed once with phosphate buffered saline (PBS) and refed. Treated cultures were either refed with complete MCDB 170 containing 25 ng/ml EGF (s) or maintained in EGF deficient MCDB 170 plus 8 µg/ml mAb 225 (n). Control cultures (l) were refed with complete MCDB 170 containing 25 ng/ml EGF. Cells were exposed to a 2 hr pulse of 5 µCi [^{3}H]thymidine (closed symbols) and 80 nCi [^{14}C]leucine (open symbols) in 1.5 ml of medium for 1 hr before and after the indicated times. Total acid insoluble counts were then determined (Stampfer *et al*, 1993a) and are presented on a per dish basis

without mAb 225. These observations suggested that the growth inhibited cells were arrested in a viable, non-cytotoxic state.

To assay protein and DNA synthesis, incorporation of ^{14}C labelled leucine and ^{3}H labelled thymidine was monitored in normal 184 HMEC exposed to EGF deficient medium plus mAb 225 for 49 hours and then restimulated with EGF containing medium (Fig. 2). Protein synthesis remained depressed as long as the antibody was present. DNA synthesis decreased 12 hours after antibody addition and was sharply decreased by 24 hours. Re-exposure to EGF led to a rapid increase in protein synthesis. DNA synthesis resumed only after 10 hours and then increased sharply to a peak around 18 hours. In control cycling cell populations, the pattern of DNA synthesis varied from experiment to experiment, depending on cell density and feeding schedules. In general, control cell populations growing at lower density showed a continuous increase in [^{3}H]thymidine incorporation, whereas cultures that were medium to subconfluent as illustrated in Fig. 2 showed rapid increases in DNA synthesis peaking 15 hours after refeeding. In either case, a steady increase in DNA synthesis could be seen immediately after exposure to fresh medium. A 1 hour exposure to EGF after mAb 225 removal was sufficient to allow the majority of cells capable of cycling to enter S phase. We have examined cells from two other reduction mammoplasty specimens and found similar results. For one individual, specimen 48, DNA synthesis following restimulation with EGF began and peaked about 2 hours earlier. Specimen 48 also showed greater synchrony exiting S phase, that is, there was less than a 10% labelling index for cells labelled at 24–26 hours after EGF restimulation. These results suggested that HMEC restimulated with EGF after the growth arrest were maintaining synchrony entering the S phase, and, at least for one individual, good synchrony could be maintained into the next cell cycle.

We next examined expression of the early response genes c-*myc,* c-*fos* and c-*jun.* Expression of these genes was detectable in normal cycling HMEC cells but was decreased while the cells were growth arrested. High levels of mRNA for all these genes were observed within 1 hour of re-exposure to EGF (Fig. 3). Synthesis of TGFA mRNA, which was also inhibited in the presence of mAb 225, was detected by 2 hours after re-exposure to EGF. Some mRNA species, such as keratin 5 and NB1, continued to be expressed during growth arrest. The pronounced induction of the early response genes at 1 hour indicates the high level of synchrony of these cell populations upon release from growth arrest.

Studies done largely with growth arrested fibroblasts have defined a G_0 state characterized by low metabolic activity, a rapid increase in levels of mRNAs for certain early response genes upon release from the growth arrest and an increase of 6–7 hours in the time required to begin DNA synthesis following release from growth arrest, relative to continuously cycling cells (Bravo 1990). These properties are all observed with these growth arrested HMEC, suggesting that HMEC growth arrest is also in a G_0 state. The HMEC differed from fibroblasts in that the levels of c-myc mRNA remained high throughout the cell cycle, and c-fos and c-jun mRNAs, although showing cycle dependent fluctuation, were readily detectable in the cycling epithelial cell populations.

We next examined the immortally transformed HMEC cell lines for the effects of blockage of EGFR signal transduction on cell cycle progression. In contrast to the normal HMEC, these lines were unable to grow in mass culture in the absence of exogenous EGF. This difference may be due to an absence of a TGFA autocrine loop in the cell lines, since a sensitive radioimmunoassay for TGFA indicated that whereas 184A1 and 184B5 synthesized as much TGFA as did normal 184 HMEC, they failed to secrete this protein (Stampfer and Yaswen, 1992). Consequently, it was not necessary to add mAb

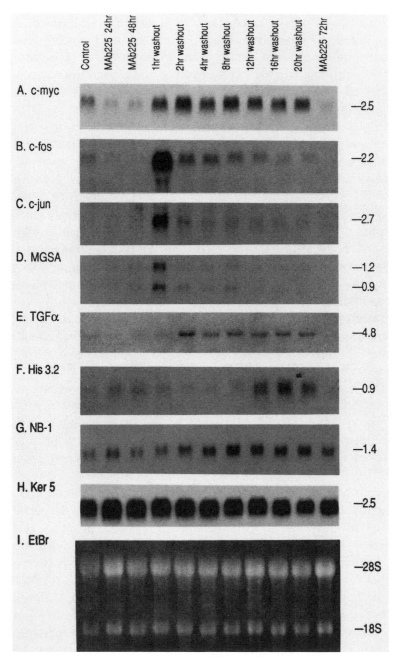

Fig. 3. Effects of blockage and restimulation of EGF receptor signal transduction on mRNA expression of normal HMEC. Cells from specimen 184 were grown in 100 mm dishes in complete MCDB 170 until midconfluence. Treated cultures were then exposed to EGF deficient MCDB 170 plus 8 μg/ml mAb 225 for 48 hr, washed once with PBS and refed with complete MCDB 170 containing 25 ng/ml EGF. Cells were harvested for RNA isolation at the indicated times. Control cultures were maintained in complete MCDB 170 and harvested 24 hr after feeding. Ten μg of total cellular RNA was fractionated on 1.3% agarose/formaldehyde gels and transferred to nylon filters (Stampfer *et al*, 1993a). The filters were sequentially probed with cDNA to (A) c-*myc*; (B) c-*fos*; (C) c-*jun*; (D) melanoma growth stimulating activity; (E) TGFA; (F) histone 3.2; (G) *NB1*; (H) keratin 5. (I) Total RNA in the original gel stained with ethidium bromide

225 to inhibit the growth of these lines; similar results were obtained when the cells were exposed to EGF deficient medium plus or minus mAb 225. In most parameters examined, the two cell lines resembled the normal 184 HMEC. 184B5 had a slightly shorter cell cycle than the normal 184 or 184A1 cells. The main difference was the absence of reduced levels of c-myc mRNA and protein and c-fos mRNA during growth arrest of 184B5. 184A1 did show some reduction in c-myc protein expression during G_0, although levels of c-myc and c-fos mRNAs were not reduced to the same extent as in the normal HMEC. These data are still too limited to attribute this difference in early response gene expression to immortal transformation. Although the cell cycle parameters thus far examined in the immortal cells are largely similar to those of cells with a finite lifespan, the existence of at least one major difference demonstrates that a given parameter should not de assumed to be the same unless shown to be so. Many recent studies have shown that malignantly transformed cells harbour differences from normal cells with respect to such cell cycle properties as cyclin, TP53 and RB function, DNA repair, growth factor requirements and sensitivity to growth inhibitors. We have not observed any differences in expression of TP53 (Lehman *et al*, 1993) and RB between normal and immortal cell lines, and we are currently examining expression of various cyclins and kinases.

These studies have indicated that blockage of EGFR signal transduction is sufficient by itself to cause normal and immortally transformed HMEC to enter a G_0 like resting state similar to the G_0 state described in fibroblasts. The arrest is rapid, efficient and readily reversible, with synchronous re-entry into the cell cycle upon re-exposure to EGF. The growth arrested cell populations have not been subjected to conditions that are cytotoxic or lead to metabolic imbalance, and they remain viable for long periods. Therefore, examination of the synthesis and activity of specific mRNA and protein species as a function of the cell cycle, and the effects of potential growth enhancers and inhibitors at different stages of the cycle, can be easily performed in these normal human epithelial cell cultures. The information obtained about the cell cycle controls present in the normal HMEC can then be compared with that seen in cells whose growth control has been altered as a consequence of immortal and malignant transformation.

An important question raised by these studies on TGFA growth control in cultured HMEC is their relationship to in vivo physiology. Studies in rodents have shown a role for TGFA and EGF in the physiology of several organs, including the mammary gland. Transcripts for both TGFA and EGF are found in the mammary glands of developing and mature mice, and implantation of these growth factors will substitute for systemic oestrogen in stimulating end bud growth in the regressed mammary glands of oophorectomized animals (Coleman *et al*, 1988; Snedeker *et al*, 1991). The localization of the TGFA transcripts in the cap cell layer (considered a stem cell population in the mouse), as well as the enrichment for the EGF receptor in this proliferating cell population, suggests that TGFA may serve as a positive growth regulator in the normal gland. Paracrine as well as autocrine stimulation may be involved in vivo, since TGFA mRNA is also found in the stromal cells adjacent to the proliferating epithelium. Unlike the proliferating epithelial cap cells, these stromal cells contain oestrogen receptors (Daniel *et al,* 1987). In human tissues, in situ hybridization studies show that the majority of mammary epithelial cells express TGFA mRNA, and that the level is increased in mid-pregnant tissues (Liscia *et al,* 1990), with high levels observed in the stromal cells. These data are supportive of a possible autocrine and/or paracrine function of TGFA in humans. The question remains whether an in vivo equivalent of a G_0 resting state due to absence of EGFR signal transduction exists. Such a state could be postulated to have a role in the mammary gland, given its cyclical proliferative activity during the menstrual cycle. However, a mechanism for disrupting the autocrine loop would be required. It is also possible that in normal, polarized mammary epithelial cells, endogenously synthesized TGFA secreted apically may not activate EGF receptors in an autocrine manner. In many organs, EGF receptors have been shown to have a basal location (Bossert *et al,* 1990; Shirasuna *et al,* 1991; Maygarden *et al,* 1992). In such a model, TGFA growth control could be exerted through paracrine function, with the stromal cells synthesizing and secreting TGFA in response to systemic physiological signals. Autocrine growth stimulation could still occur in tumour cells, where normal polarity and cell-cell organization are disrupted.

EFFECTS OF TGFB ON NORMAL AND TRANSFORMED HMEC

Transforming growth factor beta (TGFB) is a potent growth inhibitor for normal epithelial cells. It has been postulated to be a significant modulator of several key physiological processes such as wound healing, tissue morphogenesis and remodelling and carcinogenesis. Malignantly transformed epithelial cells may show escape from TGFB induced growth inhibition—a property suggested to aid in tumour development. Because of the multifunctional action of TGFB in vivo, and its possible role in carcinogenesis, we have focused attention on HMEC responses to this pleiotropic cytokine. Our initial studies (Hosobuchi and Stampfer, 1989) indicated that normal HMEC are growth inhibited by TGFB. Although some HMEC strains displayed continued growth for one to two passages following TGFB exposure, all normal HMEC examined were ultimately growth arrested by TGFB. Cells closer to senescence showed more rapid growth inhibition in vitro at lower TGFB concentrations than did younger cells. Analysis by flow activated cell sorting and by incorporation of [^{3}H]thymidine into DNA indicated that cells arrested in the late G_1 phase of the cell cycle and that the growth inhibition was at least partially reversible (Stampfer MR, unpublished data). The extent of reversibility decreased with cell passage in vitro and was relatively asynchronous. Normal HMEC showed distinctive morphological changes in the presence of TGFB, characterized by an elongated, flattened appearance.

The HMEC transformed to immortality or malignancy had altered growth responses to TGFB (Hosobuchi and Stampfer, 1989). The 184B5 line maintained active proliferation in the presence of TGFB, although it showed some decrease in growth rate at TGFB concentrations greater than 3 ng/ml and displayed some morphological alterations. We have been able to isolate a clonal variant of 184B5 (B5T1) that is severely growth inhibited by TGFB. Other clonal isolates have shown pronounced morphological alterations and reduction in growth rates while still maintaining steady proliferation. The 184A1 line showed a complex response to TGFB: most cells were growth inhibited, but all cultures contained a minority population that continued growth indefinitely in the presence of TGFB, allowing us to isolate 184A1 variants that could maintain growth in the presence of TGFB. This minority population did not simply represent genetic heterogeneity, since four out of four single cell clonal isolates of 184A1 showed the same heterogeneity as the parental population. The plasticity in expression of TGFB growth responses in these HMEC lines has led us to suggest that epigenetic, as well as genetic, mechanisms may play a part in resistance to TGFB induced growth inhibition.

Although growth responses to TGFB vary among the normal and immortalized HMEC lines, all of these HMEC showed a similar profile of $TGFB_1$ receptors, and all expressed specialized responses to TGFB (Stampfer *et al*, 1993b). In particular, these HMEC exhibited strong induction of extracellular matrix associated mRNA and protein species (such as fibronectin, collagen IV and laminin), two proteases (type IV collagenase and urokinase type plasminogen activator) and the protease inhibitor, plasminogen activator inhibitor 1 (Fig. 4, Table 1). The level of overall protein synthesis, especially secreted proteins, was increased following TGFB exposure, even where cell growth was inhibited. Therefore, the HMEC growth inhibited by TGFB were not in a resting state. These results indicate that the effects of TGFB on cell growth can be dissociated from its effects on specialized responses. Thus, within this one cell type, there must be at least two independent pathways for TGFB activity, one that leads to cessation of proliferation and one that induces a specific set of cellular responses that are likely to have a role in glandular remodelling, homoeostasis and/or wound healing. Since both the normal and transformed HMEC express a variety of TGFB responses, this cell system provides a useful experimental model for further studies on the mechanism(s) of these specialized TGFB induced responses.

The immortal cell lines, with their variant cells that display a range of growth responses to TGFB, allow us to compare closely related cells that do and do not retain proliferative capacity in the presence of TGFB. These cells can be used to elucidate the pathway specifically responsible for TGFB growth sensitivity separate from the pathway leading to induction of specialized functions. For example, preliminary studies have shown that the levels of c-myc mRNA and protein are decreased in synchronized populations of normal HMEC exposed to TGFB. However, there is no correlation in myc expression and extent of growth inhibition when 84A1 and 184B5 variants with widely

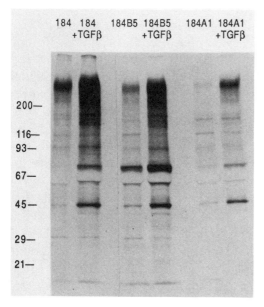

Fig. 4. Effect of TGFB on secreted proteins in normal and immortally transformed HMEC. Sparse to midconfluent cultures of 184, 184B5 and 184A1 cells were exposed to 3 ng/ml of human recombinant $TGFB_1$ for 72 hr. Control cells received no TGFB. For the last 24 hr, cells received [^{14}C]leucine (10 μCi in 1.4 ml). Fifteen μl of conditioned medium from each culture was analysed by 4–20% sodium dodecyl sulphate-polyacrylamide gel electrophoresis followed by fluorography (Stampfer *et al*, 1993b). The prominent band at 220 kDa is fibronectin, as verified by immunoprecipitation with antibodies to human fibronectin. The band at 47 kDa probably represents the 47 kDa PAI-1 protein

different levels of TGFB growth inhibition are compared. In these same cell populations, the extent of RB phosphorylation correlates closely with the extent of growth inhibition (unpublished data). Since escape from TGFB induced growth inhibition is associated with carcinogenesis, an understanding of this mechanism in the immortally transformed HMEC, and its relationship to the other growth control pathways in the cell, might provide useful insights into breast cancer development.

ISOLATION AND CHARACTERIZATION OF THE NB1 GENE/CALMODULIN LIKE PROTEIN

One approach we have taken to characterize the differences between normal and transformed HMEC has been to identify genes that are expressed in the normal HMEC but that are downregulated in the immortal and malignantly transformed cells. Towards this end, selected normal HMEC cDNAs were identified and cloned using probes enriched by subtractive hybridization between the normal 184 cell cDNA and both 184B5 and B5KTu (the 184B5 derivative malignantly transformed by Ki-*ras*) cell mRNA (Yaswen *et al*, 1990; Stampfer and Yaswen, 1992). Several genes preferentially expressed in normal

TABLE 1. Effects of TGFB on growth and on expression of extracellular matrix associated mRNA and proteins

Cell type	184		184A1		184B5	
Growth effect of TGFB	Inhibited		Majority inhibited, some resistant		Maintains growth	
	TGFB −	TGFB +	TGFB −	TGFB +	TGFB −	TGFB +
Fibronectin mRNA and protein	++	+++++	±	++	+	+++
Procollagen a1(IV) mRNA	+	++++	+	++++	+	++
Laminin B1 mRNA	+	++++	+	+++	++	+++
Procollagenase type IV (72 kDa)	++	++++	++	++++	−	±
Urokinase type plasminogen activator (PU/ml)	20	60	52	130	0.26	0.86
Plasminogen activator inhibitor 1 (ng/ml)	190	420	80	260	200	840

Midconfluent cultures received TGFB (3–5 ng/ml) for 48–72 hr before assay. Cells were assayed for mRNA by northern blot. Fibronectin protein in conditioned medium was measured by immunoprecipitation of ^{14}C labelled protein. Procollagenase IV in conditioned medium was visualized by gelatin zymogram; urokinase type plasminogen activator was assayed by radial caseinolysis. Plasminogen activator inhibitor 1 in conditioned medium was measured by enzyme linked immunosorbent assay (Stampfer et al, 1993)

184 cells were isolated with this method, including those for fibronectin, keratin 5 and vimentin. In addition, one 350 bp cDNA fragment was isolated which initially showed no similarity to any sequence reported in GenBank. This cDNA hybridized specifically to a 1.4 kb mRNA, designated NB1, which was expressed in the normal HMEC but was downregulated or undetectable in the transformed cell lines. Sequence analysis of a full length NB1 clone revealed a 447 bp open reading frame with extensive similarity (70%, 71% and 80%) at the nucleic acid level to the three known human genes coding for the ubiquitous calcium binding protein, calmodulin. The similarity between the translated aminoacid sequence of NB1 and human calmodulin was 85% over the length of the entire protein.

With northern and polymerase chain reaction (PCR) analyses, NB1 mRNA has thus far been found only in normal epithelial cells and tissues from human breast, prostate, cervix and skin. It has not been found in normal epithelial cells other than those from stratified or pseudostratified tissues. It was not detectable in non-epithelial cells and tissues, nor in any of the mammary epithelial tumour cell lines that we have examined. Human breast cells obtained from lactational fluids were also negative for NB1 expression with PCR analysis. Expression of NB1 mRNA is not significantly decreased when cells are growth arrested by exposure to anti-EGFR antibodies or in senescing cells where proliferation is minimal, but it is increased in cells growth arrested by

TGFB. Expression of NB1 is reduced in HMEC grown on reconstituted extracellular matrix material (Stampfer and Yaswen, 1992).

Recombinant NB1 protein (designated CLP or calmodulin like protein) from bacterial transformants migrated slightly faster than authentic or recombinant calmodulin in denaturing polyacrylamide gels (Yaswen *et al*, 1992). Like calmodulin, CLP was stable to heat denaturation and bound to phenyl-Sepharose in a calcium dependent manner. Purified recombinant protein was used to develop polyclonal antisera in rabbits, and these antisera displayed a strong preference for CLP over calmodulin. Virtually all remaining calmodulin cross reactivity could be removed by preabsorption of the antisera with calmodulin-agarose. On the evidence of titrations carried out with recombinant protein, the level of endogenous CLP in 184 HMEC was approximately 100–200 ng/10^6 cells, a level similar to the estimated level of calmodulin in other cultured cell lines (Chafouleas *et al*, 1984). The majority of the protein was present in non-ionic detergent soluble cellular fractions.

Using the NB1 specific antisera, we have shown that the relative abundance of CLP reflects relative NB1 mRNA levels in various cell types, being most highly expressed in normal HMEC, lower or undetectable in the immortally transformed cell lines and virtually undetectable in tumorigenic breast and prostate cell lines as well as in normal breast fibroblasts. By contrast, levels of calmodulin protein were nearly constant in the same cell extracts (Fig. 5).

Indirect immunofluorescence was used to study the distribution of CLP in HMEC of normal finite lifespan and immortalized HMEC (Yaswen *et al*, 1992). In normal interphase cells, CLP was present diffusely throughout the cytoplasm and, to varying degrees, in the nuclei as well. During mitosis, CLP immunofluorescence was particularly bright in regions around mitotic spindles. In 184B5, CLP expression was heterogeneous both among different cells and within individual cells. No significant CLP immunofluorescence above control levels was observed in 184A1.

The distribution of CLP in surgical specimens from histologically normal and malignant tissues was compared by means of immunohistochemistry (Yaswen *et al*, 1992). In benign breast specimens from non-pregnant, non-lactating women, the majority of the basal epithelial cells in small ducts stained intensely positive (Fig. 6A). Luminal cells in the small ducts also stained specifically, although not as intensely as the basal cells. In larger ducts, staining was mainly confined to the basal cell layer and was generally less intense than in the small ducts. In all cases, distribution of the protein appeared to be uniformly intracellular. Thus, CLP appears to be predominantly associated with the basal cell phenotype in breast cells in vivo. In contrast to normal breast tissue, sections from six infiltrating ductal breast carcinomas were consistently negative for CLP (Fig. 6B). Serial sections of the normal and tumour tissues all showed abundant calmodulin expression. In normal prostate, nearly all the epithelial cells were stained to a similar degree by CLP antiserum, whereas staining was reduced in tumour derived issues (Fig. 6C,D). In normal cervix and skin, no

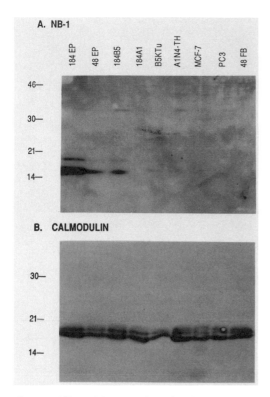

Fig. 5. Differential expression of endogenous (A) NB1 protein (CLP) and (B) calmodulin in normal and transformed cells. Immunoblots of heat stable cell lysates (10 µg) obtained from confluent cultures of normal HMEC strains (184 EP, 48 EP), immortally transformed HMEC lines (184B5, 184A1), malignantly transformed HMEC lines (B5KTu, A1N4-TH), a breast tumour derived cell line (MCF-7), a prostate tumour derived cell line (PC3) and normal breast fibroblasts (48 FB) are shown (Yaswen *et al* 1992)

staining was observed in the basal cell layer (Fig. 6E,G). In the cervix, suprabasal cells were intensely CLP positive, with the degree of staining diminishing in the more distant upper layers. In the skin, the intensity of CLP staining increased from the suprabasal layer to the stratum corneum, which itself was not stained. Thus, in the four different tissues examined, CLP has shown distinct patterns of expression. These results suggest that the role of CLP may be defined by the differentiated state of the cells in which it is expressed, perhaps being involved in the initiation or maintenance of certain differentiated responses.

The initial characterization of genomic DNA corresponding to the NB1 transcript indicated the unexpected absence of introns. All vertebrate cal modulin genes studied to date contain five similarly placed introns (Koller *et al*, 1990). A literature search revealed the existence of a previously reported human calmodulin "pseudogene" *hGH6*, which shared identity with *NB1* cDNA (Koller and Strehler, 1988). This gene was designated a pseudogene since the authors were unable to demonstrate the existence of a corresponding

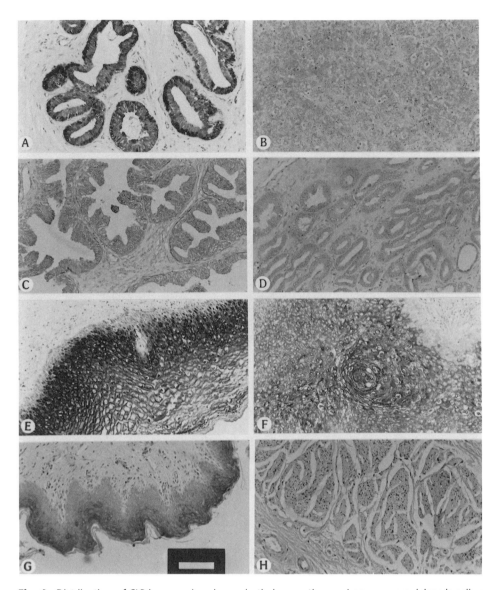

Fig. 6. Distribution of CLP in normal and neoplastic human tissues. Immunoperoxidase localization of CLP in histologically normal breast (A), ductal carcinoma of the breast (B), normal prostate (C), prostate carcinoma (D), normal cervix (E), squamous carcinoma of the cervix (F), normal foreskin (G), epidermoid carcinoma of the cervix (H). Bar equals 106 μm. Paraffin embedded tissue sections were deparaffinized and examined as described by Yaswen *et al* (1992)

mRNA. Our evidence of expression of *NB1* at both the mRNA and protein levels suggests that *NB1* may be a rare example of an expressed retroposon (Brosius, 1991).

External calcium concentration affects the proliferative potential and differentiated states of some cultured epithelial cells, including rodent and human keratinocytes and mammary epithelial cells (Boyce and Ham, 1983; Soule and McGrath, 1986; Yuspa *et al*, 1989). In normal keratinocytes, increasing calcium concentrations can lead to cessation of proliferation and to expression of markers of terminal differentiation. Loss of response to the calcium induced differentiation signal has been shown to correlate with the early stages of transformation in rodent keratinocyte cultures (Yuspa and Morgan, 1981). Therefore, the observation that expression of this calmodulin like protein is strictly regulated in human epithelial cells as a function of the state of differentiation and transformation leads us to consider the hypothesis that CLP may have a role in calcium regulation of these states. Current studies are examining the function of CLP in the cultured HMEC and how this function could be relevant to the questions regarding the interface of differentiation and transformation in human epithelial cells. In particular, could the downregulation of CLP expression observed after in vitro and in vivo transformation of HMEC reflect a consequence of transformation (ie the transformed state may be incompatible with high expression of CLP) or a requirement of transformation (ie a particular state of differentiation is required for transformation to occur). These questions pertaining to the modulation of CLP are also relevant to the observations that breast tumour cells display the phenotype of the mature luminal cells and do not express basal cell properties.

DISCUSSION AND FUTURE DIRECTIONS

The HMEC system described above has been developed to a level that permits its widespread use in addressing some of the broad questions concerning control of proliferation and differentiation. Thus, abundant quantities of well characterized HMEC of normal finite lifespan from different individuals can be generated in uniform cell batches. These cells grow rapidly for many population doublings in a serum free medium. The HMEC are sensitive to specific growth factors thought to be active in vivo, such as TGFA, TGFB, glucocorticoids and insulin like growth factor 1 (Milazzo *et al*, 1992). Excellent cell synchrony can be obtained by using gentle, non-cytotoxic methods. In addition, syngeneic immortally transformed cell lines are available for comparison. These lines display many of the properties seen in normal HMEC and do not have characteristics of malignantly transformed cells other than some karyotypic abnormalities. Variants in growth factor responsiveness can be isolated from these cell lines. The immortal lines can also be used to determine what further changes, for example exposure to specific oncogenes, can render them malignantly transformed.

Although questions concerning the changes that occur as these cells age in vitro and become senescent have not been the focus of our laboratory, we believe that this HMEC system offers many advantages for those wishing to study human cellular senescence. We have carefully characterized the reproductive lifespan of HMEC from 18 individuals ranging in age from 16 to 80 years. All the normal HMEC senesce after a reproducible number of population doublings. Since tumour derived, but not normal, human epithelial cells have the capacity to escape the growth control of cellular senescence, an understanding of the normal mechanisms that confer finite lifespan should also advance understanding of the aberrant processes that occur during malignant transformation.

The existence of syngeneic normal and immortally transformed HMEC allows us to address questions concerning the nature of the changes that occur in cells that escape from senescence. Presumably, the errors that give rise to immortality will be manifest in changes in the pathway of cell cycle progression and DNA synthesis. Alterations in early response gene, RB, TP53, cyclin kinase and phosphatase activity have been observed in some cases of immortal transformation. However, these changes could be secondary to the initiation of errors occurring in a wide range of cellular processes, including DNA integrity and repair processes. Our laboratory and others have begun experiments to define the differences between finite lifespan and immortal HMEC. Our intention is to focus first on the changes that can be detected in cell cycle parameters and then use that information to trace back possible causative errors. So far, we and other groups have seen that the immortal cells show some karyotypic instability, increased mutation frequency (Eldridge and Gould, 1992), reduced DNA repair during the G_2 phase (Sanford et al, 1992), reduced intercellular communication (Eldridge et al, 1989), some changes in growth factor responses (eg resistance to TGFB induced growth inhibition, loss of requirement for specific growth factors), reduced synthesis of fibronectin and a calmodulin like protein, the ability to be malignantly transformed with specific oncogenes and some changes in expression of early response genes during G_0 arrest. We have not observed differences in TP53 or RB expression. Although normal and immortal HMEC differ in expression of other properties (keratins, PEM, vimentin, three dimensional structure formation when grown on extracellular matrix material [Stampfer et al, 1993b]), these differences are more to be likely due to their different state of maturation than to an intrinsic property of immortal transformation.

Although HMEC can and have been used to study changes correlated with malignant transformation, we believe that neither this system nor any other system currently available has all the features needed to understand this process. Part of the problem has been the absence of easy methods to identify and isolate malignant human breast epithelial cells; the other main problem has been the difficulty in growing breast tumour cells in vitro. Other laboratories have been investigating ways to circumvent these difficulties (Petersen et al, 1992; Ethier et al, 1993), to allow direct comparison of early passage normal and tumour cells in vitro. A consequence of these problems is that most malignant human breast cells studied are also immortally transformed. Although immortal transformation is associated with malignant transformation in vivo, only rarely does a cell from a human breast tumour display indefinite lifespan in vitro (Smith et al, 1987). Thus, any use of immortally transformed cell lines as models of tumour cells runs the risk of confounding properties associated with immortality with those connected to malignancy. Also, most of the oncogenes used by our laboratory and others to confer malignancy on breast cells in culture are not known to be associated with human breast cancer (eg mutated *ras*, mutated *erbB2*, papillomaviruses, SV40 T antigen). Therefore, the comparisons that have been made between cultured non-malignant and malignantly transformed HMEC may not accurately reflect what happens in vivo. Given these reservations, these comparisons have thus far shown differences in expression of anchorage independent growth, growth factor synthesis and requirements (Clark *et al*, 1988; Li and Shipley, 1991), responsiveness to insulin (Milazzo *et al*, 1992), tropomyosin expression (Bhattacharya *et al*, 1990), cellular invasive and metastatic behaviour (Thompson *et al*, in press) and E-cadherin and vimentin expression (Sommers *et al*, 1989; Thompson *et al*, in press).

To answer many questions about the interface between differentiation and transformation, we believe that significant improvements will need to be made to the HMEC culture system. Obviously, mammary epithelial cells in the body do not exist as two dimensional objects growing on impermeable surfaces. Rather, they form three dimensional structures in which there is cell-cell communication between polarized epithelial cells, and they have cell surfaces that face either a permeable basement membrane or a lumen. They also have two way communication with the connective tissue of the breast as well as the rest of the body via nutrients, ion exchange, growth factors, hormones and other small molecules. It is reasonable to assume that key aspects of growth control and differentiation, and thus also carcinogenesis, will be intimately connected to the interactions that occur as a result of this three dimensional, inter-communicative system. Certainly, one of the hallmarks of cancer in the body is the disruption of normal cell-cell and cell-basement membrane interactions. Abnormality in three dimensional architecture is a key criterion used by pathologists to determine whether a tumour is malignant.

We therefore believe that a better understanding of the processes involved in human breast carcinogenesis will require development of culture systems that allow for expression of cellular polarity, epithelial-stromal interaction and three dimensional architecture. Culture systems that incorporate these features could be useful not only in defining the mechanisms controlling expression of differentiated properties and the differences between normal and transformed cells, but also in facilitating induction of in vitro transformation. In particular, if a specific state of maturation or cell-cell or cell-matrix interaction rendered cells more susceptible to transformation, mimicking that configuration in vitro might allow for in vitro transformation. Given the current extreme difficulty in obtaining transformation of human epithelial cells in vitro by any physical carcinogen, any improvements would be very valuable. Studies to determine what factors in what combinations can induce human transformation, and what factors can inhibit transformation might then be feasible.

We have initiated studies to determine the effects of differing calcium concentrations, growth factors, serum, extracellular matrix material and three dimensional support systems on expression of properties associated with breast epithelial cell maturation and functional differentiation (eg expression of keratins, CLP, PEM, lactoferrin, casein) in both normal HMEC and the 184B5 cell line. Preliminary studies have indicated that the maturation phenotype can be readily modulated in preselection normal HMEC, but we have yet to define conditions that allow expression of the fully mature luminal phenotype in the postselection cell populations. Ideally, we would like to define three dimensional culture conditions that could permit systematic evaluation of the effects of cell polarity, epithelial-epithelial and epithelial-stromal cell interactions, individual extracellular matrix components and specific growth factors and small molecules on expression of HMEC proliferation and differentiation, and the capacity of HMEC to transform in vitro.

SUMMARY

The progressive changes that occur as human epithelial cells transform to malignancy involve derangements in the normal processes of cellular proliferation and differentiation. These changes manifest in altered cell-cell and cell-basement membrane interactions. Since it is impossible to examine these events systematically as they occur in vivo, development of in vitro cell systems that can as accurately as possible reflect the in vivo state offer the next best alternative for determining the molecular mechanisms underlying human carcinogenesis. We have developed a human mammary epithelial cell system that permits long term growth of normal finite lifespan cells in a serum free medium. These cells have been transformed in vitro to immortality and malignancy. We have shown that signal transduction of the EGF receptor is essential for the normal HMEC to maintain growth. Blockage of this signal leads to a G_0 arrest, and reversal of this blockage leads to a synchronous re-entry into the cell cycle. Transforming growth factor beta is a potent inhibitor of normal HMEC growth, but the transformed cell lines are capable of escaping TGFB growth inhibition while retaining physiological responses such as synthesis of extracellular matrix components. This cell system is being used to examine the differences between normal and transformed cells in expression of cell cycle and differentiation related properties. Further improvements in the cell culture system will facilitate studies on the interrelation between differentiation and carcinogenesis.

Acknowledgements

This work was supported by National Institutes of Health grants CA-24844 and CA-54247 and the Office of Energy Research, Office of Health and Environmental Research, US Department of Energy under Contract No. DE-AC03-76SF00098.

References

Bartek J, Durban EM, Hallowes RC and Taylor-Papadimitriou J (1985a) A subclass of luminal epithelial cells in the human mammary gland, defined by antibodies to cytokeratins. *Journal of Cell Science* **75** 17–33

Bartek J, Taylor-Papadimitriou J, Miller N and Millis R (1985b) Pattern of expression of keratin 19 as detected with monoclonal antibodies to human breast tumors and tissues. *International Journal of Cancer* **36** 299–306

Bartley JC, Bartholomew JC and Stampfer MR (1982) Metabolism of benzo(a)pyrene in human mammary epithelial and fibroblast cells: Metabolite pattern and DNA adduct formation. *Journal of Cell Biochemistry* **18** 135–148

Bates SE, Valverius E, Ennis BW *et al* (1990) Expression of the TGFα/EGF receptor pathway in normal human breast epithelial cells. *Endocrinology* **126** 596–607

Bhattacharya B, Prasad GL, Valverius EM, Salomon DS and Cooper HL (1990) Tropomyosins of human mammary epithelial cells: consistent defects of expression in mammary carcinoma cell lines. *Cancer Research* **50** 2105–2112

Bossert NL, Nelson KG, Ross KA, Takahashi T and McLachlan JA (1990) Epidermal growth factor binding and receptor distribution in the mouse reproductive tract during development. *Developmental Biology* **142** 75–85

Boukamp P, Petrussevka RT, Breitkreutz D *et al* (1988) Normal keratinization in a spontaneously immortalized aneuploid human keratinocyte cell line. *Journal of Cell Biology* **106** 761–771

Boyce ST and Ham RG (1983) Calcium regulated differentiation of normal human epidermal keratinocytes in chemically defined clonal culture and serum-free serial culture. *Journal of Investigative Dermatology* **81** 33–40

Bravo R (1990) Genes induced during the G_0/G_1 transition in mouse fibroblasts. *Cancer Biology* **1** 37–46

Briand P, Petersen OW and Van Deurs B (1987) A new diploid nontumorigenic human breast epithelial cell line isolated and propagated in chemically defined medium. *In Vitro Cellular and Developmental Biology* **23** 181–188

Brosius J (1991) Retroposons—seeds of evolution. *Science* **251** 753

Chafouleas JG, Lagacé L, Bolton WE, Boyd AEI and Means AR (1984) Changes in calmodulin and its mRNA accompany reentry of quiescent (G0) cells into the cell cycle. *Cell* **36** 73–81

Chang SE and Taylor-Papadimitriou J (1983) Modulation of phenotype in cultures of human milk epithelial cells and its relation to the expression of a membrane antigen. *Cell Differentiation* **12** 143–154

Clark R, Stampfer M, Milley B *et al* (1988) Transformation of human mammary epithelial cells by oncogenic retroviruses. *Cancer Research* **48** 4689–4694

Coleman S, Silberstein GB and Daniel CW (1988) Ductal morphogenesis in the mouse mammary gland: evidence supporting a role for epidermal growth factor. *Developmental Biology* **127** 304–315

Daniel CW, Silberstein GB and Strickland P (1987) Direct action of 17β-estradiol on mouse mammary ducts analyzed by sustained release implants and steroid autoradiography. *Cancer Research* **47** 6052–6057

Dulbecco R, Allen RA, Bologna M and Bowman M (1986) Marker evolution during development of the rat mammary gland: stem cells identified by markers and the role of myoepithelial cells. *Cancer Research* **46** 2449–2456

Dutrillaux B, Gerbault-Seureau M and Zafrani B (1990) Characterization of chromosomal anomalies in human breast cancer. *Cancer Genetics and Cytogenetics* **49** 203–217

Eldridge SR and Gould MN (1992) Comparison of spontaneous mutagenesis in early-passage human mammary cells from normal and malignant tissues. *International Journal of Cancer* **50** 321–324

Eldridge SR, Martens TW, Sattler CA and Gould MN (1989) Association of decreased intercellular communication with the immortal but not the tumorigenic phenotype in human mammary epithelial cells. *Cancer Research* **49** 4326–4331

Ethier S, Mahacek M, Gullick W, Frank T and Weber B (1993) Differential isolation of normal luminal mammary epithelial cells and breast cancer cells from primary and metastatic sites using selective media. *Cancer Research* **53** 627–635

Finch C and Hayflick L (1976) *The Handbook of the Biology of Aging*, Van Nostrand Reinhold, New York

Guelstein VI, Tchypysheva TA, Ermilova VD et al (1988) Monoclonal antibody mapping of keratins 8 and 17 and of vimentin in normal human mammary gland, benign tumors, dysplasias and breast cancer. *International Journal of Cancer* **42** 147–153

Hammond SL, Ham RG and Stampfer MR (1984) Serum-free growth of human mammary epithelial cells: rapid clonal growth in defined medium and extended serial passage with pituitary extract. *Proceedings of the National Academy of Sciences of the USA* **81** 5435–5439

Hosobuchi M and Stampfer MR (1989) Effects of transforming growth factor-β on growth of human mammary epithelial cells in culture. *In Vitro Cellular and Developmental Biology* **25** 705–712

Koller M and Strehler EE (1988) Characterization of an intronless human calmodulin-like pseudogene. *FEBS Letter* **239** 121–128

Koller M, Schnyder B and Strehler EE (1990) Structural organization of the human CaMIII calmodulin gene. *Biochimica et Biophysica Acta* **1087** 180–189

Lehman T, Modali R, Boukamp P et al (1993) p53 mutations in human immortalized epithelial cell lines. *Carcinogenesis* **14** 833–839

Li W and Shipley GD (1991) Expression of multiple species of basic fibroblast growth factor mRNA and protein in normal and tumor-derived mammary epithelial cells in culture. *Cell Growth & Differentiation* **2** 195–202

Liscia DS, Merlo G, Ciardiello F et al (1990) Transforming growth factor-α messenger RNA localization in the developing adult rat and human mammary gland by *in situ* hybridization. *Developmental Biology* **140** 123–131

Maygarden SJ, Strom S and Ware JL (1992) Localizaton of epidermal growth factor receptor by immunohistochemical methods in human prostatic carcinoma, prostatic intraepithelial neoplasia, and benign hyperplasia. *Archives of Pathological Laboratory Medicine* **116** 269–273

Milazzo G, Giorgino F, Damante G et al (1992) Insulin receptor expression and function in human breast cancer cell lines. *Cancer Research* **52** 3924–3930

Petersen O'Ronnov-Jessen L, Howlett A and Bissell M (1992) Interaction with basement membrane serves to rapidly distinguish growth and differentiation patterns of normal and malignant human breast epithelial cells. *Proceedings of the National Academy of Sciences of the USA* **89** 9064–9068

Petersen OW, Hoyer PE and van Deurs B (1987) Frequency and distribution of estrogen receptor-positive cells in normal, non-lactating human breast tissue. *Cancer Research* **47** 5748–5751

Pierce JH, Arnstein P, DiMarco E et al (1991) Oncogenic potential of *erb*B-2 in human mammary epithelial cells. *Oncogene* **6** 1189–1194

Ricketts D, Turnbull L, Ryall G et al (1991) Estrogen and progesterone receptors in the normal human breast. *Cancer Research* **51** 1817–1822

Rudland PS and Hughes CM (1989) Immunocytochemical identification of cell types in human mammary gland: variations in cellular markers are dependent on glandular topography and differentiation. *Journal of Histochemistry and Cytochemistry* **37** 1087–1100

Sanford KK, Price FM, Rhim JS, Stampfer MR and Parshad R (1992) Role of DNA repair in malignant neoplastic transformation of human mammary epithelial cells in culture. *Carcinogenesis* **13** 137–141

Shirasuna K, Hayashido Y, Sugiyama M, Yoshioka H and Matsuya T (1991) Immunohistochemical localization of epidermal growth factor (EGF) and EGF receptor in human oral mucosa and its malignancy. *Virchows Archiv A Pathological Anatomy and Histopathology* **418** 349–353

Smith HS, Wolman SR, Dairkee SH *et al* (1987) Immortalization in culture: occurrence at a late stage in the progression of breast cancer. *Journal of the National Cancer Institute* **78** 611–615

Snedeker SM, Brown CF and DiAugustine RP (1991) Expression and functional properties of transforming growth factor a and epidermal growth factor during mouse mammary gland ductal morphogenesis. *Proceedings of the National Acadamy of Sciences of the USA* **88** 276–280

Sommers CL, Walker-Jones D, Heckford SE *et al* (1989) Vimentin rather than keratin expression in some hormone-independent breast cancer cell lines and in oncogene-transformed mammary epithelial cells. *Cancer Research* **49** 4258–4263

Soule HD and McGrath CM (1986) A simplified method for passage and long-term growth of human mammary epithelial cells. *In Vitro Cellular and Developmental Biology* **22** 6–12

Soule HD, Maloney TM, Wolman SR *et al* (1990) Isolation and characterization of a spontaneously immortalized human breast epithelial cell line, MCF-10. *Cancer Research* **50** 6075–6086

Stampfer MR (1982) Cholera toxin stimulation of human mammary epithelial cells in culture. *In Vitro* **18** 531–537

Stampfer MR and Bartley JC (1985) Induction of transformation and continuous cell lines from normal human mammary epithelial cells after exposure to benzo(a)pyrene. *Proceedings of the National Academy of Sciences of the USA* **82** 2394–2398

Stampfer MR and Bartley JC (1988) Human mammary epithelial cells in culture: differentiation and transformation In: Dickson R and Lippman M (eds). *Breast Cancer: Cellular and Molecular Biology*, pp 1–24, Kluwer Academic Publishers, Norwell, Massachusetts

Stampfer MR and Yaswen P (1992) Factors influencing growth and differentiation of normal and transformed human mammary epithelial cells in cultures, In: Milo GE, Castro BC and Shuler C (eds). *Transformation of Human Epithelial Cells: Molecular and Oncogenetic Mechanisms*, pp 117–140, CRC Press, Boca Raton, Florida

Stampfer MR, Hallowes R and Hackett AJ (1980) Growth of normal human mammary epithelial cells in culture. *In Vitro* **16** 415–425

Stampfer MR, Bartholomew JC, Smith HS and Bartley JC (1981a) Metabolism of benzo(a)-pyrene by human mammary epithelial cells: toxicity and DNA adduct formation. *Proceedings of the National Academy of Sciences of the USA* **78** 6251–6255

Stampfer MR, Vlodavsky I, Smith HS *et al* (1981b) Fibronectin production by human mammary cells. *Journal of the National Cancer Institute* **67** 253–261

Stampfer MR, Pan CH, Hosoda J, Bartholomew J, Mendelsohn J and Yaswen P (1993a) Blockage of EGF receptor signal transduction causes reversible arrest of normal and transformed human mammary epithelial cells with synchronous reentry into the cell cycle. *Experimental Cell Research* **208** 175–188

Stampfer MR, Yaswen P, Alhadeff M and Hosoda J (1993b) TGFβ induction of extracellular matrix associated proteins in normal and transformed human mammary epithelial cells in culture is independent of growth effects. *Journal of Cellular Physiology* **155** 210–221

Taylor-Papadimitriou J, Millis R, Burchell J *et al* (1986) Patterns of reaction of monoclonal antibodies HMFG-1 and -2 with benign breast tissues and breast carcinomas. *Journal of Experimental Pathology* **2** 247–260

Taylor-Papadimitriou J, Stampfer MR, Bartek J, Lane EB and Lewis A (1989) Keratin expression in human mammary epithelial cells cultured from normal and malignant tissue: relation to in vivo phenotypes and influence of medium. *Journal of Cell Science* **94** 403–413

Thompson E, Torri J, Sabol M *et al* Oncogene- induced basement membrance invasiveness in human mammary epithelial cells. *Clinical and Experimental Metastastes* (in press)

Valverius E, Bates SE, Stampfer MR *et al* (1989) Transforming growth factor alpha production and EGF receptor expression in normal and oncogene tranformed human mammary epithelial cells. *Molecular Endocrinology* **3** 203–214

VanBerkum MFA and Means AR (1991) Three amino acid substitutions in domain I of calmodulin prevent the activation of chicken smooth muscle myosin light chain kinase. *Journal of Biological Chemistry* **266** 21488–21495

Walen K and Stampfer MR (1989) Chromosome analyses of human mammary epithelial cells at stages of chemically-induced transformation progression to immortality. *Cancer Genetics and Cytogenetics* **37** 249–261

Wolman SR, Smith HS, Stampfer M and Hackett AJ (1985) Growth of diploid cells from breast cancer. *Cancer Genetics and Cytogenetics* **16** 49–64

Yaswen P, Smoll A, Peehl DM, Trask DK, Sager R and Stampfer MR (1990) Down-regulation of a calmodulin-related gene during transformation of human mammary epithelial cells. *Proceedings of the National Academy of Sciences of the USA* **87** 7360–7364

Yaswen P, Smoll A, Hosoda J, Parry G and Stampfer MR (1992) Protein product of a human intronless calmodulin-like gene shows tissue-specific expression and reduced abundance in transformed cells. *Cell Growth & Differentiation* **3** 335–345

Yuspa SH and Morgan DL (1981) Mouse skin cells resistant to terminal differentiation associated with initiation of carcinogenesis. *Nature* **293** 72–74

Yuspa SH, Kilkenny AE, Steinert PM and Roop DR (1989) Expression of murine epidermal differentiation markers is tightly regulated by restricted extracellular calcium concentrations in vitro. *Journal of Cell Biology* **109** 1207–1217

Zhai Y-F, Beittenmiller H, Wang B *et al* (1993) Increased expression of specific protein tyrosine phosphatases in human breast epithelial cells neoplastically transformed ny the neu oncogene. *Cancer Research* **53** 2272–2278

The authors are responsible for the accuracy of the references.

Oncogenes, Tumour Suppressor Genes and Growth Factors in Breast Cancer: Novel Targets for Diagnosis, Prognosis and Therapy

ROBERT CALLAHAN[1] • DAVID S SALOMON[2]

[1]Oncogenetics and [2]Tumor Growth Factor Sections, Laboratory of Tumor Immunology and Biology, National Cancer Institute, Bethesda, Maryland 20892

INTRODUCTION

Breast cancer is one of the more prevalent types of cancer in women especially in the USA and Western countries. Approximately one of nine women will develop breast cancer during their lifetime (Kelsey and Berkowitz, 1988). Therefore, identification of environmental, biochemical and genetic factors that might contribute to the aetiology and progression of this disease is essential in terms of improving prevention, diagnosis and therapy. However, our knowledge of molecular markers that define the developmental pathway of mammary epithelial cells and the consequences that these markers may have on the interactions that occur between mammary epithelial, stromal and adipose tissues is clearly limited. To begin to address these issues, a major effort has been made over the past decade in identifying and delineating at a molecular level the changes that occur in mammary tissue during the development of the mammary gland as well as the genetic alterations that might contribute to the progression from normal growth through malignancy to metastasis.

It seems likely that several factors such as menstrual and family history, long term treatment with oestrogens, diet and previous atypical benign breast disease either provide the selective environment for the clonal outgrowth of cells with a particular somatic mutation or induce and/or suppress the expression of specific genes that leads to deregulated growth and differentiation of the mammary epithelium (Harris et al, 1982; Gompel and van Kerkem, 1983; Lynch et al, 1984). This has provided the potential clinical rationale for identifying the changes that are predictive of disease outcome and the gene products that might represent potential targets for therapeutic intervention in breast cancer management. Two approaches, which are not necessarily mutually exclusive and are probably complementary, have been taken to elucidate at a molecular level the process of malignant progression of human breast cancer. One approach has focused on the genetic cataloguing of somatic mutations that are frequently found in primary breast tumours (Callahan et al, 1993; Walker and Varley, 1993), and the other approach has focused on the identification of specific gene products whose expression is perturbed in primary breast tumours or breast cancer cell lines (Greig et al, 1988). An effort has been made to link these alterations to clinical parameters in the patient's history and physiological status, the characteristics of the tumour or the patient's overall prognosis. In this chapter, we briefly summarize the current status of each approach. Although substantial progress has been made in these areas, it seems clear that we are only at the beginning of a learning curve in understanding at a molecular level the consequences of the various somatic mutations and the aberrant expression of specific growth factors and their cognate receptors that might contribute to the normal and pathogenic development of the mammary gland. Nevertheless, some prospective candidate targets for therapeutic intervention have been identified.

GROWTH FACTORS AND THEIR RECEPTORS IN BREAST CANCER

One phenotypic property that is universally exhibited by transformed mesenchymal and epithelial cells is their ability to proliferate in an unrestrained manner. This property in vitro is reflected by a decreased serum requirement for growth of these cells. This is in part due to a partial or complete relaxation of the growth factor requirements that are necessary for maintaining the proliferation of these cells. Eventually, transformed cells may progress to a state where there is a total loss in the requirement for specific sets of exogenous in vivo host derived or in vitro serum derived growth factors. This

TABLE 1. Growth factors and growth inhibitors in mammary epithelial or stromal cells

Growth factors	Growth inhibitors
Epidermal growth factor (EGF)	Transforming growth factor beta 1 (TGFB1)
Transforming growth factor alpha (TGFA)	TGFB2
Heregulin α (HRGA)	Mammastatin
Amphiregulin (AREG)	Mammary derived growth inhibitor (MDGI)
Cripto 1 (CR 1)	
Insulin like growth factor 1 (IGF1)	
IGF2	
Platelet derived growth factor (PDGF)	
Fibroblast growth factor 2 (FGF2)	
Keratinocyte growth factor (KGF)	
FGF5)	
Kaposi's growth factor (KFGF/HST1)	
Hepatocyte growth factor (HGF)	
Mammary derived growth factor 1 (MDGF1)	

autonomous situation may be due in part to the ability of these transformed cells to overexpress and to secrete their own endogenous growth factors and to respond to these peptides in an autocrine, juxtacrine or intracrine dependent fashion (Sporn and Roberts, 1992). Alternatively, transformed cells may become hypersensitive to very low concentrations of growth factors due to overexpression of growth factor receptors (Sporn and Roberts, 1992).

Normal and malignant mammary epithelial cells and surrounding stromal cells are able to respond to a number of different growth factors and in some cases to synthesize some of these peptides (Table 1) (Salomon *et al*, 1992). In this regard, an autocrine role has been formally demonstrated for the oestrogen inducible growth factors, transforming growth factor alpha (TGFA) and insulin like growth factor 2 (IGF2), in several different human breast cancer cell lines (Bates *et al*, 1988; Osborne *et al*, 1989). In addition, growth inhibitors such as TGFB1 and TGFB2 are increased in response to anti-oestrogens both in vitro and in vivo and may mediate in part the growth inhibitory effects of these compounds (Butta *et al*, 1992). Furthermore, TGFB has been showed to downregulate TGFA expression in vitro and in vivo as well as function as an autocrine negative growth regulator in several human breast cancer cell lines. Its expression has also been detected in primary human breast cancers (Arteaga *et al*, 1990).

There is evidence showing that stromal cells within the normal mammary gland or surrounding breast tumours are able to elaborate growth factors such as IGF1, IGF2 and various members of the fibroblast growth factor (FGF) family of peptides such as acidic FGF (FGF1) and basic FGF (FGF2) and growth inhibitors such as TGFB1 which might function in a paracrine manner to influence the proliferation of adjacent normal and/or malignant mammary epithelial cells (Clarke *et al*, 1992). Therefore, there is a reciprocal cross communication occurring between the mammary epithelium and stroma as mediated by different growth factors via the extracellular matrix. Components of the extracellular matrix such as proteoglycans containing heparan sulphate can also function as a storage site for a number of different heparin binding growth factors such as FGF2, amphiregulin (AREG), heparin binding epidermal growth factor (HB-EGF) and TGFB1 (Ruoslahti and Yamaguchi, 1991). Some of these epithelial or stromal derived peptides such as TGFA and FGF2 are likely to contribute to angiogenesis in the developing mammary gland and during tumorigenesis. Transformed mammary epithelial cells might also escape from normal growth regulatory constraints by constitutively over-expressing cell surface receptors for specific growth factors. The epidermal growth factor (EGF) receptor (c-erbB1), *c-erbB2*, which is the human homologue of the rat c-*neu* gene, and the IGF1 receptor are cell surface glycoproteins that contain an intracellular tyrosine kinase domain and that are frequently overexpressed in a subset of breast cancers (Gullick, 1990b). The EGF receptor tyrosine kinase and c-erbB2 tyrosine kinase function as the receptors for the EGF/TGFA related peptides and for the heregulin family of peptides such as heregulin alpha (HRGA), respectively (Barker and Vinson, 1990; Holmes *et al*, 1992). Overexpression of these growth factors or their cognate receptors are probably important factors in the pathogenesis of breast cancer.

SOMATIC MUTATIONS IN BREAST CANCER

The quantitative activation of expression of certain growth factors, growth factor receptors and nuclear proteins occurs as a direct consequence of gene amplification in tumour cells. These loci include the c-*myc* proto-oncogene on chromosome 8q24-qter (Escot *et al*, 1986), an amplicon on chromosome 11q13 that contains the INT2 (FGF3), HST1 (FGF4) (Lidereau *et al*, 1988; Ali *et al*, 1989; Liscia *et al*, 1989), *PRAD1* and *EMS1* genes (reviewed in Lammie and Peters, 1991) and the c-*erbB2* proto-oncogene on chromosome 17q (Ali *et al*, 1988). In addition, *BEK* (bacterial expressed kinase) and *FLG* (FMS like gene), two members of the FGF receptor (*FGFR*) gene family, are amplified in 11.5% and 12.7% of breast cancers, respectively (Adnane *et al*, 1990). However, it is not known at present whether amplification of these two genes also leads to their overexpression. Since the involvement and probable contribution of the amplified genes to breast cancer have been extensively reviewed (Lammie and Peters, 1991; Callahan *et al*, 1992; Walker and Varley, 1993), we only discuss their potential as targets for therapy in subsequent sections of this chapter.

By far the most frequent type of mutation found in primary breast tumours is loss of heterozygosity (LOH) (Callahan *et al*, 1992). This is a common feature of many kinds of malignancies (Seemayer and Cavenee, 1989; Weinberg, 1991) and occurs as a consequence of either interstitial deletions, chromosome loss or aberrant mitotic recombinational events. It is thought that LOH reveals within the affected region of the genome the presence of a recessive mutation in the remaining allele of a "tumour suppressor" gene(s) (reviewed in Knudson, 1989; Hollingsworth and Lee, 1991). Tumour suppressor genes are believed to be involved in the normal suppression of cellular proliferation during development (Knudson, 1989). At present, 20 of the 41 chromosome arms in the human genome have been shown to be affected by LOH in primary breast tumours. However, only two of the putative target genes for LOH have been identified, *TP53* on chromosome 17p12 (Osbourne *et al*, 1991) and *RB1* on chromosome 13q14 (Lee *et al*, 1988). It seems likely that this could change in the not too distant future due to the increasing density of polymorphic loci that span each chromosome arm and has provided the momentum for this work (Group, 1992; Weissenbach *et al*, 1992). A major effort is currently being focused on chromosome 17q21, the location of the hereditary breast and breast/ovarian cancer loci (BRCA1) (Hall *et al*, 1990, 1992; Narod *et al*, 1991). Another contributing factor will be the probable commonality of some target genes (ie *TP53* and *RB1*) in malignancies of different tissues.

One conclusion from the current status of this work is that the complexity of somatic mutations that are selected during tumour progression is probably an underestimate. More recent studies have focused on defining the regions of each chromosome arm that contain the putative target tumour suppressor genes, and this has led to the recognition that there are probably multiple target genes on some chromosome arms. For instance, on chromosome 1p, there are two distinct regions (1p13–p21 and 1p32–pter) affected by LOH (Bieche *et al*, 1993). Similarly, on chromosome 17, there are at least four regions (17p13.3, 17p12, 17q21 and 17q23-qter) that are independently affected by LOH (Cropp *et al*, 1990; Sato *et al*, 1991; Andersen *et al*, 1992; Merlo *et al*, 1992; Merlo GM, Cropp C and Callahan R, unpublished). A second contributing factor is that most studies of somatic mutations in breast cancer have focused on invasive ductal carcinomas; very few studies have been done on less common histopathological types of breast carcinomas.

It has been argued that much of the LOH found in breast carcinomas is a consequence of, rather a contributing factor to, malignant progression (McGuire and Naylor, 1989). Because target genes for the regions affected by LOH are lacking, it is difficult to address this issue at present. However, if this were true, one could expect that LOH at different regions of the genome would occur independently of one another. This seems not to be the case. In our own studies, we have been able to stratify the tumour panel into two groups of tumours based on the particular regions of the genome that were affected by LOH or gene amplification (Cropp *et al*, 1990; Callahan *et al*, 1993). Other laboratories have reported similar findings (Devilee *et al*, 1989; Sato *et al*, 1991; Andersen *et al*, 1992). Collectively, these findings suggest that particular factors in the patient's history and/or physiological status most likely provide the selective pressure for the outgrowth of cells with particular sets of somatic mutations. Clearly, much larger studies will be required to confirm this conclusion and to determine which sets of mutations are linked to particular clinical parameters.

NEW APPROACHES AND TARGETS IN THE DIAGNOSIS, DETERMINATION OF PROGNOSIS AND TREATMENT OF BREAST CANCER

Analysis of Serum, Urine and Pleural Effusions for Growth Factors or Growth Factor Receptors

Quantitative or qualitative differences in the level of expression of growth factors, their cognate cell surface receptors or specific intracellular signal transduction proteins offer the potential for establishing novel diagnostic and prognostic markers for breast cancer in either the early or the later stages of this disease and for developing creative and selectively non-toxic modalities for therapy (Greig *et al*, 1988; Gullick, 1990a; Siegfried, 1992). Measurement of growth factors or shed extracellular domains (ECDs) of growth factor receptors in serum, pleural effusions or urine may provide additional information with respect to the early diagnosis of breast cancer and for following up the response to chemotherapy or endocrine therapy with respect to tumour recurrence. In this regard, TGFA has been found in the serous effusions of nearly 200 cancer patients (Ciardiello *et al*, 1989; Osborne and Arteaga, 1990; Stromberg *et al*, 1991). The presence of TGFA activity in the pleural effusions was directly correlated with tumour burden, patient performance status and reduced survival (Osborne and Arteaga, 1990). In breast cancer, the presence of TGFA in pleural effusions was directly associated with the number of involved lymph nodes, premenopausal patients and oestrogen receptor (ER) and progesterone receptor (PgR) negative tumours. In addition, levels of TGFA were significantly higher in the pleural effusions obtained from breast cancer patients than in effusions from non-cancer patients (Ciardiello *et al*, 1989; Kamiya *et al*, 1993; Stromberg *et al*, 1991). A 43 kDa EGF related protein that is probably derived from a portion of the EGF precursor has also been found in the urine of breast cancer patients (Eckert *et al*, 1991). The level of this protein was also found to correlate with axillary lymph node involvement, ER negative tumours, tumour size, tumour stage and grade of differentiation of the primary tumour. Breast cancer patients with progressive disease showed higher urinary levels of this protein, and the levels declined after removal of the primary tumour or after preoperative chemotherapy but increased in the urine of patients who had local recurrence, metastasis or failed to respond to chemotherapy. Plasma levels of platelet derived growth factor are also substantially elevated in stage IV breast cancer patients and are generally associated with a higher metastatic frequency and shorter survival (Ariad *et al*, 1991). A 130 kDa glycoprotein that is biochemically and immunologically related to the ECD of p185[erbB2] has been detected in the conditioned medium obtained from several human breast cancer cell lines (Lin and Clinton, 1991). Likewise, an antigen that is immunologically related to the p185[erbB2] protein and probably related to a 75 kDa glycoprotein that is derived from the ECD of the p185[erbB2] protein can be detected and quantified in the serum from nude mice which are bearing ovarian and breast tumour xenografts that are over expressing c-*erbB2* (Langton *et al*, 1991). Serum immunoassays may therefore be useful in early diagnosis and for monitoring the response to therapy in a subset of breast cancer patients that have c-*erbB2* overexpressing tumours. In this respect, elevated levels of the ECD of the p185[erbB2] protein have been detected in primary breast tumours and in the corresponding serum in 20–50% of breast cancer patients (Breuer *et al*, 1993; Hosono *et al*, 1993). Moreover, there is a decline in serum levels of this protein to normal values after surgical removal of the tumour or after chemotherapy (Breuer *et al*, 1993; Hosono *et al*, 1993).

Anti-oestrogens, Transforming Growth Factor Beta and Tyrosine Kinase Inhibitors

A second area that can be potentially exploited is the identification of breast cancer populations with different prognoses based on the patterns of growth factor α and/or growth factor receptor expression in primary breast tumours. Overexpression of the *EGF* receptor and/or c-*erbB2* are already known to be associated with reduced patient survival and with failure to respond to endocrine therapy (Barker and Vinson, 1990; Gullick, 1990b; Nicholson *et al*, 1990; Dati *et al*, 1991; Koenders *et al*, 1991, 1993; Lofts and Gullick, 1991; Klijn *et al*, 1992; Wright *et al*, 1992). More recently, two additional EGF related peptides, AREG and cripto 1 (CR 1), have been found to be expressed in nearly 80% of breast carcinomas (Qi *et al*, in press). CR 1 was more restricted in its distribution as only 13% of non-involved, adjacent breast epithelium expressed this peptide, whereas 43% of epithelial cells that were adjacent to carcinoma expressed AREG, suggesting that CR 1 may be a novel breast tumour marker.

Oestrogen receptor status is one of the more reliable prognostic markers in breast cancer for predicting disease free survival and response to anti-oestrogens. Loss of ER expression or detection can be due to multiple causes and generally occurs during disease progression. Recently, several ER variants have been identified that result from genetic alterations due to basepair insertions, transitions and deletions (McGuire *et al*, 1991). Restoration of ER function by correcting or silencing these defects may provide a mechanism for therapy. Likewise, identification of these lesions in primary breast tumours may be informative with respect to predicting patient response to tamoxifen. Tamoxifen can also function in certain cases independently of the ER since it can enhance the expression of TGFB1 in the stroma of breast tumours that are both ER positive and ER negative. This demonstrates that part of the anti-tumour effects of this compound are mediated via stromal elaboration of an epithelial growth inhibitor through a paracrine mechanism (Wakefield *et al*,

1990; Butta *et al*, 1992; Dickens and Coletta, 1993). These data suggest that ER negative tumours may in certain cases be appropriate targets for anti-oestrogen therapy. In addition to tamoxifen, gestodene, a synthetic progesterone that is growth inhibitory for several human breast cancer cell lines and retinoids, can also induce an increase in the expression of active TGFB1 and/or TGFB2 in human breast cancer cells, suggesting that other steroidal compounds that have anti-tumour activity may also be operating through such a pathway (Wakefield *et al*, 1990; Dickens and Coletta, 1993). Expression of TGFB is also observed in malignant breast epithelial cells in primary breast tumours, and the level of expression is positively associated with nodal status and with disease progression (Gorsch *et al*, 1992; Walker and Dearing, 1992). In addition to its ability to modulate the expression of TGFB, tamoxifen can also enhance the expression of c-*erbB2* in ER positive breast cancer cells (Antoniotti *et al*, 1992). The expression of c-*erbB2* is normally downregulated like TGFB in response to oestrogens (Dati *et al*, 1990; Warri *et al*, 1991). This may explain the observation that breast carcinomas which possess an amplified c-*erbB2* gene do not respond favourably to anti-oestrogen therapy and generally have higher recurrence rates (Lofts and Gullick, 1991; Antoniotti *et al*, 1992; Hosono *et al*, 1993).

Other pharmacological compounds besides anti-oestrogens, progestins or retinoids that may prove to be beneficial in the treatment of breast cancer are agents that can specifically inhibit the tyrosine kinase activity of growth factor receptors. Receptors that are activated in breast cancer and that are potential targets for such drugs include the EGF receptor, the HRGA receptor (c-*erbB2*) and the IGF1 receptor. The tyrosine kinase inhibitors include erbstatin, genistein and the tyrphostins (Enright and Booth, 1991; Osherov *et al*, 1993; Peterson and Barnes, 1991). In this regard, there are several recently developed analogues of tyrphostin that can selectively inhibit either the EGF receptor tyrosine kinase or the c-erbB2 tyrosine kinase activity (Osherov *et al*, 1993). More importantly, it has recently been demonstrated that the use of some of these compounds may be efficacious in breast cancer since an analogue of tyrphostin was able to inhibit the EGF receptor tyrosine kinase activity in several human breast cancer cell lines and to antagonize significantly EGF or TGFA induced proliferation in these cells (Reddy *et al*, 1992). This compound was also found to block the mitogenic response to insulin, IGF1 and IGF2 in these cells, suggesting that other growth factor receptor tyrosine kinases were probably being targeted by this agent. Finally, this tyrphostin analogue was able to inhibit markedly oestrogen induced proliferation of oestrogen responsive breast cancer cells, suggesting that the compound was blocking the autocrine action of an oestrogen inducible peptide(s) such as TGFA or IGF2 that was functioning through these growth factor receptor tyrosine kinases. Another potential mechanism to perturb receptor function would be to design specific receptor dimerization inhibitors that would prevent receptor oligomerization, which is a necessary prerequisite for ligand induced activation of the cytoplasmic tyrosine kinase activity (Gullick, 1990a).

Ligand Antagonists, Ligand Toxins and Inhibitors of Intracellular Signal Transduction Proteins

Ligand antagonists have also proved to be successful in blocking the biological effects of peptide hormones. In this respect, synthetic peptide antagonists have been developed for bombesin, gastrin, substance P, bradykinin, somatostatin and luteinizing hormone releasing hormone (Grieg et al, 1988; Gullick, 1990a; Osborne and Arteaga, 1990; Siegfried, 1992). Site directed mutagenesis of growth factor genes, chemical modification of short regions of the protein molecule or obtaining peptide antagonists from epitope libraries that are involved in receptor recognition and binding could be useful in the acquisition of novel receptor blocking agents (Greig et al, 1988; Scott, 1992; Siegfried, 1992). In addition, peptidomimetic analogues that contain non-peptide hydrophobic regions or the screening of natural products might be efficacious in obtaining pure growth factor α antagonists (Rieman et al, 1992). In this context, a synthetic, acetyl-diethyl-homoarginine 10-mer peptide corresponding to residues 34–43 in the third disulphide loop of human TGFA was found to inhibit EGF, TGFA and oestrogen induced proliferation of MCF7 human breast cancer cells but not IGF1 induced growth (Eppstein et al, 1989). Although this peptide did not block the binding of EGF to the EGF receptor, it probably was involved in modifying receptor dimerization or internalization. Another approach for the treatment of breast cancer cells that are overexpressing the EGF or c-erbB2 receptors would be to target selectively toxins or drugs by conjugating them to EGF receptor ligands such as TGFA or AREG or to erbB2 ligands such as HRGA (FitzGerald and Pastan, 1989; Mesri et al, 1993, Theuer et al, 1993). Such an approach has already proved to be successful in vitro in the selective killing of EGF receptor overexpressing human breast bladder, ovarian and squamous cell carcinoma cell lines using a recombinant chimeric molecule consisting of the *Pseudomonas* exotoxin A chain linked to TGFA (Mesri et al, 1993; Theuer et al, 1993).

Growth factors might also be selectively sequestered from interacting with their appropriate receptors by agents that can bind to specific regions of the peptide. In this context, suramin, which is a polysulphonated naphthylurea, and more recently the heparinoid pentosan polysulphate are two new anti-tumour agents that can inhibit the in vitro growth and in vivo xenograft growth of several human breast cancer cell lines (Vignon et al, 1992; Zugmaier et al, 1992; Stein, 1993). These compounds have several different metabolic effects, but one important property that probably contributes to their anti-tumour activity is their ability to inhibit the binding of a number of different heparin binding growth factors such as FGF2, IIB-EGF, AREG, HRGA, PDGF, TGFA and TGFB to their cognate receptors. This effect appears to be due to the ability of these molecules to function as heparin analogues and thereby bind to peptides that would normally interact to various degrees with proteoglycans containing heparin or heparan sulphate either in the extracellular matrix or on the cell surface of target cells (Klagsbrun and Baird, 1991; Ruoslahti and Yamaguchi, 1991). This latter possibility may be important since proteoglycans containing heparan sulphate may serve as cell surface presentation molecules to respective receptors for growth factors such as FGF2, AREG, HB-EGF and TGFB (Klagsbrun and Baird, 1991). In addition, these compounds can frequently facilitate dissociation of some of these growth factors after they are bound to their receptors. Another possible mechanism to entrap growth factors so they cannot interact with their receptors is to infuse specific growth factor binding proteins or pharmacological analogues that perform a similar function. These serum binding proteins frequently can neutralize the mitogenic effects of specific families of growth factors. Such an approach has already proved to be feasible using the IGF1 binding protein 1 in blocking the mitogenic effects of exogenous IGF1 on MCF-7 human breast cancer cells (McGuire et al, 1992).

Finally, it is now possible to design specific pharmacological agents that can inhibit the action of proteins that are involved in the intracellular signal transduction pathway for a number of growth factors. For example, the p21^{ras} protein is positioned at a central point in a pathway that is activated by several different growth factor receptor tyrosine kinases, including the EGF and HRGA receptors (Satoh et al, 1992). Stimulation of growth factor receptors by their respective ligands leads to a rapid and transient increase in the active GTP bound form of p21^{ras} due to a stimulation in the association of GRB2-mSOS, a signal transduction protein complex, with the autophosphorylated receptor, thereby positioning this complex in proximity to and facilitating the exchange of GDP with GTP on the p21^{ras} protein (Buday and Downward, 1993). The p21^{ras} protein must associate with the plasma membrane for this event to occur and for it to exert biological activity. Attachment of p21^{ras} to the inner aspect of the plasma membrane is due in large part to the farnesylation of the protein at its carboxyl terminus at the CAAX box by farnesyltransferase (Der and Cox, 1991). Recently, a series of new drugs have been isolated that can specifically inhibit this farnesyltransferase activity (Travis, 1993). Treatment of cells that are transformed by point mutated, oncogenic forms of the p21^{ras} protein with these inhibitors of farnesylation blocks cellular transformation. It is certainly conceivable that breast cancer cells that may have a constitutively active p21^{ras} protein in the GTP bound state due to chronic autocrine growth factor induced receptor activation may be particularly sensitive to this class of compounds.

Anti-growth Factor α and Anti-receptor Monoclonal Antibodies

Cell surface molecules such as growth factor receptors or transmembrane growth factor precursors might serve as accessible targets for monoclonal antibodies that could be used for radioimaging and for immunotherapy in breast cancer. In this regard, EGF, TGFA, AREG, HB-EGF and HRGA are initially synthesized as glycosylated, transmembrane proteins that are biologically active. Several different monoclonal antibodies have been developed that can bind to and neutralize the biological activity of EGF, TGFA and IGF1 and that can significantly inhibit the in vitro proliferation and/or tumorigenicity of some human breast, colon, squamous cell, lung and ovarian adenocarcinoma cell lines (Grieg *et al*, 1988; Gullick, 1990; Osborne and Arteaga, 1990; Siegfried, 1992). However, the most promising clinical data for the use of such immunoreagents come from the use of antibodies directed against the extracellular domains of the EGF receptor, c-erbB2 and the IGF1 receptor (Osborne and Arteaga, 1990; Shepard *et al*, 1991; Mendelsohn, 1992). In general, monoclonal antibodies against either EGF, TGFA, AREG, CR1 or several different growth factor receptors such as the EGF, HRGA or IGF2 receptors have been successfully used to immunocytochemically detect and localize these proteins in either frozen or formalin fixed paraffin embedded sections of various human breast lesions (Gullick *et al*, 1987; Gullick, 1990b; Ennis *et al*, 1991; Lofts and Gullick, 1991; Shepard *et al*, 1991). Therapeutic uses of anti-receptor blocking or anti-growth factor neutralizing monoclonal antibodies may be achieved by using unconjugated antibodies to prevent the binding of autocrine growth factors such as TGFA, AREG, HRGA or IGF1 to their respective receptors by steric inhibition. In addition, these antibodies can be chemically or genetically linked to radionuclides, therapeutic drugs or bacterial toxins to selectively deliver these agents to breast cancer cells that are overexpressing these different receptors or membrane associated growth factor precursors.

Several anti-EGF receptor monoclonal antibodies have been characterized with respect to their ability to inhibit the in vitro growth of MCF-7, ZR75-1 and MDA-MB-468 human breast cancer cells and to arrest the growth of MDA-MB-468 xenografts in nude mice (Ennis *et al*, 1991; Mendelsohn, 1992). The in vivo growth inhibitory effect of these monoclonal antibodies is directly correlated with the number of EGF receptors that are expressed on these target cells, with the intrinsic growth potential of these different cell lines and with the ability of these immunological reagents to inhibit the binding of EGF related peptides such as TGFA or AREG to the EGF receptor. The growth inhibition produced by the anti-EGF receptor antibodies against MDA-MB-468 cells, which contain approximately 3×10^5 EGF receptor sites per cell, could be converted into a selective cytotoxic effect after conjugating the antibodies to recombinant ricin A chain (Taetle *et al*, 1988). These immunoconjugates were only minimally toxic for breast cancer cells expressing less than 5×10^4 EGF receptor sites per cell. Anti-EGF receptor monoclonal antibodies have also been successively used for radioimaging MDA-MB-468 tumour xenografts in nude mice after conjugation to indium-111 labelled pentetic acid (DTPA) (Goldenberg *et al*, 1989; Mendelsohn, 1992). The ^{111}In labelled DPTA–anti-EGF receptor antibody was found to accumulate in the breast tumour xenografts by a factor of fourfold over the antibody distribution in other mouse tissues, as calculated by tissue localization indices. The labelled antibody was unable to localize MCF-7 tumour xenografts as these cells only express 5×10^3 EGF receptor sites per cell. Preclinical studies have been performed with chimpanzees and no toxicity was observed with intravenous antibody doses of up to 650 mg (Goldenberg *et al,* 1989, Mendelsohn, 1992). Phase I trials with patients with stage III or IV adenocarcinoma of the lung showed no toxicity after the administration of nearly 300 mg of the monoclonal anti-EGF receptor antibody. Imaging studies demonstrated that primary lung lesions could be successfully visualized and that metastatic deposits of more than 1 cm could be detected. Interferon gamma has been shown to upregulate the expression of several tumour associated cell surface antigens in vitro and in vivo (Greiner *et al,* 1990). Interferon gamma can also enhance the expression of EGF receptors in human breast cancer cells in vitro, suggesting that this cytokine may be useful for upregulating growth factor receptor expression and density in vivo for the purpose of increasing the sensitivity for radioimaging or for immunotherapy (Hamburger and Pinnamaneni, 1991).

The $p185^{c-erbB2}$ protein may offer an even more selective target for immunotherapy in breast cancer since this protein, unlike the EGF receptor, is rarely expressed in normal tissues and if so is generally expressed at a very low level (Gullick *et al,* 1987; Gullick, 1990b; Lofts and Gullick, 1991). In addition, 10–30% of human breast tumours overexpress the $p185^{c-erbB2}$ protein due in most cases to gene amplification. A series of monoclonal antibodies has been generated against either the rat c-neu or the human c-erbB2 protein and which recognizes various carbohydrate epitopes in the ECD of these proteins (Drebin *et al,* 1988; Langton *et al,* 1991; Sarup *et al,* 1991; Shepard *et al,* 1991, Stancovski *et al,* 1992). These antibodies can cytostatically inhibit the in vitro monolayer growth and anchorage independent clonogenicity of several human breast and ovarian carcinoma cell lines that are overexpressing the p185 c-neu/erbB2 protein. More importantly, these antibodies can significantly inhibit the growth of different breast and ovarian carcinoma xenografts that are overexpressing c-erbB2 (Hancock *et al,* 1991; Sarup *et al,* 1991; Shepard *et al,* 1991). The minimal effective level of expression of the $p185^{c-erbB2}$ protein was found to be 1×10^5 receptor sites per cell for these antibodies to have a significant cytostatic effect. The cytostatic effects of these antibodies, like the anti-EGF receptor antibody effects, are reversible and require the continuous presence of the antibody. One mechanism by which some of these anti-erbB2 antibodies could exert their anti-proliferative effects might be due to the induction of terminal differentiation or apoptosis in selected subpopulations of tumour cells that are overexpressing this gene. In this respect, several growth inhibitory anti-erbB2 monoclonal antibodies have been shown to promote the differentiation of human breast cancer cell lines as assessed by the appearance of β and κ caseins and the development of lipid droplets (Bacus *et al,* 1992). These events were accompanied by growth arrest of the cells at late S or early G_2 phase of the cell cycle. In addition to inhibiting cell proliferation and, with certain antibodies, promoting differentiation, some of the growth inhibitory anti-EGF receptor or anti-erbB2 monoclonal antibodies can function as weak or partial receptor agonists since they can enhance the autophosphorylation of the EGF receptor or $p185^{c-erbB2}$ protein and since they can facilitate the internalization and downregulation of these receptors (Sarup *et al,* 1991; Stancovski *et al*, 1992). Certain anti-erbB2 antibodies can also block or compete with HRGA for receptor binding, thus providing a modality for blocking the autocrine growth of a subset of breast tumours (Sarup *et al*, 1991; Stancovski *et al*, 1992). Although the majority of anti-erbB2 monoclonal antibodies are cytostatic, these antibodies can synergistically enhance the cytoxicity to cytokines such as tumour necrosis factor alpha (TNFA) and to certain drugs such as cisplatin (Hudziak *et al*, 1989; Hancock *et al*, 1991). In general, erbB2 overexpressing cells are more resistant to the effects of TNFA and to the cytotoxic effects of drugs such as cisplatin, 5-fluorouracil, melphalam, mitomycin C and the anti-oestrogen tamoxifen (Hudziak *et al*, 1989). Sensitization of tumour cells to the toxic response of particular drugs is not unique to anti-erbB2 antibodies since similar effects with cisplatin have also been observed with antibodies generated against the EGF receptor. Finally, an anti-IGF1 receptor blocking monoclonal antibody has been generated that is capable of blocking the in vitro and in vivo growth of human breast cancer cells (Osborne and Arteaga, 1990).

Mutated TP53: A Target for Immunotherapy

Two major studies have shown that accumulation of the TP53 protein in primary breast tumours is a highly significant predictor of shortened disease free and overall survival of the patient (Allred *et al*, 1992; Thor *et al*, 1992). Accumulation of the TP53 protein is primarily caused by missense mutations that increase the half life of the protein (Levine *et al*, 1991). Our own studies on *TP53* mutations in invasive ductal carcinomas of the breast are consistent with these findings in that the mutation of this gene is associated with tumours with a high proliferative index (Merlo *et al*, 1993). A high tumour proliferative index is also an independent predictor of poor disease outcome. Moreover, this association was primarily linked to tumours with a mutation in exons 5 or 6. Crawford *et al* (1984) first showed that a small proportion of breast cancer patients raise a humoural response to the TP53 protein. In a small study of primary breast tumours, Davidoff *et al* (1992) have shown that patients raising a humoural response to TP53 had tumours containing mutations primarily in exons 5 and 6 of the *TP53* gene. More recently, Schlichtholz *et al* (1992) found a significant association between breast cancer patients who raised a humoural response to the TP53 protein and patients whose tumours had a high histological grade and were hormone receptor negative. In addition, they showed that the humoural response was primarily directed at epitopes at the amino and carboxyl termini of the protein (Schlichtholtz *et al*, 1992). Taken together, these studies suggest that the humoural response to TP53 protein could be used to identify lymph node negative patients who may be at risk for relapse as well as an early indicator of relapse. In addition, it seems reasonable to ask whether the patients who raised a humoural response to the TP53 protein can also be stimulated to mount a cell mediated response to the tumour, including delayed type hypersensitivity. One promising report addressing this question showed that TP53 specific CD8+ cytotoxic T lymphocytes (CTL) could be generated by immunizing Balb/c mice with spleen cells from mice previously inoculated with a peptide encompassing a mutant TP53 gene product from a human lung carcinoma cell line (Yanuck *et al*, 1993). Significantly, the CTL response of the immunized mice was specific for cells expressing the corresponding mutated protein and not wild type or different mutated forms of the TP53 protein. These results therefore provide an experimental basis for clinical trials on breast cancer patients to determine the efficacy of immunization with either peptides encompassing a mutated TP53 protein or a vaccinia virus based expression vector expressing the mutated protein. Of course, this approach will depend on determining the identity of the point mutation in each tumour and the development of the appropriate peptide or vector. In the long term, the products of at least some of the other target genes for LOH may also present as potential targets for this type of immunotherapy.

Chorionic Gonadotrophin: A Pregnancy Dependent Hormone as a Tumoristatic Agent

It is known that the development of breast cancer is heavily influenced by the reproductive history of the patient such that parous women who have an early pregnancy are at lower risk for developing breast cancer than nulliparous women (MacMahon *et al*, 1973). It is thought that pregnancy provides this protective effect as a consequence of the differentiation of the mammary gland induced by ovarian, pituitary and placental hormones. To begin to understand this phenomenon, Russo and Russo have studied the rat model for breast cancer and have shown that, like pregnancy, treatment of rats with exogenous chorionic gonadotrophin (CG) has a protective effect against both the initiation and progression of 7,12-dimethyl-benz(a)anthracene (DMBA) induced mammary tumorigenesis (reviewed in Russo and Russo, 1993). Chorionic gonadotrophin is a placental polypeptide hormone, which, when administered exogenously, affects multiple endocrine organs. It seems that its main effect on the mammary gland is mediated through its stimulation of the ovaries to produce oestrogens and progesterone as well as inhibin, a member of the TGFB gene family. However, the protective effect CG exerts on the mammary gland also occurs in oophorectomized animals, suggesting that this hormone can also act directly on mammary epithelium. In fact, CG induced inhibin expression can be detected in alveolar cells, but not ductal cells, of the rat mammary gland (Alvarado *et al*, 1993). Moreover, treatment of the spontaneously immortalized, non-tumorigenic human MCF-10F mammary epithelial cell line and MCF-7 breast cancer cells with human CG inhibits the growth of these cells in a dose dependent manner and induces the expression of inhibin (Russo and Russo, 1993). Since treatment of virgin rats with exogenous CG gave no evidence of measurable toxicity to the animals, it seems very appropriate to consider human trials, particularly with women who are at high risk for the development of breast cancer (Russo *et al*, 1990).

Anti-sense Oligodeoxynucleotides and Anti-sense mRNA Expression Vectors against Growth Factors and Growth Factor Receptors

Anti-sense oligodeoxynucleotides and expression of anti-sense mRNAs have been successfully utilized to inhibit the expression of various oncogenes (Neckers *et al,* 1992; Carter and Lemoine, 1993). In this context, a c-*neu* anti-sense expression vector has been demonstrated to be effective in blocking the soft agar growth of c-*neu* overexpressing cells (Shaw *et al,* 1993). More recently, the ability to block the expression of specific growth factor receptors such as the EGF receptor or growth factors such as FGF, IGF1, TGFB2 and TGFA has also been accomplished using similar approaches (Moroni *et al,* 1992; Murphy *et al,* 1992; Sizeland and Burgess, 1992; Trojan *et al,* 1992; Jachimczak *et al,* 1993; Kenney *et al,* 1993). In most of these cases, oligodeoxynucleotide analogues have been used in which the phosphodiester backbone is replaced by a modified internucleotide phosphate residue of methylphosphonates, phosphorothioates, phosphoroamidates or phosphate esters (Murphy *et al,* 1992; Jachimczak *et al,* 1993). Anti-sense unmodified or phosphorothioate oligodeoxynucleotides (S-oligos) against FGF2 and TGFA have proved to be effective in inhibiting the in vitro growth of human glioma, astrocytoma, colon carcinoma and breast carcinoma cells (Murphy *et al,* 1992; Sizeland and Burgess, 1992). In addition, anti-sense mRNA expression vectors that can block the expression of EGF receptors, IGF1 or TGFA have been successfully used to inhibit the in vitro and/or in vivo growth of human epidermoid carcinoma, glioma and breast carcinoma cells (Moroni *et al,* 1992, Trojan *et al,* 1992; Kenney *et al,* 1993). In the case of breast cancer cells, an amphotropic replication defective, retroviral expression vector that contained a human TGFA cDNA oriented in the reverse 3′ to 5′ direction was able to generate a functional TGFA anti-sense mRNA. This vector was used to infect several different human breast cancer cell lines and when expressed was capable of significantly inhibiting the expression of endogenous TGFA and partially blocking the basal and oestrogen stimulated proliferation of these cells (Kenney *et al,* 1993). One could envision the use of specific anti-sense S-oligos in vivo possibly to treat breast cancer cells. Anti-sense S-oligos could be encapsulated into liposomes that contain a phospholipid membrane into which a specific monoclonal antibody has been incorporated (Akhtar *et al,* 1991). The antibody could be against a specific growth factor precursor, growth factor receptor or another tumour associated cell surface antigen. This could provide a mechanism for selectively targeting the injected, anti-sense S-oligo containing liposomes to tumours that are overexpressing these antigens (Greig *et al,* 1988).

SUMMARY

The complexity of growth factors and growth factor receptors that are aberrantly expressed, as well as the mutational events that either directly cause or influence the expression of these and other gene products, should provide in the near future multiple diagnostic, prognostic indicators or targets for therapeutic intervention. It seems reasonable to expect that soon the search for aberrantly expressed gene products in breast cancer cells will merge with the search and characterization of somatic mutations that are selected during tumour progression. Clearly, the current rapid development of new molecular biological methodologies aimed at detecting and cloning of RNA sequences that are aberrantly expressed in breast tumour cells, as well as molecular probes and reagents to detect and physically map mutated genes on affected chromosomes, should accelerate the effort to identify targets for therapeutic intervention. We are at the beginning of this learning curve, but already several potential target gene products have been identified. A major challenge will be to sort out those approaches and reagents that appear efficacious on the basis of results from in vitro and in vivo model systems that will actually have an impact on the treatment of the disease in the clinic. Reagents that target some of these gene products are currently in clinical trials; however, there are others such as immunotherapy against the mutated TP53 protein and human CG treatment of high risk breast cancer patients that warrant testing in this context.

References

Adnane J, Gaudray P, Dionne CA et al (1990) BEK and FLG, two receptors to members of the FGF family, are amplified in subsets of human breast cancers. *Oncogene* **6** 659–663

Akhtar S, Basu S, Wickstrom E and Juliano RL (1991) Interactions of antisense DNA oligonucleotide analogs with phospholipid membranes (liposomes). *Nucleic Acids Research* **19** 5551–5559

Ali IU, Campbell G, Lidereau R and Callahan R (1988) Lack of evidence for the prognostic significance of c-erbB-2 amplification in human breast carcinoma. *Oncogene Research* **3** 139–146

Ali IU, Merlo G, Lidereau R and Callahan R (1989) The amplification unit on chromosome 11q13 in aggressive primary human breast tumors contains the *bcl*-1, *int*-2, and *hst* loci. *Oncogene* **4** 89–92

Allred DC, Clark GM, Elledge R et al (1992) Association of p53 protein expression with tumor cell proliferation rate and clinical outcome in node-negative breast cancer. *Journal of the National Cancer Institute* **85** 200–206

Alvarado MV, Russo J and Russo IH (1993) Immunolocalization of inhibin in the mammary gland of rats treated with hCG. *Journal of Histochemistry and Cytochemistry* **41** 29–34

Andersen TI, Gaust ad A, Ottestad L et al (1992) Genetic alterations of the tumour suppressor gene regions 3p, 11p, 13q, 17p, and 17q in human breast carcinomas. *Genes, Chromosomes & Cancer* **4** 113–121

Antoniotti S, Maggiora P, Dati C and De Bortoli M (1992) Tamoxifen up-regulates c-erbB-2 expression in oestrogen-responsive breast cancer cells in vitro. *European Journal of Cancer* **28** 318–321

Ariad S, Seymour L and Bezwoda WR (1991) Platelet-derived growth factor (PDGF) in plasma of breast cancer patients: Correlation with stage and rate of progression. *Breast Cancer Research and Treatment* **20** 11–17

Arteaga CL, Coffey RJ, Dugger TC, McCutchen CM, Moses HL and Lyons RM (1990) Growth stimulation of human breast cancer cells with anti-transforming growth factor β antibodies:

evidence for negative autocrine regulation by transforming growth factor β. *Cell Growth and Differentiation* **1** 367–374

Bacus SS, Stancovski I, Huberman E *et al* (1992) Tumor-inhibitory monoclonal antibodies to the HER-2/neu receptor induce differentiation of human breast cancer cells. *Cancer Research* **52** 2580–2589

Barker S and Vinson GP (1990) Epidermal growth factor in breast cancer. *International Journal of Biochemistry* **22** 939–945

Bates SE, Davidson NE, Valverius EM *et al* (1988) Expression of transforming growth factor α and its messenger ribonucleic acid in human breast cancer: its regulation by estrogen and its possible functional significance. *Molecular Endocrinology* **2** 543–555

Bieche I, Champeme MH, Matifas F, Cropp CS, Callahan R and Lidereau R (1993) Two distinct regions involved in 1p deletion in primary human breast cancer. *Cancer Research* **53** 1990–1994

Breuer B, Luo J-C, DeVito I *et al* (1993) Detection of elevated c-*erb*B-2 oncoprotein in the serum and tissue in breast cancer. *Medical Science Research* **21** 383–384

Buday L and Downward J (1993) Epidermal growth factor regulates p21*ras* through the formation of a complex of receptor, Grb2 adapter protein, and sos nucleotide exchange factor. *Cell* **73** 611–620

Butta A, MacLennan K, Flanders KC *et al* (1992) Induction of transforming growth factor β_1 in human breast cancer in vivo following tamoxifen treatment. *Cancer Research* **52** 4262–4264

Callahan R, Cropp CS, Merlo GR, Liscia DS, Cappa APM and Lidereau R (1992) Somatic mutations and human breast cancer: a stus report. *Cancer* **69** 1582–1588

Callahan R, Cropp C, Merlo GR *et al* (1993) Genetic and molecular heterogeneity of breast cancer cells. *Clinica Chimica Acta* **217** 63–73

Carter G and Lemoine NR (1993) Antisense technology for cancer therapy: does it make sense. *British Journal of Cancer* **67** 869–876

Ciardiello F, Kim N, Liscia DS *et al* (1989) mRNA expression of transforming growth factor alpha in human breast carcinomas and its activity in effusions of breast cancer patients. *Journal of the National Cancer Institute* **81** 1165–1171

Clarke R, Dickson RB and Lippman ME (1992) Hormonal aspects of breast cancer: growth factors, drugs and stromal reactions. *Critical Reviews in Oncolgy/Hematology* **12** 1–23

Crawford LV, Pim DC and Lamb P (1984) The cellular protein p53 in human tumors. *Molecular Biology and Medicine* **2** 261–272

Cropp C, Lidereau R, Campbell G, Champene M-H and Callahan R (1990) Loss of heterozygosity on chromosome 17 and 18 in breast carcinoma: two new regions identified. *Procedings of the National Academy of Sciences of the USA* **87** 7737–7741

Dati C, Antoniotti S, Taverna D, Perroteau I and De Bortoli M (1990) Inhibition of c-*erb*B-2 oncogene expression by estrogens in human breast cancer cells. *Oncogene* **5** 1001–1006

Dati C, Muraca R, Tazarte s O *et al* (1991) c-*erb*B-2 and *ras* expression levels in breast cancer are correlated and show a co-operative association with unfavorable clinical outcome. *International Journal of Cancer* **47** 833–838

Davidoff AM, Iglehart JD and JR Marks (1992) Imunne response to p53 is dependent upon p53/HSP70 complexes in breast cancers. *Procedings of the National Academy of Sciences USA* **89** 3439–3442

Der CJ and Cox AD (1991) Isoprenoid modification and plasma membrane association: critical factors for ras oncogenicity. *Cancer Cells* **3** 331

Devilee P, van den Broek M, Kuipers-Dijkshoorn N *et al* (1989) At least four different chromosomal regions are involved in loss of heterozygosity in human breast carcinoma. *Genomics* **5** 554–560

Dickens T-A and Coletta AA (1993) The pharmacological manipulation of members of the transforming growth factor beta family in the chemoprevention of breast cancer. *BioEssays* **15** 71–74

Drebin JA, Link VC and Greene MI (1988) Monoclonal antibodies reactive with distinct domains of the *neu* oncogene-encoded p185 molecule exert synergistic anti-tumor effects in vivo. *Oncogene* **2** 273–277

Eckert K, Granetzny A, Fischer J and Grosse R (1991) Relationship between 43 kDa epidermal growth factor-related clonogenic activity and clinical parameters for breast cancer. *Anticancer Research* **11** 2125–2130

Ennis BW, Lippman ME and Dickson RB (1991) The EGF receptor system as a target for antitumor therapy. *Cancer Investigation* **9** 553–562

Enright WJ and Booth P (1991) Specificity of inhibitors of tyrosine kinases. *Focus* **13** 79–83

Eppstein DA, Marsh YV, Schryver BB and Bertics PJ (1989) Inhibition of epidermal growth factor/transforming growth factor-α-stimulated cell growth by a synthetic peptide. *Journal of Cellular Physiology* **141** 420–430

Escot C, Theillet C, Lidereau R *et al* (1986) Genetic alterations of the c-*myc* proto-oncogene in human primary breast carcinomas. *Proceedings of the National Academy of Sciences of the USA* **83** 4834–4838

FitzGerald D and Pastan I (1989) Targeted toxin therapy for the treatment of cancer. *Journal of the National Cancer Institute* **81** 1455–1463

Goldenberg A, Masui H, Divgi C, Kamrath H, Pentlow K and Mendelsohn J (1989) Imaging of human tumor xenografts with an indium-111-labeled anti-epidermal growth factor receptor monoclonal antibody. *Journal of the National Cancer Institute* **81** 1616–1625

Gompel G and van Kerkem C (1983) The breast, In: Silverberg S (ed). *Principles of Surgical Pathology*, pp 245–255, Wiley Medical, New York

Gorsch SM, Memoli VA, Stukel TA, Gold LI and Arrick BA (1992) Immunohistochemical staining for transforming growth factor $\beta_1$1 associates with disease progression in human breast cancer. *Cancer Research* **52** 6949–6952

Greig R, Dunnington D, Murthy U and Anzano M (1988) Growth factors as novel therapeutic targets in neoplastic disease. *Cancer Surveys* **7** 653–674

Greiner J, Guadagni F, Horan-Hand P *et al* (1990) Augmentation of tumor antigen expression by recombinant human interferons: enhanced targeting of monoclonal antibodies to carcinomas, In: Goldenberg DM (ed). *Cancer Imaging with Radiolabeled Antibodies*, pp 413–432, Kluwer Academic, Boston

Group NCM (1992) A comprehensive genetic linkage map of the human genome. *Science* **258** 67–86

Gullick WJ (1990a) Inhibitors of growth factor receptors, In: Carney D and Sikora K (eds). *Genes and Cancer*, pp 263–273, John Wiley, New York

Gullick WJ (1990b) The role of the epidermal growth factor receptor and the c-erbB-2 protein in breast cancer. *International Journal of Cancer* **5** 55–61

Gullick WJ, Berger MS, Bennett PLP, Rothbard JB and Waterfield MD (1 987) Expression of the c-*erb*B-2 protein in normal and transformed cells. *International Journal of Cancer* **40** 246–254

Hall JM, Lee MK, Newman B *et al* (1990) Linkage of early-onset familial breast cancer to chromosome 17q21. *Science* **250** 1684–1689

Hall JM, Friedman L, Guenther C *et al* (1992) Closing in on a breast cancer gene on chromosome 17q. *American Journal of Genetics* **50** 1235–1242

Hamburger AW and Pinnamaneni GD (1991) Increased epidermal growth factor receptor gene expression by γ-interferon in a human breast carcinoma cell line. *British Journal of Cancer* **64** 64–68

Hancock MC, Langton BC, Chan T *et al* (1991) A monoclonal antibody against the c-*erb*B-2 protein enhances the cytotoxicity of cis-diamminedichloroplatinum against human breast and ovarian tumor cell lines. *Cancer Research* **51** 4575–4580

Harris JR, Hellman S, Canellos GP and Fisher B (1982) Cancer of the breast, In: DeVita VT and Rosenberg SA (eds). *Cancer Principles and Practice of Oncology*, pp 1119–1178, JB Lippincott, Philadelphia

Hollingsworth RE and Lee W-H (1991) Tumor suppressor genes: new prospect for cancer research. *Journal of the National Cancer Institue* **83** 91–96

Holmes WE, Sliwkowski MX, Akita RW *et al* (1992) Identification of heregulin, a specific activator of p185*erb*B2. *Science* **256** 1205–1210

Hosono M, Saga T, Sakahara H *et al* (1993) Construction of immunoradiometric assay for circulating c-*erb*B-2 protooncogene product in advanced breast cancer patients. *Japanese Journal of Cancer Research* **84** 147–152

Hudziak RM, Lewis GD, Winget M, Fendly BM, Shepard MH and Ullrich A (1989) p185[HER2] monoclonal antibody has antiproliferative effects in vitro and sensitizes human breast tumor cells to tumor necrosis factor. *Molecular and Cellular Biology* **9** 1165 –1172

Jachimczak P, Bogdahn U, Schneider J *et al* (1993) The effect of transforming growth factor-β_2-specific phosphorothioate-anti-sense oligodeoxynucleotides in reversing cellular immunosuppression in malignant glioma. *Journal of Neurosurgery* **78** 944–951

Kamiya Y, Ohmura E, Murakami H *et al* (1993) Transforming growth factor-alpha activity in effusions: comparison of radioimmunoassay and radioreceptorassay. *Life Sciences* **52** 1381–1386

Kelsey JL and Berkowitz GS (1988) Breast cancer epidemiology. *Cancer Research* **48** 5615–5623

Kenney NJ, Saeki T, Gottardis M *et al* (1993) Expression of transforming growth factor α (TGFα) antisense mRNA inhibits the estrogen-induced production of TGFα and estrogen-induced proliferation of estrogen-responsive human breast cancer cells. *Journal of Cellular Physiology* **156** 497–514

Klagsbrun M and Baird A (1991) A dual receptor system is required for basic fibroblast growth factor activity. *Cell* **67** 229–231

Klijn JG, Berns PM, Schmitz PI and Foekens JA (1992) The clinical significance of epidermal growth factor receptor (EGF-R) in human breast cancer: a review of 5232 patients. *Endocrine Reviews* **13** 3–17

Knudson AG (1989) Hereditary cancers: clue to mechanisms of carcinogenesis. *British Journal of Cancer* **59** 661–666

Koenders PG, Beex LVAM, Geurts-Moespot A, Heuvel JJTM, Kienhuis CBM and Benraad TJ (1991) Epidermal growth factor receptor-negative tumors are predominantly confined to the subgroup of estradiol receptor-positive human primary breast cancer. *Cancer Research* **51** 4544–4548

Koenders PG, Beex LVAM, Kienhuis CBM, Kloppenborg PWC and Benraad TJ (1993) Epidermal growth factor receptor and prognosis in human breast cancer: a prospective study. *Breast Cancer Research and Treatment* **25** 21–27

Lammie GA and Peters G (1991) Chromosome 11q13 abnormalities in human cancer. *Cancer Cells* **3** 413–420

Langton BC, Crenshaw MC, Chao LA, Stuart SG, Akita RW and Jackson JE (1991) An antigen immunologically related to the external domain of gp185 is shed from nude mouse tumors overexpressing the c-*erb*B-2 (HER-2/*neu*). *Cancer Research* **51** 2593–2598

Lee E, To H, Shew J, Bookstein R, Scully P and Lee WH (1988) Inactivation of the retinoblastoma susceptibility gene in human breast cancers. *Science* **241** 218–221

Levine AJ, Momand J and Finlay CA (1991) The p53 tumour suppressor gene. *Nature* **351** 453–456

Lidereau R, Callahan R, Dickson C *et al* (1988) Amplification of the *int*-2 gene in primary human breast tumors. *Oncogene Research* **2** 285–291

Lin YJ and Clinton GM (1991) A soluble protein related to the HER-2-proto-oncogene product is released from human breast carcinoma cells. *Oncogene* **6** 639–643

Liscia DS, Merlo G, Garrett C, French D, Mariani-Costantini R and Callahan R (1989) Expression of *int*-2 mRNA in human tumors amplified at the *int*-2 locus. *Oncogene* **4** 1219–1224

Lofts FJ and Gullick WJ (1991) c-*erb*B2 amplification and overexpression in human tumors, In: Dickson RB and Lippman ME (eds). *Genes, Oncogenes, and Hormones: Advances in Cel-*

lular and Molecular Biology of Breast Cancer, pp 161–179, Kluwer Academic, Boston

Lynch HT, Albano WA, Danes S *et al* (1984) Genetic predisposition to breast cancer. *Cancer* **53** 612–622

McGuire WL and Naylor SL (1989) Loss of heterozygosity in breast cancer: cause or effect. *Journal of the National Cancer Institute* **81** 1764–1765

McGuire WL, Chamness GC and Fuqua SA (1991) Estrogen receptor variants in clinical breast cancer. *Molecular Endocrinology* **5** 1571–1577

McGuire WL Jr, Jackson JG, Figueroa JA, Shimasaki S, Powell DR and Yee D (1992) Regulation of insulin-like growth factor-binding protein (IGFBP) expression by breast cancer cells: use of IGFBP-1 as an inhibitor of insulin-like growth factor action. *Journal of the National Cancer Institute* **84** 1336–1341

MacMahon B, Cole P and Brown J (1973) Etiology of human breast cancer: a review. *Journal of the National Cancer Institute* **50** 21–42

Mendelsohn J (1992) Epidermal growth factor receptor as a target for therapy with antireceptor monoclonal antibodies. *Journal of the National Cancer Institute Monographs* **13** 125–131

Merlo G, Venesio T, Bernardi A *et al* (1992) Loss of heterozygosity on chromosome 17p13 in breast carcinomas identifies tumors with a high proliferation index. *American Journal of Pathology* **140** 215–223

Merlo GM, Bernardi, A, Diella, F *et al* (1993) In primary human breast carcinomas mutations in exons 5 and 6 of the p53 gene are associated with a high S-phase index. *International Journal of Cancer* **54** 531–535

Mesri EA, Kreitman RJ, Fu YM, Epstein SE and Pastan I (1993) Heparin-binding transforming growth factor alpha-pseudomonas exotoxin A: a heparan sulfate-modulated recombinant toxin cytotoxic to cancer cells and proliferating smooth muscle cells. *Journal of Biological Chemistry* **268** 4853–4862

Moroni MC, Willingham MC and Beguino L (1992) EGF-R antisense RNA blocks expression of the epidermal growth factor receptor and suppresses the transforming phenotype of a human carcinoma cell line. *Journal of Biological Chemistry* **267** 2714–2722

Murphy PR, Sato Y and Knee RS (1992) Phosphorothioate antisense oligonucleotides against basic fibroblast growth factor inhibit anchorage-dependent and anchorage-independent growth of a malignant glioblastoma cell line. *Molecular Endocrinology* **6** 877–884

Narod SA, Feunteun J, Lynch HT *et al* (1991) Familial breast-ovarian cancer locus on chromosome 17q12-q23. *Lancet* **338** 82–83

Neckers L, Whitesell L, Rosolen A and Geselowitz DA (1992) Antisense inhibition of oncogene expression. *Critical Reviews in Oncogenesis* **3** 175–231

Nicholson S, Wright C, Sainsbury RC *et al* (1990) Epidermal growth factor receptor (EGFr) as a marker for poor prognosis in node-negative breast cancer patients: neu and tamoxifen failure. *Journal of Steroid Biochemistry and Molecular Biology* **37** 811–814

Osborne CK and Arteaga CL (1990) Autocrine and paracrine growth regulation of breast cancer: clinical implications. *Breast Cancer Research and Treatment* **15** 3–11

Osborne CK, Coronado EB, Kitten LJ *et al* (1989) Insulin-like growth factor-II (IGF-II): a potential autocrine/paracrine growth factor for human breast cancer acting via the IGF-I receptor. *Molecular Endocrinology* **3** 1701–1709

Osbourne RJ, Merlo GR, Mitsudomi T *et al* (1991) Mutations in the p53 gene in primary human breast cancers. *Cancer Research* **51** 6194–6198

Osherov N, Gazit A, Gilon C and Levitzki A (1993) Selective inhibition of the epidermal growth factor and HER2/neu receptors by tyrphostins. *Journal of Biological Chemistry* **268** 11134–11142

Peterson G and Barnes S (1991) Genistein inhibition of the growth of human breast cancer cells: independence from estrogen receptors and the multi-drug resistance gene. *Biochemical and Biophysical Research Communications* **179** 661–667

Qi C-F, Liscia DS, Normanno N *et al* Expression of transforming growth factor α, amphiregulin and cripto-1 in human breast carcinomas. *British Journal of Cancer* (in press)

Reddy KB, Mangold GL, Tandon AK *et al* (1992) Inhibition of breast cancer cell growth in vitro by a tyrosine kinase inhibitor. *Cancer Research* **52** 3636–3641

Rieman DJ, Anzano MA, Chan GW *et al* (1992) Antagonism of TGF-α recept or binding and TGF-α induced stimulation of cell proliferation by methyl pheophorbides. *Oncology Research* **4** 193–200

Ruoslahti E and Yamaguchi Y (1991) Proteoglycans as modulators of growth factor activities. *Cell* **64** 867–869

Russo IH and Russo J (1993) Chorionic gonadotropin: a tumoristatic and preventive agent in breast cancer, In: Teicher BA (ed). *Drug Resistance in Oncology*, pp 537–560, Marcel Dekker, New York

Russo IH, Kozalka M, Gimotty PA and Russo J (1990) Protective effect of chorionic gonadotropin on DMBA-induced mammary carcinogenesis. *British Journal of Cancer* **62** 243–247

Salomon DS, Dickson RB, Normanno N *et al* (1992) Interaction of oncogenes and growth factors in colon and breast cancer, In: Spandidos DA (ed). *Current Perspectives on Molecular & Cellular Oncology*, pp 211–260, JAI Press, London

Sarup JC, Johnson RM, King KL *et al* (1991) Characterization of an anti-p85^HER2 monoclonal antibody that stimulates receptor function and inhibits tumor growth. *Growth Regulation* **1** 72–82

Sato T, Akiyama F, Sakamoto G, Kasumi F and Nakamura Y (1991) Accumulation of genetic alterations and progression of primary breast cancer. *Cancer Research* **51** 5794–5799

Satoh T, Nakafuku M and Kaziro Y (1992) Function of ras as a molecular switch in signal transduction. *Journal of Biological Chemistry* **267** 24149–24152

Schlichtholtz B, Legros Y, Gillet D *et al* (1992) The imunne response to p53 in breast cancer patients is directed against immunodominant epitopes unrelated to the mutational hot spot. *Cancer Research* **52** 6380–6384

Scott JK (1992) Discovering peptide ligands using epitope libraries. *Trends in Biochemical Sciences* **17** 10–15

Seemayer TA and Cavenee WE (1989) Biology of disease: molecular mechanisms of oncogenesis. *Laboratory Investigation* **60** 585–599

Shaw Y-T, Chang S-H, Chiou S-T, Chang W-C and Lai M-D (1993) Partial reversion of transformed phenotype of B104 cancer cells by antisense nucleic acids. *Cancer Letters* **69** 27–32

Shepard HM, Lewis GD, Sarup JC *et al* (1991) Monoclonal antibody therapy of human cancer: taking the HER2 protooncogene to the clinic. *Journal of Clinical Immunology* **11** 117–127

Siegfried JM (1992) Strategies for identification of peptide growth factors. *Pharmacology and Therapeutics*, pp 233–245, Pergamon Press, New York

Sizeland AM and Burgess AW (1992) Anti-sense transforming growth factor α oligonucleotides inhibit autocrine stimulated proliferation of a colon carcinoma cell line. *Molecular Biology of the Cell* **3** 1235–1243

Sporn MB and Roberts AB (1992) Autocrine secretion—10 years later. *Annals of Internal Medicine* **117** 408–414

Stancovski I, Peles E, Levy RB *et al* (1992) Signal transduction by the *neu/erbB*-2 receptor: a potential target for anti-tumor therapy. *Journal of Steroid Biochemistry and Molecular Biology* **43** 95–103

Stein CA (1993) Suramin: a novel antineoplastic agent with multiple potential mechanisms of action. *Cancer Research* **15** 2239–2248

Stromberg K, Duffy M, Fritsch C *et al* (1991) Comparison of urinary transforming growth factor-α in women with disseminated breast cancer and healthy control women. *Cancer Investigation* **15** 277–283

Taetle R, Honeysett JM and Houston LL (1988) Effects of anti-epidermal growth factor (EGF) receptor antibodies and an anti-EGF receptor recombinant-ricin A chain immunoconjugate on growth of human cells. *Journal of the National Cancer Institute* **80** 1053–1054

Theuer CP, Fitzgerald DJ and Pastan I (1993) A recombinant form of pseudomonas exotoxin A containing transforming growth factor alpha near its carboxyl terminus for the treatment of bladder cancer. *Journal of Urology* **149** 1626–1632

Thor AD, Moore DH, Edgerton SM *et al* (1992) Accumulation of p53 tumor suppressor gene protein is an independent marker of prognosis. *Journal of the National Cancer Institute* **84** 845–855

Travis J (1993) Novel anticancer agents move closer to reality. *Science* **260** 1877–1878

Trojan J, Blossey BK, Johnson TR *et al* (1992) Loss of tumorigenicity of rat glioblastoma directed by episome-based antisense cDNA transcription of insulin-like growth factor I. *Proceedings of the National Academy of Sciences of the USA* **89** 4874–4878

Vignon F, Prebois C and Rochefort H (1992) Inhibiton of breast cancer growth by suramin. *Journal of the National Cancer Institute* **84** 38–42

Wakefield L, Kim S-J, Glick A, Winokur T, Colletta A and Sporn M (1990) Regulation of transforming growth factor-β subtypes by members of the steroid hormone superfamily. *Journal of Cell Science Supplement* **13** 139–148

Walker RA and Dearing SJ (1992) Transforming growth factor beta$_1$ in ductal carcinoma in situ and invasive carcinomas of the breast. *European Journal of Cancer* **28** 641–644

Walker RA and Varley JM (1993) The molecular pathology of human breast cancer. *Cancer Surveys* **16** 31–57

Warri AM, Laine AM, Majasuo KE, Alitalo KK and Harkonen PL (1991) Estrogen suppression of *erb*B2 expression is associated with increased growth rate of ZR-75-1 human breast cancer cells in vitro and in nude mice. *International Journal of Cancer* **49** 616–623

Weinberg RA (1991) Tumor suppressor genes. *Science* **254** 1138–1146

Weissenbach J, Gyapay G, Dib C *et al* (1992) A second-generation linkage map of the human genome. *Nature* **359** 794–801

Wright C, Nicholson S, Angus B *et al* (1992) Relationship between c-erbB-2 protein product expression and response to endocrine therapy in advanced breast cancer. *British Journal of Cancer* **65** 118–121

Yanuck M, Carbone DP, Pendleton CD *et al* (1993) A mutant p53 tumor suppressor protein is a target for peptide-induced CD8+ cytotoxic T-cells. *Cancer Research* **53** 3257–3261

Zugmaier G, Lippman ME and Wellstein A (1992) Inhibition by pentosan polysulfate (PPS) of heparin-binding growth factors released from tumor cells and blockage by PPS of tumor growth in animals. *Journal of the National Cancer Institute* **84** 1716–1724

The authors are responsible for the accuracy of the references.

The Role of TP53 in Breast Cancer Development

R A EELES[1] • J BARTKOVA[2] • D P LANE[3] • J BARTEK[2]

[1]Section of Molecular Carcinogenesis, Institute of Cancer Research, 15 Cotswold Road, Sutton, Surrey SM2 5NG and CRC Academic Unit of Radiotherapy, Royal Marsden Hospital, Sutton, Surrey SM2 5PT; [2]Danish Cancer Society, Division for Cancer Biology, Strandboulevarden 49, Dk-2100, Copenhagen; [3]CRC Laboratories, University of Dundee, Dundee DD1 4HN

Introduction
Role of the TP53 protein
Role of the *TP53* gene in inherited predisposition to breast cancer
Detection of TP53 overexpression in breast tumours: Immunohistochemical
    and molecular data
Spectrum of *TP53* mutations in invasive breast cancers
TP53 as a prognostic factor in breast tumours
Summary

INTRODUCTION

The TP53 protein was described in 1979 (DeLeo *et al*, 1979; Lane and Crawford, 1979; Linzer and Levine, 1979), when it was found to complex with the large T viral antigen of SV40. Since then, the *TP53* gene has been found to be the most commonly altered oncogene in human tumours (Hollstein *et al*, 1991; de Fromentel *et al*, 1992). It is involved in the development of both sporadic and some hereditary breast tumours and in its unmutated form acts as a tumour suppressor gene, but it can lose its negative growth control properties or even acquire oncogenic activation when mutated (Jenkins *et al*, 1985; Lane and Benchimol, 1990). Although germline mutations in the *TP53* gene carry a high risk of early onset breast cancer, and the gene is mutated somatically in a proportion of preinvasive and invasive breast cancers, it is not usually the initiating genetic event in most breast tumours. It does, however, seem to be an independent prognostic factor for survival that might prove useful in clinical management of patients with breast cancer.

ROLE OF THE TP53 PROTEIN

When the *TP53* gene was first isolated, genomic and cDNA clones of *TP53* immortalized cells in culture (Jenkins *et al*, 1984) or transformed primary fibroblasts in co-operation with ras, suggesting that *TP53* was a dominant oncogene (Eliyahu *et al*, 1984; Parada *et al*, 1984). These clones are now known to have been mutant, and wild type *TP53* does not have these activities (Eliyahu *et al*, 1988; Hinds *et al*, 1989). In fact, it negatively regulates the growth of some cells (Mowat *et al*, 1985; Baker *et al*, 1989; Finlay *et al*, 1989) and eliminates the tumorigenic potential of a cell line in culture (Chen *et al*, 1990); loss of the normal allele has been associated with mutation of the other allele in breast tumours (Prosser *et al*, 1990) and many other cancers (Hollstein *et al*, 1991), suggesting a tumour suppressor action.

The human *TP53* gene spans a 20 kb region of DNA at 17p13.1 (Benchimol *et al*, 1985). It is composed of 11 exons, exons 2–11 coding for a 53 kDa protein (hence its name) of 393 aminoacids. In humans, the gene has five conserved domains, the first in exon 1 (codons 13–19) and the remainder encompassed by codons 117–142, 171–181, 234–258 and 270–286. These domains are highly conserved across many species, indicating that these regions of *TP53* may be critical for its function. Domains II–V are within exons 4–9 (Soussi *et al*, 1990) and contain most of the mutations reported to occur in tumours. The TP53 protein has a *trans*-action activation site (aminoacids 20–42) at the highly charged acidic amino terminus that can act as a transcriptional activating domain even when fused to another DNA binding protein (Fields and Jang, 1990; O'Rourke *et al*, 1990; Raycroft *et al*, 1990). There is an interior highly conserved hydrophobic proline rich domain between residues 76 and 290 that appears to be important for maintaining the overall structure of the protein (Levine *et al*, 1991) and probably contains the sequence specific binding domain (Prives C, personal communication). A highly charged basic region at the carboxyl terminus between aminoacids 344 and 393 can form alpha helical structures and helix-turn-helix motifs (Pennica *et al*, 1984). This terminal is necessary for the formation of homologous *TP53* complexes (Iwabuchi *et al*, 1993), which are dimers and tetramers. A nuclear transport sequence centred around aminoacids 316–325 helps to direct the protein into the nucleus (Shaulsky *et al*, 1990). There are two SV40 large T antigen binding sites (aminoacids 169–204 and 256–289) and phosphorylation sites (cdc2, a serine at position 315, phosphorylated by $p34^{cdc2}$ kinase, and CK2, a serine at position 392 phosphorylated by casein kinase II).

Wild type *TP53* has a half life of 6–20 minutes in normal cells, but the mutant form is more resistant to proteolysis, and its half life is therefore longer (about 2–12 hr). The conformation of *TP53* with a mutation between aminoacids 135 and 175 is different from that of wild type: as has been shown with monoclonal antibodies and in rodent systems, it binds to the heat shock protein, hsc70 (Hinds *et al*, 1990). Different mutants have varying binding properties: those that bind to heat shock protein do not bind to SV40 (Hinds *et al*, 1987). Mutants at codon 273 have a normal or little altered conformation. More research is needed to correlate the various *TP53* mutations with conformational change.

Loss of *TP53* tumour suppressor activity is associated with a failure to halt the transition from G_1 to S in the cell cycle in cells that have accumulated

DNA damage (Kastan *et al,* 1991). Normal, but not mutant, TP53 binds to DNA and acts as a transcriptional activator (Kern *et al,* 1991; Scharer and Iggo, 1992). The DNA binding region recognizes a motif containing two contiguous or close monomers of the sequence (purine)$_3$-C(A/T)(A/T)G (pyrimidine)$_3$ (El-Deiry *et al,* 1992; Zambetti *et al,* 1992). A particular DNA element (*TP53* CON; GGACATGCCCGGGCATGTCC) can activate the transcription of the luciferase gene when bound by wild type TP53 (Funk *et al,* 1992). Using this system and testing specific mutants in *TP53* null cells, Zhang *et al* (1993) have shown that the ability to bind to this DNA sequence varies between different mutant TP53 proteins and that binding is not necessarily related to transcriptional activation. Some mutants fail to be activated by casein kinase II, resulting in a loss of their DNA binding activity (Hupp *et al,* 1993). The wild type protein is bound by the large T antigen of SV40, the E1B antigen of adenovirus and E6 of the papillomavirus (Werness *et al,* 1990). Such binding inactivates the ability of TP53 to act as a transcription factor. The cellular oncogene, *mdm2,* also binds to TP53, abolishing its transcription factor action (Momand *et al,* 1992). There is also evidence for the binding of replication protein A (RPA) to TP53 (Dutta *et al,* 1993): RPA is required for unwinding DNA origins, and its binding to single stranded DNA may be the initial step in DNA replication. It is therefore clear that many proteins bind to TP53, but their relative importance and sequence of events need to be elucidated.

In some instances, mutant TP53 proteins appear to act in a dominant negative fashion, forming oligomeric complexes with wild type TP53 that block its normal function (Milner and Metcalf, 1991). This may be effected by preventing normal TP53 in the cytoplasm from migrating into the nucleus (Martinez *et al,* 1991). This would explain the growth advantage seen in heterozygous mutant fibroblasts (Srivastava *et al,* 1993) and is called a "dominant loss of function" mutation. In animals, mutant *TP53* cDNA introduced into normal cells without any normal TP53 protein expression enhances the tumorigenicity of these cells, indicating that mutant *TP53* also has a gain of function (Dittmer *et al,* 1993). It is clear, however, that not all mutants have this effect, for example the 248W mutant TP53 protein, which has been identified as an inherited mutation in some cases of the Li-Fraumeni syndrome, does not affect the conformation of the wild type protein (Milner and Metcalf, 1991) or DNA binding (Bargonetti *et al,* 1992).

There has been interest in the role of *TP53* as part of a damage control pathway. It seems to have a role in apoptosis induced by radiation and DNA damaging agents. Null mice without a *TP53* gene are viable and fertile and have normal development, so *TP53* is not essential for development; however, these mice have a propensity to develop certain tumours (Donehower *et al,* 1992). Increased TP53 levels can also be induced by DNA damage due to radiation, and this has led to the hypothesis that *TP53* is part of a damage control pathway (Kuerbitz *et al,* 1992). Thymocytes from *TP53* knockout mice show normal apoptosis in response to glucocorticoids but are resistant to radiation induced apoptosis, indicating that there are at least two apoptotic pathways and that TP53 is needed for only one of them (Clarke *et al*, 1993; Lowe *et al*, 1993). Levels of TP53 rise in response to some DNA damaging agents, and this arrests cells before entry into S phase, possibly enabling DNA repair to occur (Lane, 1992). Cells lacking wild type TP53 cannot arrest in G_1 (Kastan *et al*, 1992). There are several models for the mechanism of the growth arrest: TP53 may act as a transcription factor and stimulate the expression of genes that suppress growth (Vogelstein and Kinzler, 1992), TP53 may inhibit the expression of *TATA* controlled genes in general (Mack *et al*, 1993) or TP53 may interact with key proteins involved in cellular replication, such as RPA. The differential effect of TP53 acting to arrest cells in G_1 to repair DNA damage and to induce apoptosis in response to DNA damage needs further investigation, and it seems to depend critically on the cell type concerned.

There is a gene dosage effect: heterozygous mice containing only one *TP53* copy have an intermediate radiosensitivity, although it is nearer the radioresistant end of the spectrum. There is some preliminary evidence that irradiated fibroblasts from patients with the Li-Fraumeni syndrome are more radioresistant than healthy people (Chang *et al*, 1987), and mouse fibroblasts containing only one or no *TP53* genes have a moderate or high degree of aneuploidy (Harvey *et al*, 1993). The presence of a *TP53* mutation may therefore result in the cell tolerating DNA damage and perpetuating it during cell division, which could then lead to cancer formation. Apoptosis induced by TP53 would normally remove such cells carrying mutations in DNA. This raises questions for the screening and treatment of patients with Li-Fraumeni and Li-Fraumeni like cancer syndromes who have a germline *TP53* mutation. It may be preferable to screen them with modalities avoiding X irradiation, such as magnetic resonance, and treatment with surgery may be preferable if it is a suitable alternative to radiotherapy. Conservative management (involving radiotherapy) of breast cancer in patients with a germline *TP53* mutation may increase their risk of second malignancy above that of other patients.

ROLE OF THE *TP53* GENE IN INHERITED PREDISPOSITION TO BREAST CANCER

The first clue that the *TP53* gene is a cancer predisposition gene came from the Li-Fraumeni familial cancer syndrome (LFS). This was first described in 1969 as an association between young onset sarcoma in the affected individual and other tumours in close relatives (Li and Fraumeni, 1969; Li *et al*, 1988). Subsequently, mutations in the *TP53* gene were investigated as a cause of this syndrome. It was a good candidate gene, since *TP53* mutations are the commonest genetic change in human cancers and are seen in all the tumours occurring in LFS. Malkin (1990) and Srivastava *et al* (1990) were the first to describe germline mutations in exon 7 of the *TP53* gene in LFS, and other groups have subsequently reported *TP53* germline mutations. The germline mutations reported to date have occurred mainly in families with classical LFS

TABLE 1. Germline *TP53* mutations published to date[a]

Types of families	No of reported mutations
Li-Fraumeni	14
Li-Fraumeni like	14
non-Li-Fraumeni	2
no family history of cancer	1
Mutations	
Exons	
4	2
5	4
6	1
7	5
8	8
9	1
Mutation type	
missense	28
Stop codons created	
insertion	2
deletion	1
Tumour types in tested carriers	**No of tumours**
sarcoma	32 (42%)
breast	25 (32%)
brain	7
colon/gastric	4
acute myeloid leukaemia	1
acute lymphocytic leukaemia	1
non-Hodgkin lymphoma	1
hepatoblastoma	1
neuroblastoma	1
lung	1
endometrial carcinoma	1
choriocarcinoma	1
thyroid	1
symptom free carriers (aged 4–74; 2 known to be >50 years)	16

[a]For references see text

or LFS like families, which have been variably defined but in general contain at least two close relatives with different tumours of the types seen in classical LFS. The *TP53* germline mutations reported to date and the tumour types in carriers are shown in Table 1 (Law *et al*, 1991; Metzger *et al*, 1991; Santibanez-Koref *et al*, 1991; Borresen *et al*, 1992; Malkin *et al*, 1992; Prosser *et al*, 1992; Sidransky *et al*, 1992; Toguchida *et al*, 1992; Brugières *et al*, 1993; Eeles *et al*, 1993; Kovar *et al*, 1993). It is now known that germline mutations in the *TP53* gene are not the sole cause of the LFS or LFS like syndromes (Barnes *et al*, 1992; Li F, Birch J, personal communication; Eeles RA, unpublished observations), but since LFS tumours include early onset breast cancer, the LFS germline data together with the data from breast tumours suggest that germline *TP53* mutations should be investigated as a cause of familial breast cancer. It is now known that germline *TP53* mutations are found in fewer than 1% of breast cancer families that do not contain any of the other

TABLE 2.   Relative risk of tumour development in gene carriers in Li-Fraumeni kindreds[a]

Tumour type	Relative risk	
	carriers aged ≤45	carriers aged >45
Breast	17.9	1.8
Sarcoma	27.8	2.1
Brain	25.5	3.6
Leukaemia	13.1	3.9
Adrenal cortex	111.1	–

[a]Reported by Garber *et al* (1991)

tumours seen in classical LFS (Prosser *et al*, 1991; Borresen *et al*, 1992; Sidransky *et al*, 1992; Warren *et al*, 1992) and are very rarely seen in patients with sporadic breast tumours (Coles *et al*, 1992; Thoralcius *et al*, 1993).

On the other hand, individuals with a germline mutation in the *TP53* gene who survive the risks of childhood cancer are at greatest risk of breast cancer in the second and third decades of life (Table 2) (Garber *et al*, 1991). Transgenic mice that overexpress mutant *TP53* have an increased incidence of lung tumours, lymphomas and osteosarcomas but not breast cancer (Lavigueur *et al*, 1989). This may be a problem with extrapolating transgenic mouse models to humans as has been seen in other diseases; for example, knockout retinoblastoma mice do not develop retinoblastoma (Jacks *et al*, 1992; Lee *et al*, 1993; discussed by Harlow, 1992). However, early onset lung cancer in non-smokers and lymphomas are seen in Li-Fraumeni families, and it is possible that different *TP53* mutations predispose to different tumour types. Srivastava *et al* (1992) have shown that both wild type and mutant alleles are expressed in fibroblasts from individuals with *TP53* germline mutations in Li-Fraumeni families, and it has been shown that at least in some of these families, the binding of wild type TP53 to DNA and SV40 T antigen is impaired (Srivastava *et al*, 1993). Predictive genetic testing for germline mutations in the *TP53* gene is already possible, but there are several areas that warrant further research before this is offered in routine clinical practice (Eeles, 1993). The optimum screening method for mutations in the gene has yet to be determined, more research is needed to correlate the *TP53* mutation with its effect at the cellular level and tumour type and the effects of the *TP53* mutation on accumulation of DNA damage and radiation sensitivity have to be found. These answers will provide better genetic counselling, safer methods of breast cancer screening in carriers and optimum cancer management in families with *TP53* mutations.

DETECTION OF TP53 OVEREXPRESSION IN BREAST TUMOURS: IMMUNOHISTOCHEMICAL AND MOLECULAR DATA

The half life of normal TP53 is so short (6–20 min) that it is not usually detectable by immunohistochemical staining, which detects increased TP53 protein

TABLE 3. Immunohistochemical staining data of invasive breast carcinomas

Reference	No of breast tumours	Antibodies[a]	% Positive
Bartek et al (1990a)	81	PAb240 and PAb 1801	50
	94		20
Bartek et al (1990b)	11 (cell lines)	PAb240	100
Bartek et al (1991)	42	CM-1	62
Cattoretti et al (1988)	88	PAb1801	46
Davidoff et al (1991a)	184	PAb1801	27
Davidoff et al (1991b)	49	PAb1801	22
Fisher et al (1990)	188	PAb1801	21–26
		PAb240	
Horak et al (1992)	111	PAb240	53
Ostrowski et al (1991)	90	PAb1801	36
Thor et al (1992)	295	PAb1801	23
	31 in situ	PAb1801	16
Varley et al (1991)	73	PAb240	58
		PAb1801	

[a]PAb246 recognizes an epitope on mouse wild type *TP53*. PAb240 only recognizes mutant *TP53* in an immunoprecipitation reaction, and the epitope has been defined as RHSVV. It is not species specific. PAb1801 monoclonal antibody recognizes mutant *TP53*, and epitope is between aminoacids 32 and 79. CM-1 is a rabbit polyclonal antibody raised against normal human TP53. DO1 anbd DO7 are mouse monoclonal antibodies raised against normal human TP53.

levels. Mutation in the *TP53* gene and protein is associated with an increased protein stability, which prolongs this half life. The incidence of TP53 immunohistochemical positivity in sporadic human breast carcinomas ranges from 20% (Bartek *et al*, 1990a) to 62% (Bartek *et al*, 1991) and is shown in Table 3. Bartek *et al* (1990a) showed that the percentage positivity is lower in formalin fixed sections than in frozen sections (20% and 50%, respectively). There is often heterogeneity of staining across the tumour, and not all breast cancer cells will stain within one tumour (Fig. 1). Some of these discrepancies have been resolved with the use of antibodies that have improved activity against formalin fixed antigen (Midgeley *et al*, 1992; Vojtesek *et al*, 1992; Bartek *et al*, 1993).

The incidence of immunohistochemical positivity is lower in in situ carcinomas of the breast than in invasive disease but is still significant, being reported as 16% (Thor *et al*, 1992) and 10–45% (Table 4) (Gusterson BA, unpublished). Gusterson's data suggest that TP53 overexpression is not seen in lobular carcinoma in situ (CIS) and is most prevalent in the comedo form of ductal CIS. The association of invasive breast carcinoma with lobular CIS has a very long natural history, and the comedo form of ductal CIS when associated with invasive disease carries a higher local recurrence risk. These data indicate that the *TP53* mutation can be an early event, at least in some breast cancers, if in situ disease is indeed the precursor lesion.

The incidence of immunohistochemical positivity is higher than the incidence of mutations detected with molecular techniques (Table 5), although a strong nuclear staining pattern in the majority of breast cancer cells still corre-

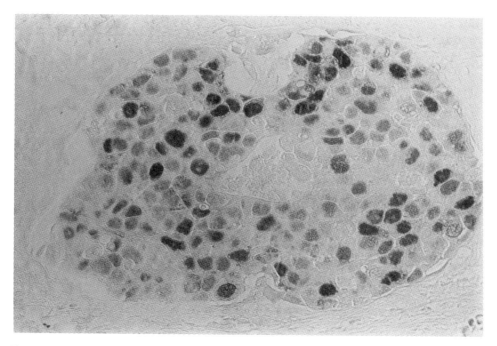

Fig. 1. Invasive breast carcinoma stained with DO1. The primary antibody is detected with secondary antibody and a biotin-streptavidin-peroxidase system (Vectastain elite kit, Vector, Burlingham, USA). 3,3′ Diaminobenzidine in 0.3% nickel sulphate is used as the chromogen. (x94)

lates almost perfectly with mutation. Immunohistochemical staining detects the presence of increased levels of the TP53 protein, and although the level can be increased when a mutant protein is present, it could also increase for other reasons, such as overexpression of the normal protein or a reduced function of a TP53 protease. The importance of the less commonly reported cytoplasmic pattern of staining is uncertain: it may, for instance, be an artefact of fixation (Gusterson *et al*, 1991). Immunohistochemical staining results therefore indicate a higher level of aberrant regulation of TP53 expression in breast cancers than molecular mutation analysis results suggest. The presence of mutation does not always result in positive immunohistochemical staining

TABLE 4. Immunohistochemical staining of carcinoma in situ (CIS) of the breast with DO7 antibody to TP53

Type of CIS	Number	% Positive with DO7
Lobular	39	0
Ductal		
comedo/solid	26	45
cribriform[a]/micropapillary	29	10
papillary	2	0
Paget's	4	25

Courtesy of Prof B Gusterson
[a]All positive cribriform tumours have pleomorphic nuclei and a high mitotic rate

TABLE 5. Molecular analyses of TP53 in breast tumours

Reference	No of breast tumours	Exons tested	% Mutant	Test used
Andersen *et al* (1993)	179	5–8	21	CDGE
Bartek *et al* (1990b)	11 cell lines, 4 tested	4–8	100	Seq
Borresen *et al* (1992)	163	5–8	21	CDGE
Coles *et al* (1992)	77	5–9	32	HOT
Davidoff *et al* (1991b)	7	4–10	100	Seq
Kovach *et al* (1991)	11	5–9	36	Seq
Mazars *et al* (1992)	96	2,5–9	18.7	SSCP
Osbourne *et al* (1991)	26	4–9	12	Seq
Prosser *et al* (1990)	60	5,6	13	HOT
Runnebaum *et al* (1991)	59	5–9	17	SSCP
	59	2–11	36	Seq
Thompson *et al* (1992)	60	5–9	28	HOT
Thoralcius *et al* (1993)	109	5,7,8	17	CDGE
Varley *et al* (1991)	53	exon 5 RFLP at codon 175	2	RFLP
	10	exon 5	10	Seq
	10	exon 8	10	Seq

SSCP = single strand conformational polymorphism. CDGE = constant denaturant gradient electrophoresis. HOT = hydroxalamine/osmium tetroxide chemical mismatch. Seq = sequencing. RFLP = restriction fragment length polymorphism

(Eeles *et al,* 1993) (Fig. 2) and vice versa (Barnes *et al,* 1992). Staining has now been described under benign conditions (Eeles *et al,* 1993), and normal TP53 overexpression can be induced in skin by DNA insults such as exposure to ultraviolet light (Hall *et al,* 1993). It is therefore now quite clear that immunohistochemical positivity does not always equate to mutation but may instead be more closely associated with the cellular environment (Vojtesek and Lane, 1993).

Molecular analyses of *TP53* mutations in invasive breast cancers are summarized in Table 5. The incidence of positivity varies from 13% to 100% (the latter are from small sample sizes; the percentage is mainly around 13–28%), and very few studies have analysed the entire coding sequence, although most have screened the conserved regions within which over 90% of *TP53* mutations are now thought to reside. There are various techniques for screening areas of a gene for point mutations and small alterations. The most commonly used are single strand conformational polymorphism (SSCP), denaturing gradient gel electrophoresis or a variant thereof (constant denaturing gradient gel electrophoresis, CDGE) and hydroxalamine–osmium tetroxide chemical mismatch (HOT). All are based on the polymerase chain reaction (PCR). Single strand conformational polymorphism is based on the fact that single stranded DNA folds into different conformations depending on its base composition, and constant denaturing gradient gel electrophoresis relies on the melting properties of DNA, which are altered by base composition; the sensitivity is increased by adding guanine cytosine clamps (runs of about 40 GCs) to the PCR

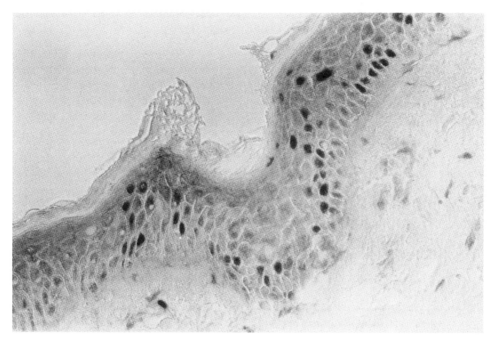

Fig. 2. Skin from a patient from an LFS like family stained with DO1. The patient has had seven independent primary tumours, including three sarcomas and bilateral breast cancer and has a germline mutation at codon 273 of the *TP53* gene (CGT—TGT). Although all cells contain the mutation, not all stain. (x94) Figure by kind permission of Elsevier. (From Eeles *et al* [1993] *Oncogene* **8** 1274)

product. Hydroxalamine–osium tetroxide mismatch involves the mixing of mutant and normal single stranded DNA, and the chemicals hydroxalamine and osmium tetroxide bind to sites of mismatch between the normal and mutant. Piperidine then cleaves at the sites of binding. In a blind study of *TP53* mutants, HOT was the most sensitive method (100%), and SSCP and CDGE sensitivities were 90% and 88%, respectively (Condie *et al*, 1992). The HOT technique can be laborious and uses hazardous chemicals, so SSCP and CDGE are more convenient for large numbers of samples. The sensitivity of CDGE can be improved by altering the setup conditions to achieve 100% sensitivity for exons 5–8. The different values for the incidence of *TP53* mutation between series could be due to differences in the screening techniques used or in the tumour populations tested. In our experience, SSCP has a satisfactory sensitivity rate (90%) and can detect the presence of mutant diluted to 1% of normal, provided the mutant band shifts are large enough to be easily distinguished from the normal position. This could be important in the analysis of breast tumours, which, even if microdissected, contain many normal stromal cells. If, as the immunohistochemical staining pattern suggests, there is considerable heterogeneity, the percentage of mutants in the sample may be low. A new method that uses a yeast reporter system to measure the functional activity of *TP53* will probably become the method of choice in the future (Ishioka *et al,* 1993).

About 10% of breast cancer patients have circulating antibodies to the TP53 protein. Davidoff (1992), in a study of 60 invasive breast cancers, found that no tumour with low level/normal TP53 expression elicited an antibody response, but 23% of those overexpressing TP53 did so. Analysis of the types of mutations revealed that those eliciting an antibody response had mutations primarily in exons 5 and 6, rather than 7 and 8, and they complexed with hsc70. Davidoff speculates that hsc70 is involved with the antigenic presentation of TP53.

SPECTRUM OF *TP53* MUTATIONS IN INVASIVE BREAST CANCERS

The *TP53* gene is an ideal reporter gene in the study of mutational spectra to ascertain the possible role of carcinogens in oncogenesis. It is mutated in over 50% of cancers and sustains a broad range of mutation, and most of the tumour associated mutations in *TP53* are point mutations resulting in missense mutations that alter, but do not truncate, the protein (Levine *et al,* 1991). These are clustered between aminoacids 120 and 290, and most are localized in four conserved regions. In breast cancer, as in lung cancer, there is over-representation of G–T transversions at CpG dinucleotides, and there is a G–T hot spot at codon 157 not seen in colon cancer or background spectra, suggesting either a mutagenic agent in the aetiology of breast cancer or less efficient DNA repair in breast than in colorectal epithelium (Fig. 3) (Biggs *et al,* 1993). The hot spots for mutation at codons 248 and 273 seen in lung cancer are absent in breast cancer. The G–T transversions in breast cancer are also more common on the coding strand. This is in contrast to colon cancer, where G:C to A:T transitions at CpG dinucleotides are more common, or non-small cell lung cancer, where G:C to T:A transversions predominate and there is a bias for the G to be on the non-transcribed strand. This may be because transversions in the transcribed strand are preferentially repaired.

The argument for an environmental factor in the aetiology of breast cancer is strong, because rates vary between countries by five- to tenfold and migrants acquire the rates of their new country within two generations (Higginson *et al,* 1992). A major risk factor for breast cancer is excess oestrogen exposure. However, this is thought to act as a promoter and therefore would not affect the mutational spectrum.

Radiation is known to increase the risk of breast cancer, especially if the patient is exposed at an early age (Higginson *et al,* 1992). Radiation induces the formation of free radicals, which may damage DNA by modifying guanine (Reid and Loeb, 1992). Although radiation may not cause a large proportion of breast cancer, it may be important in the aetiology of the disease in women carrying the gene for ataxia telangiectasia (AT). The radiation sensitivity of AT heterozygotes and their prevalence in the population is controversial. Swift *et*

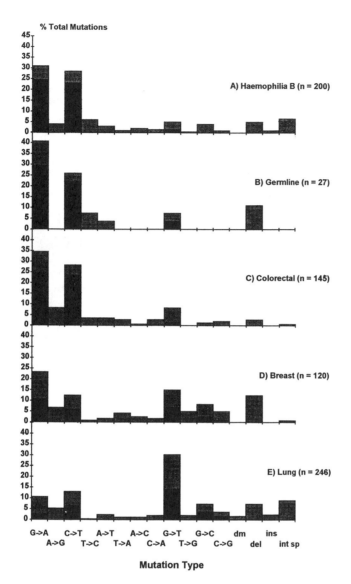

Mutation Type

Fig. 3. The mutational spectra of *TP53* in breast, lung and colorectal cancers. The haemophilia B spectrum represents the background spectrum and the spectrum of germline mutations in *TP53* is shown. The first four columns in each graph are transition mutations, the middle eight are transversions and the last four are other changes (dm=double mutant; del=deletion; ins=insertion; int sp=intron splice). The black shading denotes the proportion of mutations at CpG dinucleotide sites. Figure by kind permission of Mr P Biggs and Oxford University Press. (From Biggs *et al* [1993] *Mutagenesis* **8** 278)

al (1991) estimate this to account for at least 10% of breast cancers, and the latter will only be elucidated when the AT gene is cloned.

Excess dietary fat has been implicated in the aetiology of breast cancer. This is based on animal data, which indicate that high fat diets increase the incidence of mammary tumours (Willet, 1989), and international correlations of per caput fat consumption and breast cancer rates. A large prospective study is now under way in Europe to study the effects of diet on cancer incidence.

TP53 AS A PROGNOSTIC FACTOR IN BREAST TUMOURS

Adjuvant chemotherapy and hormonal therapy improve survival in breast cancer patients with involvement of regional lymph nodes (Early Breast Cancer Trialists' Collaborative Group, 1992). Disease free survival has been reported to be prolonged in node negative women given adjuvant therapy, but this has yet to translate into an improvement in survival and so is not given by all oncologists. It is likely that a subset of node negative women will benefit from adjuvant therapy, but they need to be identified. Mazars *et al* (1992) have shown that the *TP53* mutation correlates with negative steroid receptor status, and Horak *et al* (1992) showed a correlation with epidermal growth factor receptor overexpression. Both of these factors are associated with more aggressive tumours. Thoralcius *et al* (1993) have shown that the *TP53* mutation correlates with negative oestrogen receptor status and negatively with survival.

Thor *et al* (1992) have shown that the *TP53* mutation correlates with positive immunohistochemical staining in frozen tissue and that positive staining is an independent prognostic factor for disease free survival and of borderline significance (p=0.052) for overall survival in 295 invasive breast carcinomas. Positive staining can be used to differentiate lymph node negative patients into two prognostic groups, those with positive TP53 staining having a worse survival.

Allred *et al* (1992) have performed a multivariate analysis on 544 frozen breast carcinomas from lymph node negative patients and found that accumulation of TP53 as determined by immunohistochemical staining is a significant adverse prognostic factor for disease free survival. Similarly, Barnes *et al* (1993) identified a group of 25% of patients who had uniform TP53 staining in their breast tumours and very significantly poorer prognosis. At the molecular level, the *TP53* mutation has been shown to be an independent prognostic factor for disease free and overall survival (Andersen *et al*, 1993). These data may be important for distinguishing patients who are lymph node negative but may still have potential benefit from adjuvant chemotherapy.

SUMMARY

The TP53 protein is proving to be central to cell cycle control after exposure to DNA damage, and every week a new feature of its role in the regulation of cell division is described. *TP53* is the most commonly altered oncogene in human tumours and is involved in the development of both sporadic and some hereditary breast tumours. Although there is no doubt that germline mutations in the *TP53* gene carry a high risk of early onset breast cancer, and the gene is mutated somatically in a proportion of preinvasive and invasive breast cancers, it is not usually the initiating genetic event in most breast tumours. It does, however, seem to be an independent prognostic factor for survival and could prove useful in clinical management of node negative breast cancer patients. There has been an explosion of reports about the function of the TP53 protein—in particular, it seems to have a central role in the monitoring of some types of DNA damage. This role may prove to be the most important aspect of its association with breast cancer development, both as a prognostic factor and as a handle for treatment.

References

Allred DC, Clark GM, Brown RW *et al* (1992) Mutation of p53 is associated with increased proliferation and early recurrence in node-negative breast cancer. *Proceedings of the American Society of Clinical Oncology* **11** 55 [Abstract]

Andersen TI, Holm R, Nesland JS, Heimdal KR, Ottestad L and Borresen A-L (1993) Prognostic significance of TP53 alterations in breast carcinoma. *British Journal of Cancer* **68** 540–548

Baker SJ, Fearon ER, Nigro JM *et al* (1989) Chromosome 17 deletions and p53 gene mutations in colorectal carcinoma. *Science* **244** 217–221

Bargonetti J, Reynisdottir I, Friedman PN and Prives C (1992) Site-specific binding of wild-type p53 to cellular DNA is inhibited by SV40 T antigen and mutant p53. *Genes and Development* **6** 1886–1898

Barnes DM, Hanby AM, Gillett CE *et al* (1992) Abnormal expression of wild type p53 protein in normal cells of a cancer family patient. *Lancet* **340** 259–263

Barnes DM, Dublin EA, Fisher CJ, Levison DA and Millis RR (1993) Immunohistochemical detection of p53 protein in mammary carcinoma: an important new independent indicator of prognosis? *Human Pathology* **24** 469–476

Bartek J, Bartkova J, Vojtesek B *et al* (1990a) Patterns of expression of the p53 tumour suppressor in human breast tissues and tumours in situ and in vitro. *International Journal of Cancer* **46** 839–844

Bartek J, Iggo R, Gannon J and Lane DP (1990b) Genetic and immunohistochemical analysis of mutant p53 in human breast cancer cell lines. *Oncogene* **5** 893–899

Bartek J, Bartkova J, Vojtesek B *et al* (1991) Aberrant expression of the p53 oncoprotein is a common feature of a wide spectrum of human malignancies. *Oncogene* **6** 1699–1703

Bartek J, Bartkova J, Lukas J, Staskova Z, Vojtesek B and Lane DP (1993) Immunohistochemical analysis of the p53 oncoprotein on paraffin sections using a series of novel monoclonal antibodies. *Journal of Pathology* **169** 27–34

Benchimol S, Lamb P, Crawford LV *et al* (1985) Transformation associated p53 protein is encoded by a gene on human chromosome 17. *Somatic Cellular and Molecular Genetics* **11** 505–509

Biggs PJ, Warren W, Venitt S and Stratton MR (1993) Does a genotoxic carcinogen contribute to human breast cancer? The value of mutational spectra in unravelling the aetiology of cancer. *Mutagenesis* **8** 275–283

Borresen A-L, Andersen TI, Garber J *et al* (1992) Screening for germline TP53 mutations in breast cancer patients. *Cancer Research* **52** 3234–3236

Brugières L, Gardes M, Moutou C *et al* (1993) Screening for germ line p53 mutations in children with malignant tumours and a family history of cancer. *Cancer Research* **53** 452–455

Cattoretti G, Rilke F, Andreola S, D'Amato L and Delia D (1988) p53 expression in breast cancer. *International Journal of Cancer* **41** 178–183

Chang EH, Pirollo KF, Zou ZQ *et al* (1987) Oncogenes in radioresistant, noncancerous skin fibroblasts from a cancer-prone family. *Science* **237** 1036–1039

Chen P-L, Chen Y, Bookstein R and Lee W-H (1990) Genetic mechanisms of tumour suppression by the human p53 gene. *Science* **250** 1576–1580

Clarke AR, Purdie CA, Harrison DJ *et al* (1993) Thymocyte apoptosis induced by p53-dependent and independent pathways. *Nature* **362** 849–852

Coles C, Condie A, Chetty U, Steel CM, Evans HJ and Prosser J (1992) p53 mutations in breast cancer. *Cancer Research* **52** 5291–5298

Condie A, Eeles RA, Borresen A-L, Coles C, Cooper CS and Prosser J (1992) Detection of point mutations in the p53 gene: comparison of SSCP, CDGE and HOT. *Human Mutation* **2** 58–66

Davidoff AM, Herndon JE, Glover NS *et al* (1991a) Relationship between p53 overexpression and established prognostic factors in breast cancer. *Surgery* **110** 259–264

Davidoff AM, Humphrey PA, Iglehart JD and Marks JR (1991b) Genetic basis for p53 overexpression in human breast cancer. *Proceedings of the National Academy of Sciences of the USA* **88** 5006–5010

Davidoff AM, Iglehart JD and Marks JR (1992) Immune response to p53 is dependent upon p53/HSP70 complexes in breast cancers. *Proceedings of the National Academy of Sciences of the USA* **89** 3439–3442

de Fromentel CC and Soussi T (1992) TP53 Tumour suppressor gene: a model for investigating human mutagenesis. *Genes, Chromosomes and Cancer* **4** 1–15

DeLeo AB, Jay G, Appella E, Dubois GC, Law LW and Old LJ (1979) Detection of a transformation related antigen in chemically induced sarcomas and other transformed cells of the mouse. *Proceedings of the National Academy of Sciences of the USA* **76** 2420–2424

Dittmer D, Pati S, Zambetti G *et al* (1993) Gain of function mutations in p53. *Nature Genetics* **4** 42–45

Donehower LA, Harvey M, Slagle BL *et al* (1992) Mice deficient for p53 are developmentally normal but susceptible to spontaneous tumours. *Nature* **356** 215–221

Dutta A, Ruppert JM, Aster JC and Winchester E (1993) Inhibition of DNA replication factor RPA by p53. *Nature* **365** 79–82

Early Breast Cancer Trialists' Collaborative Group (1992) Systematic treatment of early breast cancer by hormonal, cytotoxic or immune therapy: 133 randomised trials involving 31 000 recurrences and 24 000 deaths among 75 000 women. *Lancet* **339** 1–15, 71–85

Eeles RA (1993) Predictive testing for germline mutations in the p53 gene: are all the questions answered? *European Journal of Cancer* **29A** 1361 –1365

Eeles RA, Warren W, Knee G *et al* (1993) Constitutional mutation in exon 8 of the p53 gene in a patient with multiple independent primary tumours: molecular and immunohistochemical findings. *Oncogene* **8** 1269–1276

El-Deiry WS, Kern SE, Pietenpol JA, Kinzler KW and Vogelstein B (1992) Definition of a consensus binding site for p53. *Nature Genetics* **1** 45–49

Eliyahu D, Raz A, Gruss P, Givol D and Oren M (1984) Participation of p53 cellular tumour antigen in transformation of normal embryonic cells. *Nature* **312** 646–649

Eliyahu D, Goldfinger N, Pinhashi-Kimhi O *et al* (1988) Meth A fibrosarcoma cells express two transforming mutant p53 species. *Oncogene* **3** 313–321

Fields S and Jang SJ (1990) Presence of a potent transcription activating sequence in the p53 protein. *Science* **249** 1046–1049

Finlay CA, Hinds PW and Levine AJ (1989) The p53 proto-oncogene can act as a suppressor of transformation. *Cell* **57** 1083–1093

Fisher CJ, Barnes DM, Gillet CE, Millis RR and Lane DP (1990) Immunohistochemical staining of mutant p53 proteins in human mammary carcinoma. *British Journal of Cancer* **62** 23 [Abstract]

Funk WD, Pak DT, Karas RH, Wright WE and Shay JW (1992) A transcriptionally active DNA-binding site for human p53 protein complexes. *Molecular and Cell Biology* **12** 2866–2871

Garber JE, Goldstein AM, Kantor AF, Dreyfus MG, Fraumeni JF Jr and Li FP (1991) Follow-up study of twenty-four families with Li-Fraumeni syndrome. *Cancer Research* **51** 6094–

6097

Gusterson BA, Anbazhagan R, Warren W *et al* (1991) Expression of p53 in premalignant and malignant squamous epithelium. *Oncogene* **6** 1785–1789

Hall PA, McKee PH, Menage HD, Dover R and Lane DP (1993) High levels of p53 protein in UV irradiated human skin. *Oncogene* **8** 203–207

Harlow E (1992) Retinoblastoma: for our eyes only. *Nature* **359** 270

Harvey M, Sands AT, Weiss R *et al* (1993) In vitro growth characteristics of embryo fibroblasts isolated from p53-deficient mice. *Oncogene* **8** 2457–2467

Higginson J, Muir CS and Munoz N (1992) *Human Cancer: Epidemiology and Environmental Causes*, pp 39–44, Cambridge University Press, Cambridge

Hinds PW, Finlay CA, Frey AB and Levine AJ (1987) Immunological evidence for the association of p53 with a heat shock protein, hsc 70, in p52-plus-ras-transformed cell lines. *Molecular and Cell Biology* **7** 2863–2869

Hinds P, Finlay CA and Levine AJ (1989) Mutation is required to activate the p53 gene for cooperation with the ras oncogene and transformation. *Journal of Virology* **63** 739–746

Hinds PW, Finlay CA, Quartin RS *et al* (1990) Mutant p53 DNA clones from human colon carcinomas cooperate with ras in transforming primary rat cells: a comparison of the hot spot mutant phenotypes. *Cell Growth and Differentiation* **1** 571–580

Hollstein MC, Sidransky D, Vogelstein B and Harris CC (1991) p53 mutations in human cancers. *Science* **253** 49–53

Horak E, Smith K, Bromley L *et al* (1992) Mutant p53, EGF receptor and c-erb B2 expression in human breast cancer. *Oncogene* **6** 2277–2284

Hupp TR, Meek DW, Midgley CA and Lane DP (1993) Activation of the cryptic DNA binding function of mutant forms of p53. *Nucleic Acids Research* **21** 3167–3174

Ishioka C, Frebourg T, Yan Y-X *et al* (1993) Screening patients for heterozygous p53 mutations using a functional assay in yeast. *Nature Genetics* **5** 124–129

Iwabuchi K, Li B, Bartel P and Fields S (1993) Use of the two-hybrid system to identify the domain of p53 involved in oligomerization. *Oncogene* **8** 1693–1696

Jacks T, Fazeli A, Schmitt EM, Bronson RT, Goodell MA and Weinberg RA (1992) Effects of an Rb mutation in the mouse. *Nature* **359** 295–300

Jenkins JR, Rudge K and Currie GA (1984) Cellular immortalisation by a cDNA clone encoding the transformation-associated phosphoprotein p53. *Nature* **312** 651–654

Jenkins JR, Rudge K, Chumakov P and Currie GA (1985) The cellular oncogene, p53 can be activated by mutagenesis. *Nature* **317** 816–818

Kastan MB, Onyekwere O, Sidransky D, Vogelstein B and Craig RW (1991) Participation of p53 protein in the cellular response to DNA damage. *Cancer Research* **51** 6304–6311

Kastan MB, Zhan Q, El-Deiry WS *et al* (1992) A mammalian cell cycle checkpoint pathway utilizing p53 and GADD45 is defective in ataxia-telangiectasia. *Cell* **71** 587–597

Kern S, Kinzler K, Bruskin A *et al* (1991) Identification of p53 as a sequence specific DNA protein. *Science* **252** 1708–1711

Kovach JS, McGovern RM, Cassady JD *et al* (1991) Direct sequencing from touch preparations of human carcinomas: analysis of p53 mutations in breast carcinomas. *journal of the National Cancer Institute* **83** 1004–1009

Kovar H, Auinger A, Jug G, Muller T and Pillwein K (1993) p53 mosaicism with an exon 8 germline mutation in the founder of a cancer-prone pedigree. *Oncogene* **7** 2169–2173

Kuerbitz SJ, Plunkett BS, Walsh WV and Kastan MB (1992) Wild type p53 is a cell cycle checkpoint determinant following irradiation. *Proceedings of the National Academy of Sciences of the USA* **89** 7491–7495

Lane DP (1992) p53, guardian of the genome. *Nature* **358** 15–16

Lane DP and Crawford LV (1979) T antigen is bound to a host protein in SV40 transformed cells. *Nature* **278** 261–263

Lane DP and Benchimol S (1990) p53: oncogene or anti-oncogene? *Genes and Development* **4** 1–8

Lavigueur A, Maltby V, Mock D, Rossant J, Pawson T and Bernstein A (1989) High incidence of lung, bone and lymphoid tumours in transgenic mice overexpressing mutant alleles of the p53 oncogene. *Molecular and Cell Biology* **9** 3982–3991

Law JC, Strong LC, Chidambaram A and Ferrell RE (1991) A germ line mutation in exon 5 of the p53 gene in an extended cancer family. *Cancer Research* **51** 6385–6387

Lee EY-HP, Chang C-Y, Hu N *et al* (1993) Mice deficient for Rb are nonviable and show defects in neurogenesis and haematopoeisis. *Nature* **359** 288–294

Levine AJ, Momand J and Finlay CA (1991) The p53 tumour suppressor gene. *Nature* **351** 453–456

Li FP and Fraumeni JF Jr (1969) Soft tissue sarcomas, breast cancer and other neoplasms: a familial cancer syndrome? *Annals of Internal Medicine* **71** 747–752

Li FP, Fraumeni JF Jr, Mulvihill JJ *et al* (1988) A cancer family syndrome in twenty-four kindreds. *Cancer Research* **48** 5358–5362

Linzer DIH and Levine AJ (1979) Characterization of a 54 000 MW cellular SV40 tumor antigen present in SV40-transformed cells and uninfected embryonal carcinoma cells. *Cell* **17** 43–52

Lowe SW, Schmitt EM, Smith SW, Osborne BA and Jacks T (1993) p53 is required for radiation-induced apoptosis in mouse thymocytes. *Nature* **362** 847–849

Mack DH, Vartikar J, Pippas JM and Laimins LA (1993) Specific repression of TATA-mediated but not initiator-mediated transcription by wild-type p53. *Nature* **363** 281–283

Malkin D, Li FP, Strong LC *et al* (1990) Germline p53 mutations in a familial syndrome of breast cancer, sarcomas and other neoplasms. *Science* **250** 1233–1238

Malkin D, Jolly KW, Barbier N *et al* (1992) Germline mutations of the p53 tumour suppressor gene in children and young adults with second malignant neoplasms. *New England Journal of Medicine* **326** 1309–1315

Martinez J, Georgoff I, Martinez J and Levine AJ (1991) Cellular localization and cell cycle regulation by a temperature-sensitive p53 protein. *Genes and Development* **5** 151–159

Mazars R, Spinardi L, Ben Cheikh M, Simony-Lafontaine J, Jeanteur P and Theillet C (1992) p53 mutations occur in aggressive breast cancer. *Cancer Research* **52** 3918–3923

Metzger AK, Sheffield VC, Duyk G, Daneshvar L, Edwards MSB and Cogen PH (1991) Identification of a germline mutation in the p53 gene in a patient with an intracranial ependymoma. *Proceedings of the National Academy of Sciences of the USA* **88** 7825–7829

Midgley CA, Fisher CJ, Bartek J, Vojtesek B, Lane DP and Barnes DM (1992) Analysis of p53 expression in human tumours: an antibody raised against human p53 expressed in *E coli*. *Journal of Cell Science* **101** 183–189

Milner J and Medcalf EA (1991) Cotranslation of activated mutant p53 with wild type drives the wild-type p53 protein into the mutant conformation. *Cell* **65** 765–774

Momand J, Zambetti G, Olsen DC, George D and Levine AJ (1992) The mdm-2 oncogene product forms a complex with the p53 protein and inhibits p53-mediated transactivation. *Cell* **69** 1237–1245

Mowat M, Cheng A, Kimura N, Bernstein A and Benchimol S (1985) Rearrangements of the cellular p53 gene in erythroleukaemia cells transformed by Friend virus. *Nature* **314** 633–636

O'Rourke RW, Miller CW, Kato GJ *et al* (1990) A potential transcription activation element in the p53 protein. *Oncogene* **5** 1829–1832

Osbourne RJ, Merlo GR, Mitsudomi T *et al* (1991) Mutations in the p53 gene in human primary breast cancers. *Cancer Research* **51** 6194–6198

Ostrowski JL, Sawan A, Henry L *et al* (1991) p53 expression in human breast cancer related to survival and prognostic factors: an immunohistochemical study. *Journal of Pathology* **164** 75–81

Parada LF, Land H, Weinberg RA, Wolf D and Rotter W (1984) Cooperation between gene encoding p53 tumour antigen and ras in cellular transformation. *Nature* **312** 649–651

Pennica D, Goeddel DV, Hayflick JS, Reich NC, Anderson CW and Levine AJ (1984) The amino acid sequence of murine p53 determined from a cDNA clone. *Virology* **134** 477–482

Prosser J, Thompson AM, Cranston G and Evans HJ (1990) Evidence that p53 behaves as a tumour suppressor gene in sporadic breast tumours. *Oncogene* **5** 1573–1579

Prosser J, Elder PA, Condie A, MacFayden I, Steel CM and Evans HJ (1991) Mutations in p53 do not account for heritable breast cancer: a study in five affected families. *British Journal of Cancer* **63** 181–184

Prosser J, Porter D, Coles C *et al* (1992) Constitutional p53 mutation in a non Li-Fraumeni cancer family. *British Journal of Cancer* **65** 527–528

Raycroft L, Wu H and Lozano G (1990) Transcriptional activation by wild type but not transforming mutants of the p53 anti-oncogene. *Science* **249** 1049–1051

Reid T and Loeb L (1992) Mutagenic specificity of oxygen radicals produced by human leukaemia cells. *Cancer Res* **52** 1082–1086

Runnebaum IG, Mahalakshmi N, Bowman M, Soto D and Sukumar S (1991) Mutations in p53 as potential molecular markers for human breast cancer. *Proceedings of the National Academy of Sciences of the USA* **88** 10657–10661

Santibanez-Koref MF, Birch JM, Hartley AL *et al* (1991) p53 germline mutations in Li-Fraumeni syndrome. *Lancet* **338** 1490–1491

Scharer E and Iggo R (1992) Mammalian p53 can function as a transcription factor in yeast. *Nucleic Acids Research* **20** 1539–1545

Shaulsky G, Goldfinger N, Ben-Ze'ev and Rotter V (1990) Nuclear accumulation of p53 protein is mediated by several nuclear localisation signals and plays a role in tumorigenesis. *Molecular and Cellular Biology* **10** 6565–6577

Sidransky D, Tokino T, Helzlsouer K *et al* (1992) Inherited p53 gene mutations in breast cancer. *Cancer Research* **52** 2984–2986

Soussi T, de Fromentel C and May P (1990) Structural aspects of the p53 protein in relation to gene evolution. *Oncogene* **5** 935–952

Srivastava S, Zou Z, Pirollo K, Blattner W and Chang EH (1990) Germline transmission of a mutated p53 gene in a cancer-prone family with Li-Fraumeni syndrome. *Nature* **348** 747–749

Srivastava S, Tong YA, Devadas K *et al* (1992) Detection of both mutant and wild-type p53 protein in normal skin fibroblasts and demonstration of a shared second hit on p53 in diverse tumours from a cancer-prone family with Li-Fraumeni syndrome. *Oncogene* **7** 987–991

Srivastava S, Wang S, Tong YA, Pirollo K and Chang EH (1993) Several mutant p53 proteins detected in cancer-prone families with Li-Fraumeni syndrome exhibit transdominant effects on the biochemical properties of the wild-type p53. *Oncogene* **8** 2449–2456

Swift J, Morrell D, Massey R and Chase C (1991) Incidence of cancer in 161 families affected by ataxia telangiectasia. *New England Journal of Medicine* **325** 1831–1836

Thompson AM, Anderson TJ, Condie A *et al* (1992) p53 allele losses, mutations and expression in breast cancer and their relationship to clinico-pathological parameters. *International Journal of Cancer* **50** 528–532

Thor AD, Moore DHII, Edgerton SM *et al* (1992) Accumulation of p53 tumour suppressor gene protein: an independent marker of prognosis in breast cancers. *Journal of the National Cancer Institute* **84** 845–855

Thoralcius S, Borresen A-L and Eyfjord JE (1993) Somatic p53 mutations in human breast carcinomas in an Icelandic population: a prognostic factor. *Cancer Research* **53** 1637–1641

Toguchida J, Yamaguchi T, Dayton SH *et al* (1992) Prevalence and spectrum of germline mutations of the p53 gene among patients with sarcoma. *New England Journal of Medicine* **326** 1301–1308

Varley JM, Brammer WJ, Lane DP, Swallow ES, Dolan C and Walker RA (1991) Loss of chromosome 17p13 sequences and mutation of p53 in human breast carcinomas. *Oncogene* **6** 413–421

Vogelstein B and Kinzler K (1992) Protein function and dysfunction. *Cell* **70** 523–526

Vojtesek B and Lane DP (1993) Regulation of p53 protein expression in human breast cancer cell lines. *Journal of Cell Science* **105** 607–612

Vojtesek B, Bartek J, Midgley CA and Lane DP (1992) An immunohistochemical analysis of human p53: new monoclonal antibodies and epitope mapping using recombinant p53. *Journal of Immunological Methods* **151** 237–244

Warren W, Eeles RA, Ponder BAJ *et al* (1992) No evidence for germline mutations in exons 5-9 of the p53 gene in 25 breast cancer families. *Oncogene* **7** 1043–1046

Werness BA, Levine AJ and Howley PM (1990) Association of human papillomavirus types 16 and 18 E6 proteins with p53. *Science* **248** 76–79

Willett W (1989) The search for the causes of breast and colon cancer. *Nature* **338** 389–394

Zambetti GP, Bargonetti J, Walker K, Prives C and Levine AJ (1992) Wild type p53 mediates positive regulation of gene expression through a specific DNA sequence element. *Genes and Development* **6** 1143–1152

Zhang W, Funk WD, Wright WE, Shay JW and Deisseroth AB (1993) Novel DNA binding of p53 mutants and their role in transcriptional activation. *Oncogene* **8** 2555–2559

The authors are responsible for the accuracy of the references.

Chromosome 11q13 Abnormalities in Human Breast Cancer

VERA FANTL • ROSALIND SMITH • SHARON BROOKES
CLIVE DICKSON • GORDON PETERS

Imperial Cancer Research Fund Laboratories, P O Box 123, Lincoln's Inn Fields, London WC2A 3PX

INTRODUCTION

Cancer cells contain structurally abnormal chromosomes, and among the aberrations that appear to be relatively specific to breast cancer is the amplification of DNA markers centred on the cytogenetically defined band q13 on the long arm of human chromosome 11. The presence of this "amplicon" in a subset of tumours implies that it has provided a selective advantage during the development of the tumour cell clone, presumably by causing the elevated expression of a specific gene or genes. From a clinical standpoint, detecting this abnormality could be a useful adjunct to the standard methods of tumour classification and may well have prognostic value. From a scientific standpoint, the challenge is to identify and characterize the critical oncogene(s) within the amplified DNA and eventually to devise ways of counteracting its effects. In this chapter, we review our current understanding of the 11q13 amplicon in terms of its frequency and potential significance in primary breast cancer and the genes it encompasses. In a curious twist of fate, the two proven oncogenes on which much of this work was originally based now appear to be silent passengers on the amplified DNA, and we discuss the status of other likely contenders for the key gene in the region.

HISTORICAL PERSPECTIVE

The discovery of the amplicon on 11q13 has its origins in three classical fields of oncogene research—retrovirology, DNA transfection and cytogenetics.

Mouse Mammary Tumorigenesis

The retroviral model for breast cancer is provided by inbred strains of mice that have a characteristically high incidence of the disease due to the milk borne transmission of mouse mammary tumour virus (MMTV). In common with many other retroviruses, the oncogenic effect of MMTV is attributable to the transcriptional activation of one or more cellular proto-oncogenes by the nearby integration of viral DNA (reviewed in Peters, 1990; Nusse, 1991). By location of the MMTV proviruses in mammary tumour DNA, several common insertion sites have been identified, each corresponding to a cellular gene (Dickson *et al*, 1984; Nusse *et al*, 1984). The best known examples are *Int-1* and *Int-2* (Dickson *et al*, 1984; Nusse *et al*, 1984), now referred to as *Wnt-1* and *Fgf-3*, respectively, to reflect more accurately the gene families to which they belong (Baird and Klagsbrun, 1991; Nusse and Varmus, 1992). Although structurally unrelated, both of these genes encode secreted growth factors that function principally during embryonic development (Peters, 1991 and references therein). The effect of the virus is therefore to activate the expression of genes that would otherwise remain silent in the mammary gland. Transgenic mice that express *Wnt-1* and/or *Fgf-3* under the control of an MMTV enhancer or promoter develop mammary hyperplasia and neoplasia (Tsukamoto *et al*, 1988; Muller *et al*, 1990; Kwan *et al*, 1992; Ornitz *et al*, 1992; Stamp *et al*, 1992).

Given the compelling evidence for their role in mouse mammary tumorigenesis, attention naturally turned to the human homologues, *WNT1* and *FGF3*, on chromosomes 12q12-13 and 11q13, respectively (van't Veer *et al*, 1984; Casey *et al*, 1986; Turc-Carel *et al*, 1987). Although there is no known viral component in human breast cancer, it is conceivable that other mechanisms might activate the corresponding genes in human tumours. No abnormalities in the *WNT1* locus have been reported thus far, but it was immediately clear that the *FGF3* gene is amplified in a substantial proportion of human breast cancers (Lidereau *et al*, 1988; Varley *et al*, 1988; Zhou *et al*, 1988).

DNA Transfection

About the same time as the initial reports of *FGF3* amplification, attention was again focused on the 11q13 region by reports of transforming sequences in human tumour DNA identified by DNA transfection techniques. As is often the case, several groups working independently and with different material uncovered the same gene and gave it different names (Sakamoto *et al*, 1986; Delli Bovi and Basilico, 1987; Adelaide *et al*, 1988). Although the common titles relate to human stomach cancer (*HST1/HSTF1*) and Kaposi sarcoma (*KS3/kFGF*), there is in fact no evidence that the gene has any role in the pathogenesis of these tumours, and the equivalent DNA from normal cells is equally potent in transformation assays (Sakamoto *et al*, 1988). When the transforming DNA was sequenced, it became clear that it encodes another member of the fibroblast growth factor family (Delli Bovi *et al*, 1987; Yoshida *et al*, 1987), subsequently designated *FGF4* (Baird and Klagsbrun, 1991). As well as being structurally and functionally related to *FGF3*, *FGF4* was found to lie adjacent to *FGF3* on human chromosome 11q13 (Adelaide *et al*, 1988; Huebner *et al*, 1988; Yoshida *et al*, 1988c). Indeed, the genes are only 40 kb apart in the human genome and less than 20 kb apart in the corresponding region of mouse chromosome 7 (Nguyen *et al*, 1988; Wada *et al*, 1988; Yoshida *et al*, 1988a; Peters *et al*, 1989; Brookes *et al*, 1992). Because of their proximity, it is hardly surprising that the DNA amplification noted for *FGF3* in human tumours applies equally to *FGF4* (Adelaide *et al*, 1988; Tsuda *et al*, 1988; Tsutsumi *et al*, 1988; Yoshida *et al*, 1988c). Along similar lines, the mouse homologue of *FGF4* can also be activated by proviral insertion in MMTV induced tumours, albeit less frequently than *FGF3* (Peters *et al*, 1989). It was therefore an attractive proposition that overproduction of one or perhaps both of these fibroblast growth factors might have an important bearing on tumour development, either directly as a growth factor or by promoting angiogenesis.

Cytogenetics

The localization of *FGF3* and *FGF4* on chromosome 11q13 also led to speculation (subsequently disproved) that these genes might be affected by the well documented chromosomal translocation, t(11;14)(q13;q32), present in certain B cell neoplasms (van den Berghe *et al*, 1979; Tsujimoto *et al*, 1984; Raffeld and Jaffe, 1991). By analogy with other reciprocal translocations that involve the immunoglobulin or T cell receptor genes, this rearrangement was thought to impinge on a cellular oncogene close to the site of chromosome breakage on 11q13. Although the breakpoint, designated *BCL1*, was cloned almost 10 years ago (Tsujimoto *et al*, 1984), it is only recently that a transcription unit has been located, at some distance from the original marker (see below). Thus, although the original *BCL1* probe is frequently cited in studies of 11q13 amplification, it is important to realize that it corresponds to a breakpoint in genomic DNA and not to a cellular gene. As illustrated in Fig. 1 and discussed in more detail

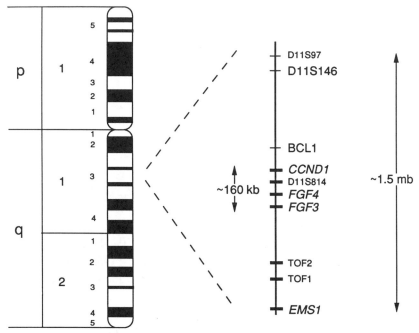

Fig. 1. Physical map of the genomic DNA adjacent to *FGF3*. The figure shows an idiogram of human chromosome 11 in which the cytogenetically visible bands on the short (p) and long (q) arms are numbered. The region centred on the *FGF3* gene in band q13 is displayed as a linear map in which CpG islands are depicted as bold lines to distinguish them from other markers/probes. Known genes are in italics. The map is based on data described by Brookes *et al* (1992, 1993)

later, it is now clear that the *BCL1* breakpoint is located approximately 250 kb centromeric of *FGF3* and *FGF4* and that there are two potential genes in the intervening DNA (Brookes *et al*, 1992).

AMPLIFICATION OF CHROMOSOME 11q13 IN BREAST CANCER

Frequency of the 11q13 Amplicon in Human Cancers

Since the original reports of 11q13 amplification, a variety of tumour types have been subjected to similar analyses. Thus, amplification of *FGF3, FGF4* and/or *BCL1* has been observed in a significant proportion of squamous cell carcinomas, particularly in the oesophagus, the head and neck region and the lung and in transitional cell tumours of the bladder (Tsutsumi *et al*, 1988; Berenson *et al*, 1989, 1990; Tsuda *et al*, 1989b; Somers *et al*, 1990; Kitagawa *et al*, 1991; Proctor *et al*, 1991; Wagata *et al*, 1991). Conversely, the amplification is very rare in haematopoietic malignancies and other solid tumours, such as stomach, renal cell, colorectal, ovarian and hepatocellular carcinomas (reviewed in Lammie and Peters, 1991). The most extensive surveys have focused on breast cancers, and the salient findings and principal references are sum-

TABLE 1. Amplification of 11q13 markers in primary human breast cancers

Centre	Numbers	% Amplified	Reference
Los Angeles	4/46	8.7	Zhou *et al* (1988)
St Cloud/Bethesda	18/110	16.4	Lidereau *et al* (1988)
Leicester	9/40	22.5	Varley *et al* (1988)
Tokyo	22/176	12.5	Tsuda *et al* (1989)
Nice/Montpellier/Marseille	36/219	16.4	Adnane *et al* (1989)
Washington	7/90	7.8	Machotka *et al* (1989)
Austin	5/100	5.0	Meyers *et al* (1990)
Paris	13/106	12.3	Tang *et al* (1990)
ICRF London	**28/183**	**15.3**	**Fantl et al (1990)**
Lund	27/311	8.7	Borg *et al* (1991)
Amsterdam	36/226	15.9	Schuuring *et al* (1992)
Rotterdam	105/704	14.9	Berns *et al* (1992)
Newcastle	12/111	10.8	Henry *et al* (1993)
		(average 13.3%)	

marized in Table 1. In our own study, highlighted in Table 1, we detected the amplification in about one in six primary tumours. Although the amplification frequencies reported by different groups are quite variable, ranging between 5% and 22.5%, many of the larger studies reach similar conclusions, and the variability is likely to reflect the way in which tumour material is processed and analysed rather than geographical or aetiological differences (Adnane *et al*, 1989).

Significance of the 11q13 Amplicon in Breast Cancer

Given the consistency of these observations, the obvious question is whether the presence of the amplification unit correlates with any clinicopathological parameters. Several studies have suggested weak links with lymph node involvement, large tumour size, early presentation, ductal morphology and lymphocyte infiltration (Adnane *et al*, 1989; Machotka *et al*, 1989; Theillet *et al*, 1989; Tsuda *et al*, 1989a; Tang *et al*, 1990; Henry *et al*, 1993), but the strongest association thus far is with hormone receptor status. In the Imperial Cancer Research Fund study (Fantl *et al*, 1990), all but one (27/28) of the tumours with DNA amplification at 11q13 had oestrogen receptor (ER) levels in excess of 10 fmol/mg ($p<0.001$), and other groups have reported similar findings (Adnane *et al*, 1989; Borg *et al*, 1991; Berns *et al*, 1992). Moreover, the mean ER levels are significantly higher in tumours with the amplification, and similar but statistically weaker trends have been noted for progesterone receptor (PR) levels (Adnane *et al*, 1989; Fantl *et al*, 1990; Borg *et al*, 1991; Berns *et al*, 1992). Thus, tumours with amplification of 11q13 represent a different cohort from those showing amplification of *HER2/erbB2*, which are primarily hormone receptor negative (reviewed in Lofts and Gullick, 1992). Neither the *ER* on 6q nor the *PR* gene on 11q22 is affected by the amplification (Gosden *et al*, 1986; Mattei *et al*, 1988).

The presence of the 11q13 amplification unit may therefore define a subclass of ER positive tumours, but it is too early to draw definite conclusions about the prognostic implications, since most of the surveys have been undertaken only in the past 5 years. Nevertheless, some groups have claimed that the amplification is associated with an adverse prognosis, as judged by relapse free or overall survival (Lidereau *et al*, 1988; Machotka *et al*, 1989; Tsuda *et al*, 1989a; Borg *et al*, 1991; Schuuring *et al*, 1992b; Henry *et al*, 1993). What is unresolved is whether the predictive value of the 11q13 amplification applies to all patients or only to particular categories defined by more traditional variables, such as lymph node or hormone receptor status (Borg *et al*, 1991; Schuuring *et al*, 1992b; Henry *et al*, 1993).

Detecting the Amplification at 11q13

Time and greater numbers of cases will eventually clarify the prognostic significance of the 11q13 amplicon, but if it does prove to be clinically useful, then a more rapid and routine assay will be needed. The variable frequencies recorded in Table 1 are likely to reflect the ways in which the DNA is isolated and analysed, rather than the pathology of the tumours. Since the degree of amplification is modest, typically between two- and fivefold, an accurate picture can require Southern blotting with multiple enzyme/probe combinations, preferably controlled internally with a non-amplified marker from elsewhere on chromosome 11. Although it would be conceivable to devise standardized protocols, DNA blotting is inherently slow and technically demanding and can provide only tissue averaged figures. Moreover, since the stromal contribution in each sample will vary, the degree and frequency of DNA amplification in the tumour cells are always likely to be underestimated with such techniques. A much more attractive proposition would be to develop an assay based on detection of a gene product, in the same way that amplification and overexpression of *HER2/erbB2* can now be determined by means of immunohistochemical staining of tumour tissue (reviewed in Lofts and Gullick, 1992). As well as being able to detect abnormal levels of protein in individual tumour cells, such an assay can identify cases in which the gene is overexpressed by mechanisms other than DNA amplification.

Lack of Correlation between Amplification and Expression

Given their background, the natural candidates for an expression based assay would appear to be *FGF3* and *FGF4*. However, in their normal embryonic setting, these genes are transcribed at relatively low levels (Jakobovits *et al*, 1986; Wilkinson *et al*, 1988; Peters et al, 1989; Velcich *et al*, 1989), and their products have proved very hard to detect except in artificial systems geared for overexpression. Even in MMTV induced tumours in which *FGF3* and *FGF4* mRNAs are readily detected, it has not been possible to visualize the respective proteins with the available antisera (our unpublished observations). More importantly, studies on the mouse system have shown that neither of these genes is expressed at a detectable level in the normal mammary gland (Jakobovits *et al*, 1986; Yoshida *et al*, 1988b; Stamp *et al*, 1992). The same appears to be true in humans, and despite determined efforts to find *FGF3* and *FGF4* transcripts in human tumours, the overwhelming weight of evidence now indicates that amplification of the 11q13 region does not lead to overexpression of either gene (Liscia *et al*, 1989; Tsuda *et al*, 1989b; Fantl *et al*, 1990; Lafage *et al*, 1990; Faust and Meeker, 1992; Schuuring *et al*, 1992a). The rare exceptions (Fantl *et al*, 1990) are most likely cases in which the amplified DNA has undergone some further perturbation, but this has yet to be confirmed. Thus, although *FGF3* or *FGF4* may have a minor role in some tumours, their presence on the amplified DNA must now be regarded as fortuitous rather than biologically relevant. In other words, it is now generally accepted that although *FGF3* and *FGF4* may have been useful indicators, some other gene on the amplified DNA must provide the impetus for amplification.

In retrospect, the lack of *FGF3* and *FGF4* expression is not surprising given that they are transcriptionally silent in the normal mammary gland. Amplification of these genes in a tumour cell is unlikely to activate their expression unless, for example, the few extra copies of DNA are enough to override the effects of negatively acting transcription factors. Although not excluded, such mechanisms assume a very delicate balance in the regulation of transcription. A much more tenable explanation is that the gene that provides the selective force for 11q13 amplification is already expressed in normal mammary epithelial cells and that amplification simply increases the number of transcriptionally active copies. Recent work has therefore focused on identifying expressed genes in the 11q13 region, and two excellent candidates have emerged, *CCND1* and *EMS1*.

CANDIDATE ONCOGENES IN THE 11q13 AMPLICON

The search for expressed genes in the region has progressed by a mixture of design and serendipity. Work in disparate fields regularly uncovers new markers that happen to map within the 11q13 region, and both *CCND1* and *EMS1* fall into this category. However, they were also isolated because of their linkage to *FGF3*, *FGF4* and *BCL1* and their overexpression in tumour cells.

The *CCND1* Gene

The name *CCND1* has now been officially adopted for the gene on 11q13 encoding cyclin D1 (Inaba *et al*, 1992; Xiong *et al*, 1992a), but the same locus has appeared in multiple guises in the recent literature. For example, it was first described as a rearranged DNA fragment in a parathyroid adenoma in which a chromosomal inversion had juxtaposed the parathyroid hormone gene on the short arm of chromosome 11 with a previously unknown locus, designated *D11S287*, at band q13 (Arnold *et al*, 1989). The rearrangement was subsequently shown to cause elevated expression of an adjacent gene, given the name *PRAD1* (Motokura *et al*, 1991; Rosenberg *et al*, 1991a). However, the frequency of the translocation in these benign lesions is quite low, and a much stronger case might be made for calling the gene *BCL1*. Although it lies approximately 110 kb from the original breakpoint (Fig. 1), the expression of *CCND1* is clearly affected by the t(11;14) translocation (Rosenberg *et al*, 1991b; Withers *et al*, 1991; Seto *et al*, 1992). A parallel for this translocation occurs in mouse lymphomas where the homologue of *CCND1* can be activated by retroviral insertion (Lammie *et al*, 1992). *CCND1* therefore has the hallmarks of a cellular oncogene, although it has not been shown to have transforming activity in cultured cells. More importantly for the purposes of this review, cDNA clones for *CCND1* were isolated by screening for sequences that are overexpressed in a squamous cell carcinoma line with amplification at 11q13 (Schuuring *et al*, 1992a).

The name *CCND1* reflects the structural similarity between the predicted gene product and members of the cyclin family (Lew *et al*, 1991; Matsushime *et al*, 1991; Motokura *et al*, 1991; Withers *et al*, 1991; Xiong *et al*, 1991). Cyclins are a group of proteins whose periodic accumulation and destruction appear to influence progress through the cell division cycle, by acting as regulatory subunits for cyclin dependent protein kinases (CDKs) (Pines, 1993). Thus, *CCND1* was identified as a human cDNA that was able to complement for G_1 phase cyclins in budding yeast (Lew *et al*, 1991; Xiong *et al*, 1991). However, it is not clear that the CCND1 product, cyclin D1, behaves as a classical cyclin. Although the expression of the gene is induced by growth factors and reaches a maximum in the late G_1 phase, the levels do not fluctuate dramatically in subsequent phases of the cycle (Matsushime *et al*, 1991; Won *et al*, 1992; Sewing *et al*, 1993). Nevertheless, recent evidence suggests that cyclin D1 does act as a regulatory subunit for members of the CDK family and is thus likely to have an important but as yet unspecified role in cell cycle control (Matsushime *et al*, 1992; Xiong *et al*, 1992b; Kato *et al*, 1993).

The *EMS1* Gene

The screen for overexpressed sequences that map to chromosome 11q13 identified a second interesting gene, *EMS1* (Schuuring *et al*, 1992a). Fortunately, we already know its location relative to other markers in the region, since the corresponding genomic DNA was recovered from a chromosome jumping library and shown to map approximately 600 kb telomeric of *FGF3* (Fig. 1) (Brookes *et al*, 1993). The sequence of the *EMS1* cDNA predicted a 550 aminoacid product with unusual tandem repeats and a so called SH3 domain, one of the hallmarks of proteins that are associated with the cytoskeleton (Schuuring *et al*, 1992a). It was also immediately clear that *EMS1* encodes the human homologue of p80/85, a protein that was characterized as a major substrate for phosphorylation by the *src* oncogene in chicken cells (Wu *et al*, 1991). Although p80/85 is located predominantly in the cytoplasm, transformation by *src* or overexpression due to gene amplification causes the protein to accumulate in podosome-like contact sites between the cell and the substratum (Wu *et al*, 1991; Schuuring *et al*, 1992a). It is therefore not difficult to imagine how this might contribute to the abnormal cell-cell interactions and invasive properties of a tumour cell.

IDENTIFYING THE CRITICAL GENE IN THE 11q13 AMPLICON

Physical Mapping of the Amplified DNA

There are of course other genes on the amplified DNA in addition to *EMS1* and *CCND1*. Since it was natural to suspect that the key gene in the region would be relatively close to *FGF3*, several groups have used genome mapping strategies to identify neighbouring genes or to saturate the entire 11q13 region with useful markers (Janson *et al*, 1991; Brookes *et al*, 1992; Ollendorff *et al*, 1992; Szepetowski *et al*, 1992a,b; Tanigami *et al*, 1992a,b; Brookes *et al*, 1993; Petty *et al*, 1993). Some of these are anonymous segments of DNA, whereas others correspond to so called CpG islands, regions rich in cytosine and guanine that remain hypomethylated in chromosomal DNA (Bird, 1986). Such features are generally associated with functional genes, and since they also correspond to sites for rare cutting restriction enzymes they are extremely useful in generating long range physical maps of genomic DNA. Figure 1 shows our current understanding of the region surrounding *FGF3*, in which we have located seven CpG islands (shown as bold lines), the *BCL1* breakpoint probe and the polymorphic markers *D11S97* (*pMS51*) and *D11S146* (*pHB159*) (Nakamura *et al*, 1988; Armour *et al*, 1989). Whereas we already know the sequences and some of the functions of *CCND1*, *FGF3*, *FGF4* and *EMS1*, the genes that may be associated with the *D11S814*, *TOF1* and *TOF2* CpG islands remain uncharacterized. Moreover, this 1500 kb segment is only a small part of band q13, which encompasses closer to 15 Mb of DNA. Although many other loci have now been located and ordered, there are still large gaps in the physical map of the entire region.

Ordering Markers by Frequency of Amplification

One of the goals is to identify every functional gene on the amplified DNA. However, a complete map will only establish the order of these genes on the chromosome, not their order of importance in tumorigenesis. The tacit assumption is that there should be a focus of amplification centred on a critical gene and conversely that the more distant a gene is from this focus the less frequently it will appear within the amplification unit. Indeed, it has been suggested that ranking markers by their frequency of amplification in breast and squamous cell tumours might be a useful way of mapping the region (Szepetowski *et al*, 1993). Taking the 11q13 region as a whole, this is clearly feasible, since genes such as *PYGM*, *PGA*, *SEA*, *PP1*-alpha and *GST* are less

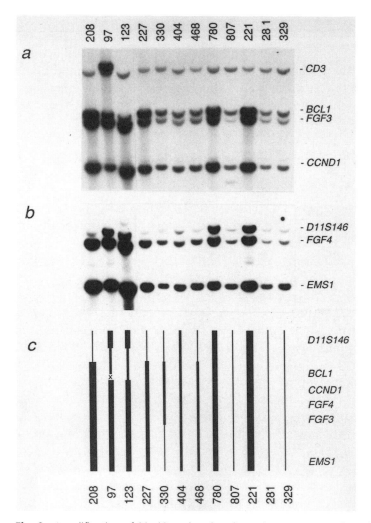

Fig. 2. Amplification of 11q13 markers in primary breast cancers. Samples of DNA from the numbered tumours were digested with *Pst*I and analysed by Southern blotting. In panel (a) the filter was hybridized simultaneously with probes for CD3-gamma, *BCL1*, *FGF3* and *CCND1*. In (b) the same blot was stripped of radioactivity and rehybridized with probes for *D11S146*, *FGF4* and *EMS1*. The methods and DNA probes have been described in detail elsewhere (Fantl *et al*, 1990; Lammie *et al*, 1991; Brookes *et al*, 1992, 1993). Panel (c) shows the amplification status of these markers relative to their order on chromosome 11q13 (see Fig. 1). The thickness of each line is proportional to the degree of amplification, ranging from approximately twofold in tumour 404 to eightfold in tumour 221. In several of these selected cases, markers were amplified to different degrees. Tumours 807, 281 and 329 are non-amplified controls. All of these DNAs have been analysed in multiple experiments and the conclusions in panel (c) are drawn from the combined data

frequently amplified than *FGF3* and *FGF4* (Lammie and Peters, 1991; Szepetowski *et al*, 1993). Although confirming that the amplification unit is centred on 11q13, such data reveal that the amplicon can be surprisingly large. However, the closer markers are to one another, the more difficult it becomes to rank their degrees or frequencies of amplification. This is illustrated in Fig.

2, which shows a Southern blot analysis of a selection of breast cancer DNAs hybridized with probes from the 11q13 region.

The order and physical distances between these loci have been established by long range mapping as discussed above (Fig. 1). In three of the tumours (404, 780 and 221), all the 11q13 markers shown here are amplified relative to CD3-gamma, the internal control that maps much more distally on the long arm of chromosome 11 (Saito *et al*, 1987). This is typical of tumours with amplification at 11q13 and suggests that the amplicon extends beyond the 1.5 Mb of DNA in the physical map. In contrast, the amplicons in tumours 208, 227 and 468 do not include *D11S146*, a polymorphic marker located centromeric of *BCL1*. Such data imply that the critical gene on the amplicon must lie telomeric to *D11S146* and all of the tumours we have analysed would be consistent with this conclusion. However, other surveys have drawn different conclusions (Ali *et al*, 1989; Theillet *et al*, 1990; Proctor *et al*, 1991; Saint-Ruf *et al*, 1991; Gaudray *et al*, 1992; Szepetowski *et al*, 1992a), and tumours 97 and 123 exemplify the difficulties with this approach. Although all the markers are amplified relative to CD3-gamma, the degree of amplification is inconsistent with the physical map (Fig. 2c). Thus, *BCL1* appears less amplified than the two adjacent markers. In tumour 97, the situation is even more complex in that a rearrangement has occurred between *BCL1* and *CCND1*, resulting in an abnormally large *CCND1* fragment.

Such complexities are open to various interpretations. The first is that there could be more than one critical gene or selective force within the 11q13 region, resulting in independent amplification units (Gaudray *et al*, 1992). In some tumours, the amplicons could be quite discrete, whereas in others they might overlap. This would explain why the degree and/or frequency of amplification can sometimes appear to be at odds with the physical map. The difficulty with this interpretation is that the higher the resolution of the analyses, the greater the number of potential target genes and amplicons that have to be postulated. Another possibility is that amplification of a large region of DNA might encompass a tumour suppressor gene whose subsequent deletion would be advantageous to the tumour cell. Finally, the apparent discontinuities in the amplicon may simply reflect rearrangement or recombination within the amplified DNA. Since current models of DNA amplification invoke inverted duplication (Fried *et al*, 1991; Toledo *et al*, 1992), genes that are normally distant from one another can become juxtaposed.

Expression of Critical Genes on 11q13

As discussed earlier, one of the criteria that the key gene(s) on the amplicon should satisfy is that it should be expressed at elevated levels as a consequence of the amplification. As previously reported and shown below, both *CCND1* and *EMS1* fulfil this requirement (Lammie *et al*, 1991; Schuuring *et al*, 1992a); *FGF3* and *FGF4* do not. Thus, Fig. 3 shows an RNA blot of a selection of primary breast tumours, of which half are known to have an amplification of

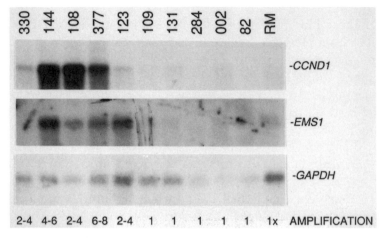

Fig. 3. Expression of *CCND1* and *EMS1* in primary breast cancers. Samples of RNA from the numbered tumours and from normal breast tissue (RM) were analysed by gel electrophoresis and blot hybridization (Lammie *et al*, 1991). The filter was hybridized sequentially with probes for *CCND1* (Lammie *et al*, 1991) and *EMS1* (Schuuring *et al*, 1992a). The *GAPDH* probe served as a control for RNA loading. Numbers below each track refer to the approximate degree amplification of the 11q13 region based on the Southern blot analysis of *FGF3*

11q13. The degree of amplification is indicated below each lane. In three of these tumours, 144, 108 and 377, *CCND1* and *EMS1* are both expressed at relatively high levels. In tumour 330, on the other hand, in which we did not see amplification of *EMS1* (Fig. 2), we similarly did not detect high levels of *EMS1* RNA. These findings point to *CCND1* as the more important player in this tumour. However, in tumour 123, in which the amplification unit breaks down between *CCND1* and *BCL1*, *EMS1* is more highly expressed. In this case, the conclusion is clouded by the fact that both genes are expressed at elevated levels relative to tumours in which the 11q13 region is unaffected. To our knowledge, there are as yet no data that definitively identify one or other of these genes as the more important player in the amplified DNA.

FUTURE PROSPECTS

Until the evidence is resolved in favour of *CCND1, EMS1* or one of the other genes in the region, these markers will continue to provide a means of detecting the amplicon in the vast majority of cases. Given the logistical difficulties with DNA analyses, current efforts are focusing on the use of antibodies to detect the respective gene products, and the preliminary results with cyclin D1 look encouraging (Gillett C, Fantl V, Smith R, Bartek J, Dickson C, Peters G and Barnes D, unpublished). If these efforts are successful, immunocytochemistry will provide a more rapid, less expensive and potentially more accurate way of scoring for abnormalities at 11q13 and may permit screening of archival material. Increased numbers should help to clarify the prognostic significance of 11q13 amplification. The incidence of breast cancer is such that, in Britain alone, there are 3000 new examples of this chromosomal abnormality each year. At the very least, the identification of these cases might refine the classification of tumours and help in the clinical management of the disease. In the longer term, a better understanding of the key gene(s) in the amplified DNA might lead to new therapeutic strategies.

SUMMARY

Amplification of markers centred on band q13 of human chromosome 11 is a consistent feature in a subset of oestrogen receptor positive breast cancers. Although the amplification was initially scored via *FGF3/INT2,* which has strong credentials as a mammary oncogene, current data suggest that some other gene on 11q13 provides the driving force for amplification. Here we have reviewed our understanding of the amplified DNA, the genes it encompasses and the evidence in favour of two candidate oncogenes, *CCND1* and *EMS1.* As well as being among the most frequently amplified markers in the region, these genes are expressed at elevated levels as a consequence of amplification, and their predicted functions would be consistent with a role in tumorigenesis. Irrespective of the final conclusions regarding their biological relevance, the overexpression of *CCND1* or *EMS1* should provide a more amenable assay for the amplification and help to clarify its clinical significance.

References

Adelaide J, Mattei M-G, Marics I *et al* (1988) Chromosomal localization of the *hst* oncogene and its co-amplification with the *int.2* oncogene in a human melanoma. *Oncogene* **2** 413–416

Adnane J, Gaudray P, Simon M-P, Simony-Lafontaine J, Jeanteur P and Theillet C (1989) Proto-oncogene amplification and human breast tumor phenotype. *Oncogene* **4** 1389–1395

Ali IU, Merlo G, Callahan R and Lidereau R (1989) The amplification unit on chromosome 11q13 in aggressive primary human breast tumors entails the *bcl*-1, *int*-2 and *hst* loci. *Oncogene* **4** 89–92

Armour JAL, Wong Z, Wilson V, Royle NJ and Jeffreys AJ (1989) Sequences flanking the repeat arrays of human minisatellites: association with tandem and dispersed repeat elements. *Nucleic Acids Research* **17** 4925–4935

Arnold A, Kim HG, Gaz RD *et al* (1989) Molecular cloning and chromosomal mapping of DNA rearranged with the parathyroid hormone gene in a parathyroid adenoma. *Journal of Clinical Investigation* **83** 2034–2040

Baird A and Klagsbrun M (1991) The fibroblast growth factor family. *Annals of the New York Academy of Sciences of the USA* **638** xiii–xvi

Berenson JR, Yang J and Mickel R (1989) Frequent amplification of the *bcl*-1 locus in head and neck squamous cell carcinomas. *Oncogene* **4** 1111–1116

Berenson JR, Koga H, Yang J *et al* (1990) Frequent amplification of the *bcl*-1 locus in poorly differentiated squamous cell carcinoma of the lung. *Oncogene* **5** 1343–1348

Berns EMJJ, Klijn JGM, van Staveren IL, Portengen H, Noordegraaf E and Foekens JA (1992) Prevalence of amplification of the oncogenes c-*myc*, HER2/neu, and *int*-2 in one thousand human breast tumours: correlation with steroid receptors. *European Journal of Cancer* **28** 697–700

Bird AP (1986) CpG-rich islands and the function of DNA methylation. *Nature* **321** 209–213

Borg A, Sigurdsson H, Clark GM *et al* (1991) Association of *INT2/HST1* coamplification in primary breast cancer with hormone-dependent phenotype and poor prognosis. *British Journal of Cancer* **63** 136–142

Brookes S, Lammie GA, Schuuring E, Dickson C and Peters G (1992) Linkage map of a region of human chromosome band 11q13 amplified in breast and squamous cell tumors. *Genes Chromosomes and Cancer* **4** 290–301

Brookes S, Lammie GA, Schuuring E *et al* (1993) Amplified region of chromosome band 11q13 in breast and squamous cell carcinomas encompasses three CpG islands telomeric of *FGF3*, including the expressed gene *EMS1*. *Genes Chromosomes and Cancer* **6** 222–231

Casey G, Smith R, McGillivray D, Peters G and Dickson C (1986) Characterization and chromosome assignment of the human homolog of *int-2*, a potential proto-oncogene. *Molecular and Cellular Biology* **6** 502–510

Delli Bovi P and Basilico C (1987) Isolation of a rearranged human transforming gene following transfection of Kaposi sarcoma DNA. *Proceedings of the National Academy of Sciences of the USA* **84** 5660–5664

Delli Bovi P, Curatola AM, Kern FG, Greco A, Ittmann M and Basilico C (1987) An oncogene isolated by transfection of Kaposi's sarcoma DNA encodes a growth factor that is a member of the FGF family. *Cell* **50** 729–737

Dickson C, Smith R, Brookes S and Peters G (1984) Tumorigenesis by mouse mammary tumor virus: proviral activation of a cellular gene in the common integration region *int-2*. *Cell* **37** 529–536

Fantl V, Richards MA, Smith R *et al* (1990) Gene amplification on chromosome band 11q13 and oestrogen receptor status in breast cancer. *European Journal of Cancer* **26** 423–429

Faust JB and Meeker TC (1992) Amplification and expression of the *bcl*-1 gene in human solid tumor cell lines. *Cancer Research* **52** 2460–2463

Fried M, Feo S and Heard E (1991) The role of inverted duplication in the generation of gene amplification in mammalian cells. *Biochimica et Biophysica Acta* **1090** 143–155

Gaudray P, Szepetowski P, Escot C, Birnbaum D and Theillet C (1992) DNA amplification at 11q13 in human cancer: from complexity to perplexity. *Mutation Research* **276** 317–328

Gosden JR, Middleton PG and Rout D (1986) Localization of the human oestrogen receptor gene to chromosome 6q24-q27 by in situ hybridization. *Cytogenetics and Cell Genetics* **43** 218–220

Henry JA, Hennessy C, Levett DL, Lennard TWJ, Westley BR and May FEB (1993) *int-2* amplification in breast cancer: association with decreased survival and relationship to amplification of c-*erb*B-2 and c-*myc*. *International Journal of Cancer* **53** 774–780

Huebner K, Ferrari AC, Delli Bovi P, Croce C and Basilico C (1988) The *FGF*-related oncogene, K-*FGF*, maps to human chromosome region 11q13, possibly near *int-2*. *Oncogene Research* **3** 263–270

Inaba T, Matsushime H, Valentine M, Roussel MF, Sherr CJ and Look AT (1992) Genomic organization, chromosomal localization, and independent expression of human cyclin D genes. *Genomics* **13** 565–574

Jakobovits A, Shackleford GM, Varmus HE and Martin GR (1986) Two proto-oncogenes implicated in mammary carcinogenesis, *int-1* and *int-2*, are independently regulated during mouse development. *Proceedings of the National Academy of Sciences of the USA* **83** 7806–7810

Janson M, Larsson C, Werelius B *et al* (1991) Detailed physical map of human chromosomal region 11q12-13 shows high meiotic recombination rate around the *MEN1* locus. *Proceedings of the National Academy of Sciences of the USA* **88** 10609–10613

Kato J, Matsushime H, Hiebert SW, Ewen ME and Sherr CJ (1993) Direct binding of cyclin D to the retinoblastoma gene product (pRb) and pRb phosphorylation by the cyclin D-dependent kinase CDK4. *Genes and Development* **7** 331–342

Kitagawa Y, Ueda M, Ando N, Shinozawa Y, Shimizu N and Abe O (1991) Significance of *int-2/hst*-1 coamplification as a prognostic factor in patients with esophageal squamous carcinoma. *Cancer Research* **51** 1504–1508

Kwan H, Pecenka V, Tsukamoto A *et al* (1992) Transgenes expressing the *Wnt-1* and *int-2* proto-oncogenes cooperate during mammary carcinogenesis. *Molecular and Cellular Biology* **12** 147–154

Lafage M, Nguyen C, Szepetowski P *et al* (1990) The 11q13 amplicon of a mammary carcinoma cell line. *Genes Chromosomes and Cancer* **2** 171–181

Lammie GA and Peters G (1991) Chromosome 11q13 abnormalities in human cancer. *Cancer Cells* **3** 413–420

Lammie GA, Fantl V, Smith R *et al* (1991) D11S287, a putative oncogene on chromosome 11q13, is amplified and expressed in squamous cell and mammary carcinomas and linked to BCL-1. *Oncogene* **6** 439–444

Lammie GA, Smith R, Silver J, Brookes S, Dickson C and Peters G (1992) Proviral insertions near cyclin D1 in mouse lymphomas: a parallel for BCL1 translocations in human B-cell neoplasms. *Oncogene* **7** 2381–2387

Lew DJ, Dulic V and Reed SI (1991) Isolation of three novel human cyclins by rescue of G1 cyclin (Cln) function in yeast. *Cell* **66** 1197–1206

Lidereau R, Callahan R, Dickson C, Peters G, Escot C and Ali I (1988) Amplification of the *int-2* gene in primary human breast tumors. *Oncogene Research* **2** 285–291

Liscia DS, Merlo GR, Garrett C, French D, Mariani-Costantini R and Callahan R (1989) Expression of *int-2* mRNA in human tumors amplified at the *int-2* locus. *Oncogene* **4** 1219–1224

Lofts FJ and Gullick WJ (1992) cERB-B2 amplification and over-expression in human tumours, In: Dickson RB and Lippman ME (eds). *Genes, Oncogenes and Hormones: Advances in Cellular and Molecular Biology of Breast Cancer*, pp 161–179, Kluwer Academic Publishers, Boston

Machotka SV, Garrett CT, Schwartz AM and Callahan R (1989) Amplification of the proto-oncogenes *int-2*, c-*erbB*-2 and c-*myc* in human breast cancer. *Clinica Chimica Acta* **184** 207–218

Matsushime H, Roussel MF, Ashmun RA and Sherr CJ (1991) Colony-stimulating factor 1 regulates novel cyclins during the G1 phase of the cell cycle. *Cell* **65** 701–713

Matsushime H, Ewen ME, Strom DK *et al* (1992) Identification and properties of an atypical catalytic subunit (p34^{PSK-J3}/cdk4) for mammalian D type G1 cyclins. *Cell* **71** 323–334

Mattei M-G, Krust A, Stropp U, Mattei J-F and Chambon P (1988) Assignment of the human progesterone receptor to the q22 band of chromosome 11. *Human Genetics* **78** 96–97

Meyers SL, O'Brien MT, Smith T and Dudley JP (1990) Analysis of the *int-1*, *int-2*, c-*myc*, and *neu* oncogenes in human breast carcinomas. *Cancer Research* **50** 5911–5918

Motokura T, Bloom T, Kim HG *et al* (1991) A novel cyclin encoded by a *bcl1*-linked candidate oncogene. *Nature* **350** 512–515

Muller WJ, Lee FS, Dickson C, Peters G, Pattengale P and Leder P (1990) The *int-2* gene product acts as an epithelial growth factor in transgenic mice. *EMBO Journal* **9** 907–913

Nakamura Y, Gillilan S, O'Connell P *et al* (1988) Isolation and mapping of a polymorphic DNA sequence pHB159 on chromosome 11 (D11S146). *Nucleic Acids Research* **16** 376

Nguyen C, Roux D, Mattei M-G *et al* (1988) The FGF-related oncogenes *hst* and *int.2*, and the *bcl.1* locus are contained within one megabase in band q13 of chromosome 11 while the *fgf.5* oncogene maps to 4q21. *Oncogene* **3** 703–708

Nusse R (1991) Insertional mutagenesis in mouse mammary tumorigenesis. *Current Topics in Microbiology and Immunology* **171** 44–65

Nusse R and Varmus HE (1992) *Wnt* genes. *Cell* **69** 1073–1087

Nusse R, van Ooyen A, Cox D, Fung YKT and Varmus H (1984) Mode of proviral activation of a putative mammary oncogene (*int-1*) on mouse chromosome 15. *Nature* **307** 131–136

Ollendorff V, Szepetowski P, Mattei M-G, Gaudray P and Birnbaum D (1992) New gene in the homologous human 11q13-q14 and mouse 7F chromosomal regions. *Mammalian Genome* **2** 195–200

Ornitz DM, Cardiff RD, Kuo A and Leder P (1992) Int-2, an autocrine and/or ultra-short-range effector in transgenic mammary tissue transplants. *Journal of the National Cancer Institute* **84** 887–892

Peters G (1990) Oncogenes at viral integration sites. *Cell Growth and Differentiation* **1** 503–510

Peters G (1991) Inappropriate expression of growth factor genes in tumors induced by mouse mammary tumor virus. *Seminars in Virology* **2** 319–328

Peters G, Brookes S, Smith R, Placzek M and Dickson C (1989) The mouse homolog of the *hst/k-FGF* gene is adjacent to *int-2* and is activated by proviral insertion in some virally induced mammary tumors. *Proceedings of the National Academy of Sciences of the USA* **86** 5678–5682

Petty EM, Arnold A, Marx SJ and Bale AE (1993) A pulsed-field gel electrophoresis (PFGE) map of twelve loci on chromosome 11q11-q13. *Genomics* **15** 423–425

Pines J (1993) Cyclins and cyclin-dependent kinases: take your partners. *Trends in Biochemical Sciences of the USA* **18** 195–197

Proctor AJ, Coombs LM, Cairns JP and Knowles MA (1991) Amplification at chromosome 11q13 in transitional cell tumours of the bladder. *Oncogene* **6** 789–795

Raffeld M and Jaffe ES (1991) *bcl*-1, t(11;14), and mantle cell-derived lymphomas. *Blood* **78** 259–263

Rosenberg CL, Kim HG, Shows TB, Kronenberg HM and Arnold A (1991a) Rearrangement and overexpression of D11S287E, a candidate oncogene on chromosome 11q13 in benign parathyroid tumors. *Oncogene* **6** 449–453

Rosenberg CL, Wong E, Petty EM *et al* (1991b) *PRAD1*, a candidate BCL1 oncogene: mapping and expression in centrocytic lymphoma. *Proceedings of the National Academy of Sciences of the USA* **88** 9638–9642

Saint-Ruf C, Malfoy B, Scholl S, Zafrani B and Dutrillaux B (1991) Gstπ gene is frequently co-amplified with INT2 and HSTF1 proto-oncogenes in human breast cancers. *Oncogene* **6** 403–406

Saito H, Koyama T, Georgopoulos K *et al* (1987) Close linkage of the mouse and human CD3γ- and δ-chain genes suggests that their transcription is controlled by common regulatory elements. *Proceedings of the National Academy of Sciences of the USA* **84** 9131–9134

Sakamoto H, Mori M, Taira M *et al* (1986) Transforming gene from human stomach cancers and a noncancerous portion of stomach mucosa. *Proceedings of the National Academy of Sciences of the USA* **83** 3997–4001

Sakamoto H, Yoshida T, Nakakuki M *et al* (1988) Cloned *hst* gene from normal human leukocyte DNA transforms NIH3T3 cells. *Biochemical and Biophysical Research Communications* **151** 965–972

Schuuring E, Verhoeven E, Mooi WJ and Michalides RJAM (1992a) Identification and cloning of two overexpressed genes, U21B31/*PRAD1* and *EMS1*, within the amplified chromosome 11q13 region in human carcinomas. *Oncogene* **7** 355–361

Schuuring E, Verhoeven E, van Tinteren H *et al* (1992b) Amplification of genes within the chromosome 11q13 region is indicative of poor prognosis in patients with operable breast cancer. *Cancer Research* **52** 5229–5234

Seto M, Yamamoto K, Iida S *et al* (1992) Gene rearrangement and overexpression of *PRAD1* in lymphoid malignancy with t(11;14)(q13;q32) translocation. *Oncogene* **7** 1401–1406

Sewing A, Bürger C, Brüsselbach S, Schalk C, Lucibello FC and Müller R (1993) Human cyclin D1 encodes a labile nuclear protein whose synthesis is directly induced by growth factors and suppressed by cyclic AMP. *Journal of Cell Science* **104** 545–554

Somers KD, Cartwright SL and Schechter GL (1990) Amplification of the *int-2* gene in human head and neck squamous cell carcinomas. *Oncogene* **5** 915–920

Stamp G, Fantl V, Poulsom R *et al* (1992) Nonuniform expression of a mouse mammary tumor virus-driven *int-2/Fgf-3* transgene in pregnancy-responsive breast tumors. *Cell Growth and Differentiation* **3** 929–938

Szepetowski P, Courseaux A, Carle GF, Theillet C and Gaudray P (1992a) Amplification of

11q13 DNA sequences in human breast cancer: D11S97 identifies a region tightly linked to BCL1 which can be amplified separately. *Oncogene* **7** 2513–2517

Szepetowski P, Simon M-P, Grosgeorge J *et al* (1992b) Localization of 11q13 loci with respect to regional chromosomal breakpoints. *Genomics* **12** 738–744

Szepetowski P, Perucca-Lostanlen D and Gaudray P (1993) Mapping genes according to their amplification status in tumor cells: contribution to the map of 11q13. *Genomics* **16** 745–750

Tang R, Kacinski B, Validire P *et al* (1990) Oncogene amplification correlates with dense lymphocyte infiltration in human breast cancers: a role for hematopoietic growth factor release by tumor cells? *Journal of Cellular Biochemistry* **44** 189–198

Tanigami A, Tokino T, Takita K, Takiguchi S and Nakamura Y (1992a) A 14-Mb physical map of the region at chromosome 11q13 harboring the MEN1 locus and the tumor amplicon region. *Genomics* **13** 16–20

Tanigami A, Tokino T, Takita K, Ueda M, Kasumi F and Nakamura Y (1992b) Detailed analysis of an amplified region at chromosome 11q13 in malignant tumors. *Genomics* **13** 21–24

Theillet C, Le Roy X, De Lapeyriere O *et al* (1989) Amplification of *FGF*-related genes in human tumors: possible involvement of *HST* in breast carcinomas. *Oncogene* **4** 915–922

Theillet C, Adnane J, Szepetowski P *et al* (1990) BCL-1 participates in the 11q13 amplification found in breast cancer. *Oncogene* **5** 147–149

Toledo F, Le Roscouet D, Buttin G and Dabatisse M (1992) Co-amplified markers alternate in megabase long chromosomal inverted repeats and cluster independently in interphase nuclei at early steps of mammalian gene amplification. *EMBO Journal* **11** 2665–2673

Tsuda T, Nakatani H, Matsumura T *et al* (1988) Amplification of the *hst*-1 gene in human esophageal carcinomas. *Japanese Journal of Cancer Research* **79** 584–588

Tsuda H, Hirohashi S, Shimosato Y *et al* (1989a) Correlation between long-term survival in breast cancer patients and amplification of two putative oncogene-coamplification units: *hst*-1/*int*-2 and c-*erb*B-2/*ear*-1. *Cancer Research* **49** 3104–3108

Tsuda T, Tahara E, Kajiyana G, Sakamoto H, Terada M and Sugimura T (1989b) High incidence of coamplification of *hst*-1 and *int*-2 genes in human esophageal carcinomas. *Cancer Research* **49** 5505–5508

Tsujimoto Y, Yunis J, Onorato-Showe L, Erikson J, Nowell PC and Croce CM (1984) Molecular cloning of the chromomal breakpoint of B-cell lymphomas and leukemias with the t(11;14) chromosome translocation. *Science* **224** 1403–1406

Tsukamoto AS, Grosschedl R, Guzman RC, Parslow T and Varmus HE (1988) Expression of the *int*-1 gene in transgenic mice is associated with mammary gland hyperplasia and adenocarcinomas in male and female mice. *Cell* **55** 619–625

Tsutsumi M, Sakamoto H, Yoshida T *et al* (1988) Coamplification of the *hst*-1 and *int*-2 genes in human cancers. *Japanese Journal of Cancer Research* **79** 428–432

Turc-Carel C, Pietrzak E, Kakati S, Kinniburgh AJ and Sandberg AA (1987) The human *int*-1 gene is located at chromosome region 12q12-12q13 and is not rearranged in myxoid liposarcoma with t(12;16)(q13;p11). *Oncogene Research* **1** 397–405

van den Berghe H, Parloir C, David G, Michaux JL and Sokal G (1979) A new characteristic karyotypic anomaly in lymphoproliferative disorders. *Cancer* **44** 188–195

van't Veer LJ, van Kessel AG, van Heerikhuizen H, van Ooyen A and Nusse R (1984) Molecular cloning and chromosomal assignment of the human homolog of *int*-1, a mouse gene implicated in mammary tumorigenesis. *Molecular and Cellular Biology* **4** 2532–2534

Varley JM, Walker RA, Casey G and Brammar WJ (1988) A common alteration to the *int*-2 proto-oncogene in DNA from primary breast carcinomas. *Oncogene* **3** 87–91

Velcich A, Delli-Bovi P, Mansukhani A, Ziff EB and Basilico C (1989) Expression of the K-*fgf* protooncogene is repressed during differentiation of F9 cells. *Oncogene Research* **5** 31–37

Wada A, Sakamoto H, Katoh O *et al* (1988) Two homologous oncogenes, HST1 and INT2, are closely located in human genome. *Biochemical and Biophysical Research Communications* **157** 828–835

Wagata T, Ishizaki K, Imamura M, Shimada Y, Ikenaga M and Tobe T (1991) Deletion of 17p and amplification of the *int-2* gene in esophageal carcinomas. *Cancer Research* **51** 2113–2117

Wilkinson DG, Peters G, Dickson C and McMahon AP (1988) Expression of the FGF-related proto-oncogene *int-2* during gastrulation and neurulation in the mouse. *EMBO Journal* **7** 691–695

Withers DA, Harvey RC, Faust JB, Melnyk O, Carey K and Meeker TC (1991) Characterization of a candidate *bcl-1* gene. *Molecular and Cellular Biology* **11** 4846–4853

Won K-A, Xiong Y, Beach D and Gilman MZ (1992) Growth-regulated expression of D-type cyclin genes in human diploid fibroblasts. *Proceedings of the National Academy of Sciences USA* **89** 9910–9914

Wu H, Reynolds AB, Kanner SB, Vines RR and Parsons JT (1991) Identification and characterization of a novel cytoskeleton-associated pp60*src* substrate. *Molecular and Cellular Biology* **11** 5113–5124

Xiong Y, Connolly T, Futcher B and Beach D (1991) Human D-type cyclin. *Cell* **65** 691–699

Xiong Y, Menninger J, Beach D and Ward DC (1992a) Molecular cloning and chromosomal mapping of *CCND* genes encoding human D-type cyclins. *Genomics* **13** 575–584

Xiong Y, Zhang H and Beach D (1992b) D type cyclins associate with multiple protein kinases and the DNA replication and repair factor PCNA. *Cell* **71** 505–514

Yoshida T, Miyagawa K, Odagiri H *et al* (1987) Genomic sequence of *hst,* a transforming gene encoding a protein homologous to fibroblast growth factors and the *int-2*-encoded protein. *Proceedings of the National Academy of Sciences USA* **84** 7305–7309

Yoshida T, Muramatsu H, Muramatsu T *et al* (1988a) Differential expression of two homologous and clustered oncogenes, *Hst1* and *int-2*, during differentiation of F9 cells. *Biochemical and Biophysical Research Communications* **157** 618–625

Yoshida T, Tsutsumi M, Sakamoto H *et al* (1988b) Expression of the *HST1* oncogene in human germ cell tumors. *Biochemical and Biophysical Research Communications* **155** 1324–1329

Yoshida MC, Wada M, Satoh H *et al* (1988c) Human *HST1* (*HSTF1*) gene maps to chromosome band 11q13 and coamplifies with the *INT2* gene in human cancer. *Proceedings of the National Academy of Sciences USA* **85** 4861–4864

Zhou DJ, Casey G and Cline MJ (1988) Amplification of human *int-2* in breast cancers and squamous carcinomas. *Oncogene* **2** 279–282

The authors are responsible for the accuracy of the references.

Inherited Susceptibility to Breast Cancer

DOUGLAS EASTON • DEBORAH FORD • JULIAN PETO

Section of Epidemiology, Institute of Cancer Research, Block D 15 Cotswold Rd, Belmont, Surrey SM2 5NG

Introduction
Genetic epidemiology of breast cancer
Breast-ovarian cancer families and the *BRCA1* gene
    Linkage to chromosome 17q
    Localization of *BRCA1*
    Genetic heterogeneity
    Cancer risks associated with *BRCA1*
    Gene frequency of *BRCA1*
    Contribution of *BRCA1* to breast and ovarian cancer incidence
    Contribution of *BRCA1* to familial breast cancer
The Li-Fraumeni syndrome and the *TP53* gene
Breast cancer and ataxia-telangiectasia
Male breast cancer
Other linkage studies
Discussion
Summary

INTRODUCTION

During the past 5 years, important progress towards understanding familial breast cancer has been made with the identification or localization of several genes responsible for inherited predisposition to the disease. An inherited component to breast cancer has long been suspected, firstly on the basis of anecdotal reports of families with many affected individuals consistent with dominant inheritance, and secondly, because of systematic epidemiological studies of familial risks, which have demonstrated that the risk of breast cancer is higher in the relatives of breast cancer patients than in the general population (eg Adami *et al*, 1980; Claus *et al*, 1990a). Results from segregation analyses based on these studies have suggested that although the majority of breast cancer cases are sporadic, some 5–10% may be due to inheritance of a highly penetrant gene (eg Claus *et al*, 1991). Now, however, molecular genetic studies have demonstrated directly that susceptibility to breast cancer is inherited in some individuals.

The main aim of this paper is to review the recent progress towards identifying the genes responsible for inherited susceptibility to breast cancer, to examine the risks of breast and other cancers conferred by these genes and to consider their likely contribution to breast cancer incidence and the familial clustering of the disease. Firstly, however, we review briefly what is known about familial breast cancer from epidemiological studies.

GENETIC EPIDEMIOLOGY OF BREAST CANCER

There have been a number of systematic studies of familial risks of breast cancer, but the largest study published is that based on the Cancer and Steroid Hormone (CASH) study conducted by the Centers for Disease Control (Claus *et al*, 1990a). This study is based on the family histories of 4730 histologically confirmed cases of breast cancer diagnosed between ages 20 and 54 and of 4688 frequency matched controls. Since the CASH study is the largest and most extensively analysed systematic study, we shall quote extensively from it, but other studies give similar results.

An important feature of familial breast cancer risks is that they are strongly related to age of diagnosis. In the CASH study, the relative risk has been estimated to be greater than fivefold in relatives of cases diagnosed below age 40 but less than twofold in relatives of cases diagnosed over age 50 (Claus *et al*, 1990a,b). Furthermore, the risk of breast cancer is much greater in women with two or more affected first degree relatives than in women with one affected relative. The familial risk is also greater in the relatives of metachronous bilateral cases than in the relatives of unilateral cases (see Bernstein *et al*, 1992).

Taken together, these observations suggest that a small proportion of breast cancer cases is due to the inheritance of a highly penetrant disease gene, the proportion of genetic cases being highest at young ages. Possible genetic models for breast cancer have been tested formally in the CASH data set using segregation analysis (Claus *et al*, 1991). Under the best fitting model, susceptibility to breast cancer is conferred by an autosomal dominant gene with population frequency .0033, such that the cumulative risk of breast cancer is 38% by age 50 and 67% by age 70 in gene carriers, compared with 1.5% by age 50 and 5% by age 70 in non-carriers. Under this model, the proportion of breast cancer cases due to the susceptibility gene falls from about 35% among cases diagnosed below age 30 to about 1% of cases diagnosed over age 80. Similar models have been obtained using other data sets (Williams and Anderson, 1984; Bishop *et al*, 1988; Newman *et al*, 1988; Iselius *et al*, 1991). Such an autosomal dominant model would be consistent with the observed pattern of disease in many anecdotal high risk families (see eg Gardner and Stephens, 1950).

One feature of the familial risks that is not well explained by an autosomal dominant gene model is that a number of studies have shown a somewhat higher risk of breast cancer in the sisters of breast cancer patients than in their mothers. The difference is fairly slight in the CASH study but more marked in other studies (eg Ottman *et al*, 1986). This difference, if real, might be an artefact due, for example, to lower fertility in susceptible individuals (although there is no evidence for such an effect). Alternatively, it could be due to the effect of shared lifestyle risk factors among sisters or to some recessive susceptibility genes.

These segregation analyses do not provide a precise description of the inherited basis for breast cancer. As we show later, it is much more likely that inherited breast cancer is determined by a number of genes conferring a range of penetrances. Nevertheless, they provide a basis for genetic counselling in multiple case families in the absence of linkage evidence.

Another important feature of familial breast cancer is its association with ovarian cancer. The risk of ovarian cancer is moderately increased, of the order 1.3–1.7-fold, in the relatives of breast cancer patients and vice versa (Schildkraut *et al*, 1989; Peto J, Easton DF, Matthews FE, Ford D and Swerdlow AJ, unpublished; Easton DF, Matthews FE, Ford D, Swerdlow AJ and Peto J, unpublished). In the CASH study, the risk of ovarian cancer has been shown to be highest in those families likely to be carrying the putative susceptibility gene (ie those families with multiple early onset breast cancer cases; Claus *et al*, in press). Moreover, there are many anecdotal reports of families with multiple cases of early onset breast cancer and ovarian cancer consistent with autosomal dominant inheritance (Lynch *et al*, 1978).

The only other cancers for which a familial association with breast cancer is well established are childhood bone and soft tissue sarcomas (Birch *et al*, 1984; Hartley *et al*, 1986). This association is probably the result of the autosomal dominant Li-Fraumeni syndrome (Li *et al*, 1988) discussed below and in Eeles *et al* (this volume). The evidence for genetic associations with other cancers is more tenuous. There is some evidence of a familial association between breast cancer and prostate cancer, both from population based studies (Cannon *et al*, 1982; Tulinius *et al*, 1992) and from anecdotal reports of high risk families (Arason *et al*, 1993). No significant association was found by Peto and colleagues (Peto J, Easton DF, Matthews FE, Ford D and Swerdlow AJ, unpublished) who found a relative risk for prostate cancer in the relatives of breast cancer patients of 1.1 based on 47 deaths. However, all the results of the systematic studies would be compatible with a relative risk for prostate cancer in first degree relatives of breast cancer patients of about 1.3. Other cancers for which a genetic association has been suggested from some studies include endometrium (Anderson *et al*, 1992; Tulinius *et al*, 1992; Peto J, Easton DF, Matthews FE, Ford D and Swerdlow AJ, unpublished), larynx (Peto J, Easton DF, Matthews FE, Ford D and Swerdlow AJ, unpublished), thyroid (Ron *et al*, 1984; Peto J, Easton DF, Matthews FE, Ford D and Swerdlow AJ, unpublished) and lung (Anderson *et al*, 1992).

BREAST-OVARIAN CANCER FAMILIES AND THE *BRCA1* GENE

Linkage to Chromosome 17q

The first convincing localization of a breast cancer susceptibility gene by genetic linkage was obtained by Hall *et al* (1990). They found significant evidence of linkage between breast cancer and the highly polymorphic marker D17S74 on chromosome 17q21 in 23 multiple case breast cancer families. Overall, the maximum LOD score in these families was 2.35 at a recombination fraction of 0.20. However, positive evidence of linkage appeared to be confined to those families with a mean age of onset of less than 46 years (LOD score 5.98 at recombination fraction 0.001). Families with older onset cases either showed evidence against linkage or were uninformative for linkage, depending on the genetic model used (Margaritte *et al*, 1992).

Confirmation of linkage to 17q21 was provided by Narod *et al* (1991) who obtained a LOD score of 2.20 at a recombination fraction of 0.20 in five breast-ovarian cancer families. This study also found significant evidence of genetic heterogeneity, with linkage apparently restricted to three of the five families tested. This cancer predisposing locus is now known as *BRCA1* (Solomon and Ledbetter, 1991).

Following these two publications and some conflicting unpublished results, an international linkage consortium, including virtually all groups conducting breast cancer linkage worldwide, was established to evaluate the linkage evidence on 17q in breast and breast-ovarian cancer families. The consortium analysed linkage data on six genetic markers on chromosome 17q in 214 families from 13 research groups (Easton *et al*, 1993) and was able to demonstrate overwhelming evidence for linkage of breast and ovarian cancer to 17q. Furthermore, this study was able to localize more precisely the *BRCA1* gene, to evaluate the extent of genetic heterogeneity and the characteristics of linked families and to estimate the penetrance of *BRCA1*.

Localization of *BRCA1*

Multipoint linkage analysis in the consortium data set was able to localize the position of *BRCA1* to an interval bounded by the markers D17S588 and D17S250. This interval has a genetic length of approximately 8 cM in males and 18 cM in females.

More recent typing of other markers in informative recombinants in linked families has substantially narrowed the region in which *BRCA1* must lie. Recombinant events have demonstrated the gene to be below *RARA* (Simard *et al*, 1993), D17S800 (Kelsell *et al*, 1993), D17S702 (Smith S, Ponder BAJ and Easton DF, personal communication) and D17S776 (Goldgar *et al*, in press a). It is unclear at this stage, however, which of these is the best proximal flanking marker. On the distal side, several groups have demonstrated that the *BRCA1* gene lies proximal to D17S579 (Bowcock *et al*, 1993; Chamberlain *et al*, 1993). *BRCA1* has also been reported to lie proximal to D17S78 (p131;

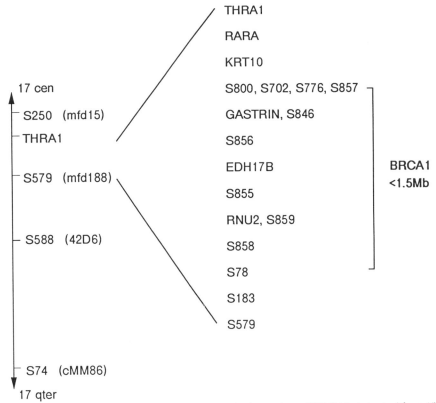

Fig. 1. Genetic map of chromosome 17q21, in the region of *BRCA1*. Adapted from King *et al* (1993)

Simard *et al*, 1993) and D17S183 (Bowcock *et al*, 1993) which lie proximal to D17S579. These results localize *BRCA1* to an interval of at most 1.5 Mb, assuming of course that all linked families are due to mutations in the same gene (Fig. 1).

Most of the known potential candidate genes for *BRCA1* in the region 17q12-q21 have now been excluded by linkage. Of the known genes that remain in the critical region, the best candidate is arguably the 17β oestradiol dehydrogenase gene *EDH17B2*. The 17β oestradiol dehydrogenase enzyme catalyses conversion between the weak oestrogen oestrone and the more potent oestradiol. This makes the gene a promising candidate for a breast cancer susceptibility gene (less so for ovarian cancer), since levels of circulating oestrogens are known to play a crucial part in breast cancer development, and oestradiol levels have been shown to be higher in breast cancers than in the normal breast (McNeill *et al*, 1986). However, Simard *et al* (1993) have sequenced the entire *EDH17B2* gene, including all the introns and over 800 bases upstream of the first exon, in four affected individuals from different linked breast-ovarian cancer families. No sequence abnormalities were detected, other than previously described polymorphisms. A similar result has been noted by Kelsell *et al* (1993) who sequenced the coding region of

EDH17B2 in three affected members of a large breast-ovarian cancer family linked to *BRCA1* and found no mutations. It is therefore unlikely that *EDH17B2* is *BRCA1*. (There is also a second gene, *EDH17B1*, within 13 kb of and strongly homologous to *EDH17B2*, which is probably a pseudogene; Kelsell *et al* [1993] did not detect any mutations in this gene either.) None of the other known genes in the candidate region appear to be good candidates, but there may of course be several dozen genes in the interval still to be identified.

Genetic Heterogeneity

A clear difference emerged in the consortium study between breast-ovarian cancer families (defined as those containing at least one ovarian cancer in addition to breast cancer cases) and those segregating breast cancer alone (see Table 1). In the multipoint heterogeneity analysis, the estimated proportion of linked breast-ovarian cancer families was 1.0, with a lower 95% confidence limit of 0.79. By contrast, the families segregating breast cancer alone showed clear evidence of heterogeneity, the estimated proportion of linked families being 0.45 with confidence limits of 0.25–0.66.

There was a suggestion in the consortium study that the proportion of linked families was higher in those families with a large number of breast cancer cases (see Table 1). In particular, there was little or no evidence of linkage among families with only two or three cases of breast cancer under age 60. There was also some confirmation of the "age at onset" effect suggested by Hall *et al* (1990). Only an estimated 67% of the families with an average age at onset of under 45 years were linked, but the proportion is lower among families with a higher average age at onset (see Table 1). The obvious interpretation of these results is that *BRCA1* mutations confer a high penetrance (see below) and that in families with only two or three cases or with higher average age at onset, the cases are more likely to be due to other genes with lower penetrance.

The proportion of "breast-ovarian" cancer families due to *BRCA1* is almost certainly not 100%, since a number of families have now been reported in which one of the affected individuals does not share the putative disease chromosome. One of the most convincing examples of an unlinked breast-ovarian cancer family was reported by Goldgar *et al* (in press b). This family contains six cases of female breast cancer diagnosed under age 50, one case of male breast cancer and four cases of ovarian cancer. In this family, at least three affected individuals are inconsistent with linkage. Unfortunately, it is not yet possible to provide a more accurate estimate of the true proportion of linked breast-ovarian cancer families including these apparently unlinked families, since the total number of families that have now been studied is uncertain.

To date, no breast cancer families containing male breast cancer cases are linked to *BRCA1*, and some families have shown clear evidence against linkage (eg Hall *et al*, 1990)

TABLE 1. Multipoint linkage analysis of breast and ovarian cancer to chromosome 17q markers, allowing for heterogeneity, and estimated proportions of linked families of different types (from Easton *et al* 1993)[a]

Group (number of families)	LOD score	Proportion linked
Breast-ovary (57)	20.79	1.00
Breast only (153)[b]	6.01	0.45
Average age of diagnosis		
<45 (54)	6.56	0.67
45–54 (63)	0.40	0.19
≥55 (36)	0.08	0.38
No. of cases diagnosed		
before age 45 years		
two or fewer (110)	1.46	0.44
three or four (36)	1.89	0.39
five or more (7)	2.88	0.72
before age 60 years		
three or fewer (98)	0.36	0.26
four or five (38)	3.29	0.60
six or more (17)	2.72	0.45

[a]Based on a multipoint analysis of D17S250, D17S588 and the disease. All estimates are at the maximum likelihood position of *BRCA1*, 9 cM proximal to D17S588 on the female map
[b]Four families with male breast cancer cases were excluded

Cancer Risks Associated with *BRCA1*

From the point of view of genetic counselling, it is important to be able to provide reliable estimates of the age specific risks of breast and ovarian cancer in *BRCA1* mutation carriers. Once the *BRCA1* gene has been identified, it will be possible to obtain these estimates from population based studies of gene carriers, but at present, the only source of data is from linked families. Such families are not ideal for estimating penetrance, because they have been selected for the occurrence of multiple cases of breast and ovarian cancer, and this ascertainment must be allowed for in the analysis. Easton *et al* (1993) overcame the problem of ascertainment by maximizing the LOD score over all possible penetrance functions. This gave an estimated penetrance of breast or ovarian cancer in female carriers of 59% by age 50 and 82% by age 70.

A rough estimate of the disease specific risks can be obtained by dividing up the overall estimated incidence by the observed age specific proportions of breast and ovarian cancer. On the basis of this analysis, the cumulative risk of breast cancer is estimated to be 49% by age 50 and 71% by age 70, and the estimated cumulative risk of ovarian cancer is 16% by age 50 and 42% by age 70.

As one would have predicted from the segregation analyses, the pattern of age specific breast cancer risks in gene carriers is very different from that in the general population. The incidence of breast cancer in gene carriers below age 30 is estimated to be about 100-fold greater than the incidence in the general population, but this ratio falls to only tenfold in the 60–69 years age group. By contrast, the relative risk for ovarian cancer in gene carriers compared with the general population declines much less markedly with age (Easton DF, Ford D, Bishop DT and Breast Cancer Linkage Consortium, unpublished).

The above results implicitly assume that the risks of breast and ovarian cancer are homogeneous across families. In fact, there is clear evidence that the risks differ substantially between families. Some of the large linked families contain no cases of ovarian cancer (eg family 1901 in Goldgar *et al* [1993], which contains ten breast cancers and no ovarian cancers), whereas other families contain more ovarian cancers than breast cancers (eg the family reported by Milner *et al* [1993], which contains three breast cancers and eight ovarian cancers). Although some of this observed heterogeneity must be the result of different ascertainment patterns in different families (some families being ascertained on the basis of multiple cases of breast cancer and others on the basis of multiple cases of ovarian cancer), it seems unlikely that this could explain the entire effect. Easton and colleagues have shown that the observed patterns of disease risks are much better explained by a model with two dif-

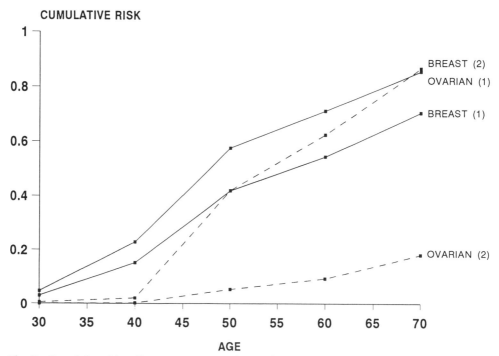

Fig. 2. Cumulative risks of breast cancer (continuous lines) and ovarian cancer (dashed lines) in *BRCA1* mutation carriers, assuming allelic heterogeneity with two susceptibility alleles indicated by (1) (high ovarian cancer risk) and (2) (moderate ovarian cancer risk)

ferent *BRCA1* susceptibility alleles, one conferring an estimated breast cancer risk of 71% by age 70 and an ovarian cancer risk of 87% and the other conferring a breast cancer risk of 86% by age 70 and an ovarian cancer risk of 18% (see Fig. 2) (Easton DF, Ford D, Bishop DT and Breast Cancer Linkage Consortium, unpublished). In this model, the first allele, conferring a high ovarian cancer risk, is estimated to account for 11% of the *BRCA1* mutations, and the second (low ovarian cancer risk) allele, the remaining 89%. Clearly, this model must be a simplification, but if this degree of allelic heterogeneity does exist, it could have an important bearing on counselling women in *BRCA1* families, particularly with regard to prophylactic oophorectomy. Once *BRCA1* has been identified, it should be possible to examine allelic heterogeneity directly by examining the types of mutation in families with different numbers of breast and ovarian cancers.

An alternative explanation for the observed differences in breast and ovarian cancer risks between different families would be that the risks in gene carriers are substantially modified by other factors, either genetic or environmental, which vary between families. This possibility cannot be ruled out, although the fact that some of the apparently high and low risk ovarian cancer pedigrees extend across many nuclear families (ie the risks appear to "breed true") would argue in favour of an effect of allelic variation.

Gene Frequency of *BRCA1*

It is not possible to estimate the gene frequency of *BRCA1*, or its contribution to breast cancer incidence, directly from the genetic linkage studies. However, reasonable estimates may be obtained by combining the penetrance estimates for *BRCA1* with the results of population based genetic epidemiological studies.

The critical observation is the excess risk of ovarian cancer in the relatives of breast cancer patients, or vice versa. Since the linkage studies suggest that nearly all high risk breast-ovarian cancer families are the result of *BRCA1*, a reasonable estimate of the gene frequency can be obtained by assuming that the excess risk of ovarian cancer in relatives of breast cancer patients is entirely accounted for by *BRCA1*.

This analysis has been performed on a systematic study of cancer mortality in the first degree relatives of 3334 breast cancer cases (Peto J, Easton DF, Matthews FE, Ford D, Swerdlow AJ, unpublished). In this study, there were 47 ovarian cancer deaths under age 70 in the first degree relatives of breast cancer patients compared with 32.1 expected at national rates—that is, an excess of 15 deaths. If this excess were entirely due to *BRCA1*, and given the penetrance estimates for *BRCA1* in Fig. 2 (ie allowing for allelic heterogeneity), the overall gene frequency of *BRCA1* can be estimated to be .0007 (Ford D, Easton DF and Peto J, unpublished). Confirmation of this result is obtained by considering the excess breast cancer mortality in a similar study of the relatives of 1203 ovarian cancer patients (Easton DF, Matthews FE, Ford D, Swerdlow AJ and Peto J, unpublished). In this study, there were 44 breast cancer deaths under age 70 compared with 31.8 expected at national rates. The same method applied to this study would also predict a gene frequency of .0007.

This gene frequency estimate is only about one fifth of the estimate of .0033 obtained in the segregation analysis of the CASH data set by Claus *et al* (1991). This may seem somewhat surprising, given that the consortium study estimated that over half of the families studied were linked to *BRCA1*. This discrepancy can be explained by the fact that the estimated penetrance of *BRCA1* is higher than that estimated by the CASH study (which presumably represents some average of the risks of all susceptibility genes). The families studied for linkage are selected on the basis of a large number of breast (and ovarian) cancers. Such families are much more likely to be segregating a highly penetrant gene, such as *BRCA1*, than genes with lower penetrance. Therefore, *BRCA1* carriers would not be expected to be as frequent (as a proportion of all susceptible individuals) in the general population as in linkage families.

Contribution of *BRCA1* to Breast and Ovarian Cancer Incidence

On the basis of the gene frequency of .0007 and the age specific penetrances for *BRCA1* (and allowing for two mutations with different risks as above), the estimated proportions of breast cancer cases due to *BRCA1* would be: 8.2% below the age of 40, 4.0% between ages 40 and 49 and 1% over age 50. The corresponding estimates for ovarian cancer are: 5.6% below age 40, 4.2% between ages 40 and 49 and 1.8% over age 50.

Contribution of *BRCA1* to Familial Breast Cancer

The above model can also be used to estimate the contribution of *BRCA1* to the overall familial clustering of breast cancer. For example, if *BRCA1* were the only breast cancer susceptibility gene, the relative risk of breast cancer at age 45 to the first degree relative of a breast cancer case aged 45 due to *BRCA1* would be predicted to be estimated to be 1.48. (The familial relative risk in parents of affected individuals due to *BRCA1* is given by: $[p(\alpha f_1^2 + (1-\alpha)f_2^2) + (1-p)(p(\alpha f_1 + (1-\alpha)f_2) + (1-p)f_0]^2/[(1-q^2)(\alpha f_1 + (1-\alpha)f_2) + q^2 f_0]^2$, where $p\alpha$ and $p(1-A)$ are the frequencies of the two mutations, $q = 1-p$, and f_0, f_1 and f_2 are the disease risks in non-carriers and in the carriers of the two types of mutation.)

The corresponding prediction at age 35 would be 2.58. The observed relative risk in the CASH study for breast cancer in relatives between ages 40 and 49 of cases between ages 40 and 49 is 2.2, and for cases under age 40 of relatives under age 40, the risk was 5.3 (derived from Claus, 1988). Thus, *BRCA1* is estimated to account for about 34% of the observed excess familial risk below age 40, and for about 40% between 40 and 49.

THE LI-FRAUMENI SYNDROME AND THE *TP53* GENE

Breast cancer is an important feature of the Li-Fraumeni syndrome, a rare autosomal dominant cancer syndrome involving childhood sarcomas, early onset breast cancer, brain tumours and a number of other cancers (Li *et al*, 1988). Some Li-Fraumeni families are now known to have germline mutations in the *TP53* gene (Malkin *et al*, 1990; Srivastavas *et al*, 1990). The proportion of Li-Fraumeni families with *TP53* mutations is not precisely known but appears to be 50% or more (Li FP, personal communication).

Germline *TP53* mutations seem to account for only a very small proportion of breast cancer incidence. Sidransky *et al* (1992) found one germline mutation in 126 unselected breast cancer cases under age 40 at diagnosis. Borresen *et al* (1992) found one germline mutation in 167 breast cancer patients unselected for age (the case was age 41) and a further case among 40 cases diagnosed below age 40. All three of the cases in which a germline mutation was identified were discovered to have a strong family history of cancer compatible with the Li-Fraumeni syndrome.

The contribution of *TP53* (or other "Li-Fraumeni genes") to familial breast cancer has not been directly assessed and is difficult to estimate indirectly because the age and site specific cancer risks in *TP53* mutation carriers are not precisely known. The recent analysis by Lustbader *et al* (1992) suggested an overall cancer risk of about 30% by age 30 and 70% by age 50 in Li-Fraumeni families, although the latter estimate is somewhat lower than previous estimates (Williams and Strong, 1985) and is an average for male and female carriers. The study by Li *et al* (1988) suggests that breast cancer accounts for about three quarters of the cancers occurring between ages 30 and 50. Taken together, these studies suggest that between 30% and 60% of female carriers will become affected with breast cancer between the ages of 30 and 50. Assuming that half of this risk occurs between ages 30 and 40 and that 1% of breast cancer cases between ages 30 and 40 are the result of a germline *TP53* mutation, the population gene frequency can be estimated very crudely as between 5×10^{-5} and 10^{-4}. The familial relative risk in the group aged 30–40 caused by *TP53* would then be between about 1.2 and 1.5—that is, 5–12% of the excess. The corresponding estimates for the group aged 40–49 would be 1.02–1.04, or 2–4% of the excess.

BREAST CANCER AND ATAXIA-TELANGIECTASIA

It is now well established that relatives of individuals affected with ataxia-telangiectasia (AT) have an excess risk of cancer in general, and breast cancer in particular (Swift *et al*, 1991). From the six published studies, Easton (1992) has estimated the relative risk of breast cancer in AT heterozygotes to be 7.8, with 95% confidence limits of 5.2 to 11.9. This breast cancer risk is substantially lower than that conferred by the *BRCA1* gene or the *TP53* gene but is nevertheless of some significance because AT heterozygotes may be relatively numerous in the population.

In contrast with *BRCA1* or *TP53,* there is little suggestion that the breast cancer risk associated with AT heterozygosity is age dependent. This cannot yet be stated with certainty, since most of the data on breast cancer risks in AT heterozygotes is based on relatively young cases. However, in the most recent study by Swift *et al* (1991), the relative risk for breast cancer in female relatives of breast cancer cases was about fourfold both above and below age 50. (This relative risk is, of course, lower than the estimated risk to heterozygotes because only a proportion of relatives are carriers.)

It is not yet possible to estimate precisely the proportion of breast cancer cases due to AT, or its contribution to familial clustering of the disease, since the *AT* gene has not been cloned and neither the breast cancer risk in AT heterozygotes nor their population frequency is known with certainty. However, it is instructive to consider what the plausible range of estimates might be. The population gene frequency for AT has been variously estimated as between 0.2% and 1%. Taking 0.5% as a "best guess" gene frequency, and a breast cancer relative risk of 8, about 7% of breast cancer cases would be attributable to AT. On the basis of these estimates, the familial relative risk of breast cancer caused by AT alone to the sister of an affected individual would be about 1.2. Taking, as a comparison, the relative risk of 2.58 observed in relatives under age 50 of cases under age 50 in the CASH study, this would represent about 13% of the observed familial risk. On the basis of the lowest plausible estimates, namely a breast cancer relative risk of 5 in AT heterozygotes and a gene frequency of .002, only about 2% of breast cancer cases would be due to AT, and the familial relative risk due to AT would be only 1.03 (about 1.5% of familial risk at young ages). At the other extreme, with a relative risk of 12 and a gene frequency of .01, about 18% of cases would be due to AT and the familial relative risk due to AT would be 1.8 (about 50% of the overall familial risk). The contribution of AT heterozygotes to breast cancer incidence in general and to familial breast cancer could therefore turn out to be relatively trivial, or quite marked.

There is, however, some evidence from linkage studies to suggest that the contribution of AT to familial breast cancer is likely to be minor. The gene (or genes) responsible for the complementation groups involved in most AT families has been localized to chromosome 11q22–q23 by genetic linkage studies (Gatti *et al,* 1988; Foroud *et al,* 1991). Wooster *et al* (1993) have conducted linkage studies in breast cancer families not linked to *BRCA1* using markers tightly linked to the *AT* locus and failed to find any evidence of linkage.

MALE BREAST CANCER

There is clear evidence from both anecdotal reports of families and systematic studies that breast cancer in men is more common in the relatives of breast cancer patients, both male and female, than in the general population. In the largest case-control study of male breast cancer published to date, Rosenblatt *et al* (1991) found a relative risk for breast cancer of 2.3 to female first degree relatives and 6.1 (based on seven cases and one control) to male first degree relatives of male breast cancer patients. In this study, the relative risks for female breast cancer appeared to increase with decreasing age of the index case and age of the relative. In other words, susceptibility to male breast cancer appears to follow a pattern similar to that of female breast cancer, and at least one of the genes conferring this susceptibility must cause the disease in both sexes.

Only one gene has been clearly associated with inherited predisposition to male breast cancer. Wooster *et al* (1992) have reported a family in which two brothers were affected with male breast cancer. In addition, both cases had hypospadias and undescended testes, features suggestive of androgen insufficiency. These cases have been shown to possess a germline mutation in the DNA binding domain of the androgen receptor gene on Xq11.2–q12. Another germline androgen receptor mutation in a patient with partial androgen insensitivity and male breast cancer has recently been reported Lobaccaro *et al* (1993). However, there is no evidence of linkage to the androgen receptor in (female) breast cancer families with or without male cases (Wooster R, Ford D, Easton DF and Stratton MR, personal communication), and indeed, the androgen receptor can be clearly excluded as the cause of certain families with multiple cases of male breast cancer by the observation of father to son inheritance (eg family 16 in Hall *et al*, 1990). Since male breast cancer does not appear to associated with either *BRCA1* or *TP53* germline mutations, all the evidence suggests that the major loci determining susceptibility to male breast cancer remain to be identified.

OTHER LINKAGE STUDIES

There is no clear evidence yet of the location of the other genes responsible for familial breast cancer. There have been reports of linkage in breast cancer families to markers on chromosome 16q (Callen *et al*, 1992) and, in one family, to the oestrogen receptor on chromosome 6q (Zuppan *et al*, 1991), but neither of these reports has yet been confirmed by other studies. There have also been a number of negative linkage reports (eg Hall *et al*, 1989; Bowcock *et al*, 1990); however, these may now have to be re-evaluated in light of the linkage to *BRCA1*.

DISCUSSION

Our understanding of inherited susceptibility to breast cancer has been transformed over the past few years, most importantly by the localization of *BRCA1*. From a genetic counselling standpoint, it is now possible to identify women in families linked to *BRCA1* and to counsel them on the basis of linkage data and reasonably precise estimates of cancer risk. It is also possible to identify high risk families not linked to *BRCA1*, and studies are now under way to localize the genes responsible for these families. Clearly, many questions about *BRCA1* remain, some of which will only be answered when the gene has been identified and sequenced. It will then be possible to provide direct estimates of the proportion of breast cancers due to *BRCA1*, and to examine allelic heterogeneity, referred to above. More importantly, it will then be possible to begin investigating the biology of *BRCA1* and its role in the cause of inherited (and perhaps also sporadic) breast and ovarian cancer. There are also some outstanding epidemiological questions relating to *BRCA1* that are being addressed by international collaborative studies being conducted by the Breast Cancer Linkage Consortium. One question under investigation is whether or not *BRCA1* confers a risk of any cancers other than breast or ovarian cancer. Another question is whether any environmental factors modify the risk of breast and ovarian cancer in *BRCA1* carriers. For example, there is already a suggestion that the risk of breast cancer at young ages associated with long term use of oral contraceptives is more pronounced in women with a family history of the disease (UK National Case–Control Study Group, 1990). If oral contraceptives were shown to have a large effect on breast cancer risk in *BRCA1* carriers, then this might explain some of the apparent secular increase in the ratio of the risk of breast cancer to ovarian cancer (for which oral contraceptives are protective) that has been noted anecdotally (Narod *et al*, 1993).

Table 2 summarizes the estimated cumulative risks of breast cancer, and of all cancers combined, due to *BRCA1, TP53* or *AT* mutations, based on the results discussed in this paper. Clearly, there is still considerable uncertainty in many of these estimates; we have not included confidence intervals since in most cases, these would be difficult to estimate. Based on the confidence limits obtained by Easton (1992), the estimates for *AT* should be accurate to within a factor of 2 in either direction. For *TP53* and *BRCA1*, the estimates are probably accurate to within about 10%, although some caution is required given that these estimates have been obtained somewhat indirectly from studies in high risk families, estimates based on prospective follow-up of gene carriers or other population based studies not being available. Moreover, although it is clear that the penetrance is high in these families, there remains the possibility (particularly for *BRCA1*) of mutations conferring a lower risk.

In Table 3, we summarize some estimates of the proportion of breast cancer cases, and of affected sister (or parent-offspring) pairs, of different ages that may be due to *BRCA1, TP53* or *AT* mutations. We emphasize that none of the estimates in Table 3, apart from the proportion of young cases due to *TP53* mutations, have been directly estimated; these are extrapolated from other estimates of penetrance, gene frequency and linkage results as described above, and therefore carry considerable uncertainty. Better estimates should be obtained from population based studies once the *BRCA1* and *AT* genes in particular have been cloned. Nevertheless, these estimates suggest that about

TABLE 2. Estimated cumulative risks of breast cancer, and of all cancers, to female carriers of germline *BRCA1*, *TP53* and *AT* mutations

Gene	Cumulative risk (%) of breast cancer by age[a]				Cumulative risk (%) of any cancer by age			
	40	50	60	70	40	50	60	70
BRCA1[b]	17	45	55	59	23	58	76	85
TP53[c]	30	40	45	–	65	80	90	–
AT[d]	3	11	20	30	5	15	30	46
CASH model	14	37	54	65	–	–	–	–

[a]Risk of breast cancer occurring as the first cancer only, allowing for the possibility that other cancers may occur first. Cumulative risks of breast cancer by the stated age in the absence of any other cancers would be higher, particularly for *TP53* and *BRCA1*. Risks of any breast cancer (including a second malignancy) would also be slightly higher
[b]From Easton DF, Ford D, Bishop DT and Breast Cancer Linkage Consortium (unpublished). Estimates assuming no allelic heterogeneity, and no risk from cancers other than breast or ovary
[c]Crude estimates based on Williams and Strong (1985), Li *et al* (1988) and Garber *et al* (1991)
[d]Assuming a relative risk of 8 for breast cancer and 2 for other cancers (which gives an overall relative risk for all cancers of about 4 below age 70, approximately the value observed by Swift *et al*, 1991)

half the familial clustering of early onset breast cancer can be explained by known genes, with *BRCA1* making by far the largest contribution. At this stage, it is unclear what genetic mechanisms underlie the familial effects not explained by known loci. The evidence from some anecdotal families suggests that some familial clustering will be explained by autosomal dominant gene(s) with high penetrance. However, it is also possible that genes with lower penetrance (as in the case of *AT*) may make an important contribution. Thus, further segregation analyses of population based studies such as the CASH study, allowing for the known effects of *BRCA1*, could be useful in defining the correct genetic model.

TABLE 3. Estimated proportion of cases, and of affected sister pairs, due to different predisposing genes[a]

Gene	Cases (%) aged			Sister pairs (%) aged		
	35	45	55	35	45	55
BRCA1	8	4	1	30	22	2
TP53	1	?	?	6	1	–
AT	7	7	6	4	7	9
Other		?		41	25	21
No inherited cause		?		19	45	68
CASH model	23	11	7	80	50	30

[a]The proportions of sibling pairs due to each gene have been calculated on the assumption that the different genes act additively. The proportions are given by $(R_{s1}-1)/R_s$, where R_s is the observed relative risk to the sibling of an affected individual, and R_{s1} is the relative risk that would be predicted if that gene were the only familial effect. (This assumes that all possible sister pairs are counted, ie sibships with more than two affected cases are counted multiple times, or alternatively that each family has just two sisters; the probabilities that a sibship with 2 out of n affected sisters, where n>2, are due to any of the genes would be lower)

It should be possible to localize further "high penetrance" genes by genetic linkage studies in multiple case families, assuming that only a limited number of genes are involved. Lower penetrance genes could, however, prove difficult to detect by linkage, as clearly shown in the case of *AT*. For example, the figures in Table 3 suggest that any remaining loci cause a relative risk of less than 2 in siblings; such an effect would be too weak to be detected by linkage studies in affected sister pairs (even if those families due to *BRCA1* could be eliminated from the analysis by mutation testing). Progress in finding these genes, if they exist, will probably be through associated phenotypic markers such as radiosensitivity (Scott and Bryant, 1992), proliferative breast disease (Skolnick *et al,* 1990) or abnormal *TP53* staining (Barnes *et al,* 1992), or by direct association studies in candidate genes.

SUMMARY

Four genes are now known to be responsible for inherited susceptibility to breast cancer: the *BRCA1* gene on chromosome 17q21, the ataxia-telangiectasia (*AT*) gene (11q22–q23), the *TP53* gene (17p13.1) and the androgen receptor (*AR*) (Xq11.2–q12). These genes, however, differ dramatically in terms of the risk of breast cancer that they confer, the proportion of breast cancer incidence that they account for and the other cancers and other phenotypes with which they are associated.

Genetic linkage studies have shown that some high risk breast cancer families, particularly those where breast cancer occurs in association with ovarian cancer, are due to a gene on chromosome 17q known as *BRCA1*. The *BRCA1* gene is estimated to confer a breast cancer risk of about 70% by age 70, and may account for about 2% of overall breast cancer incidence, although a higher proportion of younger cases.

Germline mutations in the *TP53* gene are responsible for a high proportion of Li-Fraumeni families, in which breast cancer occurs in association with childhood sarcomas and other cancers. In such families, the risk of breast cancer is over 50% by age 50, and the risk of all cancers is nearly 100%; germline *TP53* mutations are, however, probably responsible for much less than 1% of all breast cancer. By contrast, heterozygotes for the *AT* gene carry a much more moderate risk of breast cancer. This gene, however, is much more common in the population and may account for 7% or more of breast cancer incidence. Finally, germline mutations in the androgen receptor are known to cause male breast cancer, but this has only been demonstrated in two families.

Evidence from linkage and population based studies suggests that these genes may account for about one half of the observed familial clustering of breast cancer; other breast cancer susceptibility genes therefore remain to be identified.

References

Adami HO, Hansen H, Jung B and Rimsten A (1980) Familiality in breast cancer: a case-control study in a Swedish population. *British Journal of Cancer* **42** 71–77

Anderson K, Easton DF, Matthews FE and Peto J (1992) Cancer mortality in the first degree relatives of young breast cancer patients. *British Journal of Cancer* **66** 599–602

Arason A, Barkadottir RB and Egilsson V (1993) Linkage analysis of chromosome 17q markers and breast-ovarian cancer in Icelandic families, and possible relationship to prostatic cancer. *American Journal of Human Genetics* **52** 711–717

Barnes DM, Hanby AM, Gillett CE *et al* (1992) Abnormal expression of wild type p53 protein in normal cells of a cancer family patient. *Lancet* **340** 259–263

Bernstein JL, Thompson WD, Risch N and Holford TR (1992) The genetic epidemiology of second primary breast cancer. *American Journal of Epidemiology* **136** 937–948

Birch JM, Hartley AL, Marsden HB, Harris M and Swindell R (1984) Excess risk of breast cancer in the mothers of children with soft-tissue sarcomas. *British Journal of Cancer* **49** 325–331

Bishop DT, Cannon-Albright L, McLellan T, Gardner EJ and Skolnick MH (1988) Segregation and linkage analysis of nine Utah breast cancer pedigrees. *Genetic Epidemiology* **5** 151–169

Borresen AL, Andersen TI, Garber J *et al* (1992) Screening for germline *TP53* mutations in breast cancer patients. *Cancer Research* **52** 3234–3236

Bowcock AM, Hall JM, Hebert JM and King M-C (1990) Exclusion of the retinoblastoma gene and chromosome 13q as the site of a primary lesion for human breast cancer. *American Journal of Human Genetics* **46** 12–17

Bowcock AM, Anderson LA, Friedman LS *et al* (1993) THRA1 and D17S183 flank an interval of <4cM for the breast-ovarian cancer gene (*BRCA1*) on chromosome 17q21. *American Journal of Human Genetics* **52** 718–722

Callen DF, Hildebrand CE and Reeders S (1992) Report of the 2nd international workshop on human chromosome 16 mapping. *Cytogenetics and Cell Genetics* **60** 158–167

Cannon L, Bishop DT, Skolnick M, Hunt S, Lyon JL and Smart CR (1982) Genetic epidemiology of prostate cancer in the Utah Mormon genealogy. *Cancer Surveys* **1** 47–69

Chamberlain JS, Boenhke M, Frank TS *et al* (1993) *BRCA1* maps proximal to D17S579 on chromosome 17q21 by genetic analysis. *American Journal of Human Genetics* **52** 792–798

Claus EB (1988) Age at onset and the inheritance of breast cancer. PhD dissertation, Yale University

Claus EB, Risch N and Thompson WD (1990a) Age of onset as an indicator of familial risk of breast cancer. *American Journal of Epidemiology* **131** 961–972

Claus EB, Risch N and Thompson WD (1990b) Using age of onset to distinguish between subforms of breast cancer. *Annals of Human Genetics* **54** 169–77

Claus EB, Risch N and Thompson WD (1991) Genetic analysis of breast cancer in the cancer and steroid hormone study. *American Journal of Human Genetics* **48** 232–241

Claus EB, Schildkraut JM, Thompson WD and Risch N An analysis of the genetic relationship between breast and ovarian cancer. *American Journal of Human Genetics* (in press)

Easton DF (1992) Some problems in the genetic epidemiology of cancer. PhD thesis, University of London

Easton DF, Bishop DT, Ford D, Crockford GP and the Breast Cancer Linkage Consortium (1993) Genetic linkage analysis in familial breast and ovarian cancer: results from 214 families. *American Journal of Human Genetics* **52** 678–701

Foroud T, Wei S, Ziv Y *et al* (1991) Localisation of an ataxia-telangiectasia locus to a 3cM interval on chromosome 11q22-q23: linkage analysis of 111 families by an international consortium. *American Journal of Human Genetics* **49** 1263–1279

Garber JE, Goldstein AM, Kantor AS, Dreyfus MG, Fraumeni JF Jnr and Li FP (1991) Follow-up study of twenty-four families with Li-Fraumeni Syndrome. *Cancer Research* **51** 6094–6097

Gardner EJ and Stephens FE (1950) Breast cancer in one family group. *American Journal of Human Genetics* **2** 30–40

Gatti RA, Berkel I, Boder E *et al* (1988) Localisation of an ataxia-telangiectasia gene to chromosome 11q22-23. *Nature* **336** 577–580

Goldgar DE, Cannon-Albright LA, Oliphent A *et al* (1993) Chromosome 17q linkage studies in 18 Utah breast cancer kindreds. *American Journal of Human Genetics* **52** 743–748

Goldgar DE, Fields P, Lewis CM *et al* A large kindred with 17q-linked breast and ovarian cancer: genetic, phenotypic and genealogical analysis. *Journal of the National Cancer Institute* (in press a)

Goldgar DE, Rowe K, Cannon-Albright L, McDonald M, Lewis CM and Skolnick M Genetic epidemiology of ovarian cancer in Utah, In: Sharp F, Mason WP, Berek JS and Blackett AD (eds). *Ovarian Cancer 3*, Chapman and Hall, London (in press b)

Hall JM, Zuppan PJ, Anderson LA, Huey B, Carter C and King M-C (1989) Oncogenes and human breast cancer. *American Journal of Human Genetics* **44** 577–584

Hall JM, Lee MK, Morrow J *et al* (1990) Linkage analysis of early onset familial breast cancer to chromosome 17q21. *Science* **250** 1684–1689

Hartley AL, Birch JM, Marsden HB and Harris M (1986) Breast cancer risk in mothers of children with osteosarcoma and chondrosarcoma. *British Journal of Cancer* **54** 819–823

Iselius L, Slack J, Littler M and Morton NE (1991) Genetic epidemiology of breast cancer in Britain. *Annals of Human Genetics* **55** 151–159

Kelsell DP, Black DM, Bishop DT, Spurr NK (1993) Genetic analysis of the BRCA1 region in a large breast/ovarian family: refinement of the minimal region containing BRCA1. *Human Molecular Genetics* **2** 1823–1828

King M-C, Rowell S and Love SM (1993) Inherited breast and ovarian cancer: what are the risks? what are the choices? *Journal of the American Medical Association* **269** 1975–1980

Li FP, Fraumeni JF Jr, Mulvihill JJ *et al* (1988) A cancer family syndrome in twenty-four kindreds. *Cancer Research* **48** 5368–5362

Lobaccaro J-M, Lumbroso S, Bedon C *et al* (1993) Androgen receptor mutation in male breast cancer. *Human Molecular Genetics* **2** 1799–1802

Lustbader ED, Williams WR, Bondy ML, Strom S and Strong LC (1992) Segregation analysis of cancer in families of childhood soft-tissue sarcoma patients. *American Journal of Human Genetics* **51** 344–356

Lynch HT, Harris RE, Guirgis HA *et al* (1978) Familial association of breast/ovarian cancer. *Cancer* **41** 1543–1549

Malkin D, Li FP, Strong LC *et al* (1990) Germline p53 mutations in a familial syndrome of breast cancer, sarcomas and other neoplasms. *Science* **250** 1233–1238

Margaritte P, Bonaiti-Pellie C and King M-C and Clerget-Darpoux F (1992) Linkage of familial breast cancer may not be restricted to early onset disease. *American Journal of Human Genetics* **50** 515–519

McNeill M, Reed MJ, Beranek PA *et al* (1986) A comparison of the in-vivo uptake and metabolism of H-3 estrone and H-3-estradiol by normal breast and breast-tumor tissues in postmenopausal women. *International Journal of Cancer* **38** 193–196

Narod SA, Feunteun J, Lynch HT *et al* (1991) Familial breast-ovarian cancer locus on chromosome 17q12-23. *Lancet* **338** 82–83

Narod SA, Lynch H, Conway T, Watson P, Feunteun J and Lenoir G (1993) Increasing incidence of breast cancer in family with *BRCA1* mutation. *Lancet* **341** 1101–1102

Newman B, Austin MA, Lee M and King M-C (1988) Inheritance of human breast cancer: evidence for autosomal dominant transmission in high risk families. *Proceedings of the National Academy of Sciences of the USA* **85** 3044–3048

Ottman R, Pike MC, King M-C, Casagrande JT and Henderson BE (1986) Familial breast cancer in a population based series. *American Journal of Epidemiology* **123** 15–21

Rosenblatt KA, Thomas DB, McTieman A *et al* (1991) Breast cancer in men: aspects of familial aggregation. *Journal of the National Cancer Institute* **83** 849–853

Schildkraut JM, Risch N and Thompson WD (1989) Evaluating the genetic association among ovarian, breast and endometrial cancer: evidence for a breast-ovarian relationship. *American Journal of Human Genetics* **45** 521–529

Scott D and Bryant PE (1992) Second L.H. Gray Workshop report. *International Journal of*

Radiation Biology **61** 293–297

Sidransky D, Tokino T, Helzlsouer K *et al* (1992) Inherited p53 mutations in breast cancer. *Cancer Research* **52** 2984–2986

Simard J, Feunteun J, Lenoir G *et al* (1993) Genetic mapping of the breast-ovarian cancer syndrome to a small interval on chromosome 17q12-21: exclusion of candidate genes *EDH17B2* and *RARA. Human Molecular Genetics* **2** 1193–1199

Skolnick MH, Cannon-Albright LA, Goldgar DA *et al* (1990) Inheritance of proliferative breast disease in breast cancer kindreds. *Science* **250** 1715–1720

Solomon E and Ledbetter DH (1991) Report of the Committee on the Genetic Constitution of Chromosome 17. *Cytogenetics and Cell Genetics* **58** 686–738

Srivastavas S, Zou ZQ, Pirollo K, Blattner W and Chang EW (1990) Germline transmission of a mutated p53 gene in a cancer family with Li-Fraumeni syndrome. *Nature* **348** 747–749

Swift M, Morrell D, Massey RB and Chase CL (1991) Incidence of cancer in 161 families affected with ataxia-telangiectasia. *New England Journal of Medicine* **325** 1831–1836

Tulinius H, Egilsson V, Olafsdottir GH and Sigvaldson H (1992) Risk of prostate, ovarian, and endometrial cancer among relatives of women with breast cancer. *British Medical Journal* **305** 855–857

UK National Case-Control Study Group (1990) Oral contraceptive use and breast cancer risk in young women: subgroup analyses. *Lancet* **335** 1507–1509

Williams WR and Anderson DE (1984) Genetic epidemiology of breast cancer: segregation analysis of 200 Danish pedigrees. *Genetic Epidemiology* **1** 7–20

Williams WR and Strong LC (1985) Genetic epidemiology of soft tissue sarcomas in children, In: Muller HR and Weber W (eds). *Familial Cancer, First International Research Conference*, pp 151–153, Karger, Basel

Wooster R, Mangion J, Eeles R *et al* (1992) A germline mutation in the androgen receptor in two brothers with breast cancer and Reifenstein syndrome. *Nature Genetics* **2** 132–134

Wooster R, Ford D, Mangion J *et al* (1993) Absence of linkage to the ataxia telangiectasia locus in familial breast cancer. *Human Genetics* **92** 91–94

Zuppan P, Hall JM, Lee MK, Ponglikitmongkol M and King M-C (1991) Possible linkage of the estrogen receptor gene to breast cancer in a family with late onset disease. *American Journal of Human Genetics* **48** 1065–1068

The authors are responsible for the accuracy of the references.

Histopathology: Old Principles and New Methods

JEFFREY T HOLT[1,2] • **ROY A JENSEN**[1,2] • **DAVID L PAGE**[1]

[1]*Departments of Pathology and* [2]*Cell Biology, Vanderbilt University School of Medicine, Nashville, Tennessee 37232*

INTRODUCTION

Breast cancer is a morphologically and genetically heterogeneous disease (Chen *et al*, 1992). Histopathology remains the benchmark and the only reliable means to diagnose breast cancer in either invasive or preinvasive stages and to identify the presence of metastatic disease. The development of breast cancer presumably involves multiple steps or stages in which the cells develop the ability to grow autonomously, become invasive, acquire a mass (angiogenesis) and metastasize (Foulds, 1957). Careful histological examination of breast biopsies has demonstrated intermediate stages that almost certainly have acquired some of these characteristics, but not others. Ductal carcinoma in situ (DCIS) is a lesion in which the cells resembling invasive cancers have grown to fill and distort the ducts and lobules but do not invade the stroma or show metastasis at presentation. This lesion can occur in at least two forms, comedo and non-comedo DCIS. Classically, comedo DCIS was a grossly palpable lesion that was considered "cancer" in the 19th and early 20th century, and larger examples progress to cancer in at least 50% of patients within 3 years without definitive therapy (Page *et al*, 1982; Ottesen *et al*, 1992). Small non-comedo DCIS lesions are detected by microscopic analysis of breast biopsies and are associated with a tenfold increased risk of invasive breast cancer, which corresponds to a 25–30% absolute risk of breast cancer within 15 years (Page *et al*, 1982; Ottesen *et al*, 1992; Ward *et al*, 1992). Widespread application of mammography for early detection has changed the relative incidence of comedo and non-comedo DCIS such that non-comedo DCIS now represents the predominant form of DCIS diagnosed in the USA (Page *et al*, 1982; Ottesen *et al*, 1992; Pierce *et al*, 1992). The strongest evidence implicating DCIS as a determinate precursor lesion is the observation that invasive cancers that develop in women with a history of DCIS tend to occur in the same region of the same breast in which DCIS was originally identified. The precursor lesions to DCIS are likely to be atypical ductal hyperplasia and proliferative disease without atypia which progress to breast cancer at lower rates but show increased risk when associated with a family history of breast cancer (Carter and Smith, 1977; Betsill *et al*, 1978; Page *et al*, 1978, 1982; Dupont and Page, 1985; Weed *et al*, 1990; Abendroth *et al*, 1991; Lawrence, 1991; Solin *et al*, 1991; Fentiman, 1992; London *et al*, 1992; Posner and Wolmark, 1992; Swain, 1992). This chapter describes the histological features that are used to diagnose invasive and preinvasive breast cancer and presents some strategies using histopathology and molecular probes as tools to study the epidemiological association of breast cancer progression from preinvasive to later stages, as well as predictive correlates of other hyperplastic lesions.

HISTOLOGICAL INDICATORS OF INCREASED BREAST CANCER RISK

Premalignant breast disease is characterized by an apparent morphological progression from atypical hyperplasia to carcinoma in situ (preinvasive cancer) to invasive cancer, which ultimately metastasizes, resulting in the death of the patient. Detailed epidemiological studies by our group and others have established that different morphological lesions have a likelihood of progressing to cancer at different rates, varying from atypical hyperplasia (low risk) to comedo ductal carcinoma in situ (which progresses to cancer in nearly 100% of patients) (Page *et al*, 1978, 1982, 1985; Page and Dupont, 1991; London *et al*, 1992). Family history is also an important risk factor in the development of breast cancer and increases the relative risk of these premalignant lesions (Dupont and Page, 1985; Dupont *et al*, 1989; London *et al*, 1992). Of particular interest is non-comedo carcinoma in situ, which is associated with an approximate tenfold increased relative risk of breast cancer compared to control groups (Betsill *et al*, 1978; Page *et al*, 1982; Ottesen *et al*, 1992). Two other observations besides this increased relative risk support the concept that DCIS is premalignant: (a) DCIS is frequently present in tissues adjacent to breast cancer (Ottesen *et al*, 1992; Schwartz *et al*, 1992) and (b) as previously mentioned, invasive breast cancers in women with DCIS generally occur in the same region of the same breast where the DCIS was found. For these reasons, DCIS probably represents a rate limiting step in the development of breast cancer.

We have been pursuing the identification of the lesions associated with the development of breast cancer since the late 1970s (Page *et al*, 1978). This effort began with attempts to refine histological and cytological criteria for hyperplastic breast lesions analogous to those of the uterine cervix and colon. Because of the availability of tissue from breast biopsies done many years previously, we followed up women for 15–20 years to determine outcome in terms of risk for development of breast cancer. This cohort included about 8000 women and over 10 000 breast biopsies (Dupont and Page, 1985). Many excellent concurrent studies evaluating lesions associated with cancer at the time of cancer diagnosis have indicated lesions of potential interest (Wellings *et al*, 1975). Our approach verified the importance of many lesions associated with elevation of breast cancer risk in a prospective and predictive fashion, beginning the search for intermediate endpoints. It is hoped that these intermediate stages in cancer development will provide sufficiently precise indicators of breast cancer development to guide prevention and intervention strategies (Lippman *et al*, 1990; Weed *et al*, 1990). Identification of intermediate lesions prior to the development of cancers capable of metastasizing would also provide the opportunity to define the molecular events associated with the development of breast cancer.

Studies of the natural history of premalignant breast disease have provided insight into different types of lesions with different implications for breast cancer risk and the process of carcinogenesis (see Table 1). We accept as premalignant breast disease any reproducibly defined condition that confers an elevated risk of breast cancer approaching double that in the general population (Komitowski and Janson, 1990). The specifically defined atypical hyperplasias and lobular carcinoma in situ confer relative risks of four to ten times that in the general population. This risk is for carcinoma to develop anywhere in either breast (Page *et al*, 1985, 1991), and the statistical significance of these observations has been sufficiently strong that the p valves derived from these studies have regularly been less than .0001. These numbers translate into absolute risk figures of a 10–25% likelihood of a woman developing invasive carcinoma over a 10–15 year period. Ductal carcinoma in situ is a very special element in this because the magnitude of risk is as high as for any other condition noted (tenfold relative risk), but more importantly, the invasive cancers that develop tend to do so in the same site in the same breast. This local recurrence and evolution to invasiveness mark these lesions as determinate precursors of invasive breast cancer (Betsill *et al*, 1978; Page *et al*, 1982). These figures are for the type of DCIS that has been detected commonly since the advent of mammography, the small and non-comedo type. It is likely that the comedo type indicates a much greater risk, but the exact implications are unknown because comedo DCIS has been regularly treated by mastectomy over the past 50 years making follow-up studies impossible.

The precision of histopathological diagnosis in this area is most convincingly demonstrated by the repetition of our findings using these same diagnostic criteria in a large prospective study (London *et al*, 1992). There has also been a

TABLE 1. Anatomical lesions types in human breast with premalignant implication

Premalignant lesions	Relative risk[a]	p value	Reference
Indicators of generalized increased risk			
atypical ductal hyperplasia	4–5 fold	<0.00001	Dupont and Page (1985)
lobular carcinoma in situ	9–10 fold	<0.00001	Page et al (1991)
Determinant lesions with regional risk			
non-comedo DCIS	10–11 fold	<.00005	Page et al (1982)

[a] The 95% confidence interval for relative risk

recent review of the reproducibility of the assignment of diagnosis by a panel of pathologists (Schnitt et al, 1992). Precision in the diagnosis of these lesions has been fostered by combining histological pattern criteria with the extent of lesion and with cytological criteria (Page et al, 1992). Classic surgical pathology criteria were predominantly derived from histological pattern only.

A further point of relevance to the importance of these histopathologically defined lesions of premalignancy in the breast is the familial relationship. A family history of breast cancer in a first degree relative confers about a doubling of breast cancer risk. However, women with the atypical hyperplasias at biopsy and family history are at nine to ten times the risk of invasive breast cancer as the general population (Dupont and Page, 1985; Dupont et al, 1989). Careful consideration of all of the above mentioned epidemiological data has led to the proposed model in Fig. 1 for progression from generalized premalignant lesions to determinant lesions to invasive cancer. This model for the induction and progression of premalignant breast disease is based on studies derived from the Nashville cohort of more than 10 000 breast biopsies (follow up rate 85%; median follow up interval 17 years; 135 women developed breast cancer).

The diagnosis of DCIS is made solely on the basis of morphological criteria that are based on the architectural and cytological features of the lesion. In addition, the extent of the process is an important determinant in assigning the diagnosis of DCIS. Non-comedo DCIS is usually a microscopic lesion that consists of intraductal cellular proliferations that fill and extend the duct, contain rigid internal architecture and often have hyperchromatic and monomorphic nuclei.

TRADITIONAL APPROACHES TO BREAST CANCER DIAGNOSIS AND CLASSIFICATION

In marked contrast to the many controversies associated with premalignant breast disease in recent years, the diagnosis and classification of breast cancers

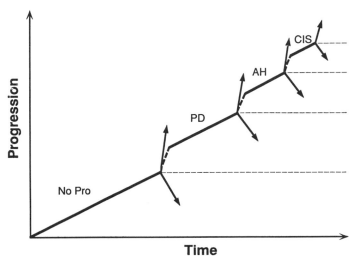

Fig. 1. Model for stochastic progression of morphological changes in breast epithelium from hyperplasia to invasive carcinoma. From Page and Dupont (1992) (used with permission of Wiley-Liss, New York). CIS = carcinoma in situ; AH = atypical hyperplasia; PD = proliferative disease without atypia; No Pro = no proliferative disease

have been a relatively tranquil area of interest. This is due primarily to the longstanding recognition by general pathologists of the utility of recognizing and separating out special types of breast cancer for prognostic purposes, and the wide acceptance of specific diagnostic criteria for these lesions.

In addition, it is our belief that there has been an inappropriate de-emphasis on the recognition of special types of breast cancer by clinicians in their pursuit of the omnipotent biochemical or immunohistochemical prognostic marker for breast cancer. In our opinion, such an approach is inherently flawed if it fails to recognize the heterogeneous clinical manifestations of breast cancer as reflected in its diverse histological appearances. Therefore, we recognize any distinct histological appearance of breast cancer as a special type cancer only if its clinical behaviour is sufficiently different from those more commonly recognized to warrant such a designation. As such, we specifically recognize invasive lobular carcinoma, medullary carcinoma, mucinous carcinoma, tubular carcinoma and invasive cribriform carcinoma as special types of breast cancer with prognoses considerably different from those that lack specific histological features. This latter group of cancers is more commonly known as infiltrating ductal carcinoma, but we prefer to call attention to the importance of making this distinction by designating these lesions as no special type tumours. This approach emphasizes their lack of specific histological features (which defines these tumours) and deflates the myth that we have determined a site of origin for these lesions. In addition to providing a means of diagnosis, histological patterns provide important biological information. Histology provides the basic evidence of whether a lesion is in situ or invasive. For hyperplastic proliferations, we have been able to identify those that are common and have little indication of elevated risk (less than double). These proliferations are recognized by specific pattern criteria, which are reflections of biological differentiation as recently evidenced by the presence of the structural protein fodrin in usual and common pattern hyperplasia (Simpson and Page, 1992). It is thought that the presence of fodrin along the lateral approximated membranes of the cells is a reflection of the maintenance of differentiation related to polarity and normal intercellular relationships in these examples of increased cell number. The presence of fodrin in an orderly fashion along the lateral membranes is lost in the atypical hyperplasias as well as in carcinomas in situ. It has long been demonstrated that a well defined myoepithelial cell layer is also lost after this stage, although many ductal carcinomas in situ may maintain myoepithelial differentiation (Bussolati *et al*, 1980).

Non-comedo and Comedo Ductal Carcinoma In Situ

One of the major separations by histology is the non-comedo and comedo DCIS, a major difference now widely accepted. This separation is similar to the difference between extensive pagetoid spread by enlarged, highly atypical melanocytes and the radial growth phase of melanoma, which is common, indolent and incapable of metastasis (Guerry *et al*, 1993). This difference between comedo and non-comedo is determined by the presence of a highly atypical nuclear pattern together with extensive necrosis. More limited (punctate by mammography) examples of calcification are regularly seen in non-comedo examples. The non-comedo examples are also marked by the usual maintenance of classic micropapillary, cribriform and solid patterns as well as the presence of lower grade nuclei. It is the concurrence of these three criteria (nuclear pattern, necrosis and histological pattern) that allows reproducible recognition of these different types of carcinoma in situ. The comedo examples of DCIS are often *TP53* positive and very frequently *neu/erbB2* positive. Expression of these oncogenes may be related to specific morphological or biological features of these lesions such as nuclear pleomorphism or cellular motility. This may also be related to the finding that Paget's disease of the nipple is regularly positive with *neu/erbB2* and one would assume that when cells of DCIS are able to reach the surface of the nipple it must be a reflection of extreme motility.

Tubular Carcinoma

Histologically, the next major reflection of biology and prognosis is of course differentiation. Anatomical differentiation forms the classical basis of the concept of tumour grade, and the presence of tubules mimicking normal glands is an excellent indicator of good prognosis when present. However, its absence is not a good negative or positive indicator of prognosis (Page, 1991). Tubular differentiation (shown in Fig. 2) is closely correlated with oestrogen receptor status and less closely correlated with progesterone receptor level. Structural proteins such as the cadherins and integrins also reflect or determine differen-

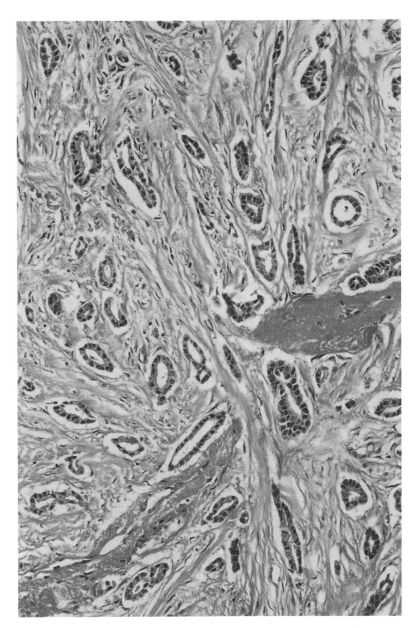

Fig. 2. Invasive tubular carcinoma showing small individual glands infiltrating dense fibrous stroma. Note the low cell density. From Page and Anderson (1987) (used with permission)

tiation, just as phenotype would be expected to reflect genotype. For the overall biological qualities of individual tumours, see Table 2.

Other Types of Carcinoma

If, as Leslie Foulds indicated decades ago (Foulds, 1957), independent factors or features of cancers sort independently, then we would expect to have some

TABLE 2. Separate qualities of malignancy[a]

Growth control
cell division
avoidance of cell deletion by
gaining vascularity
avoiding necrosis
avoiding cell deletion by apoptosis
Invasion
involves cell motility and stromal interaction
Metastatic capacity
probably a rare event relative to tumour cell mass
Cellular mass at time of diagnosis
a reflection of natural history–large means more events
cell density is a central but negelected element

[a]Modified from Foulds (1957)

cancers that have a rapid growth rate, but rarely metastasize distantly. This is characterized by the medullary special type of breast cancer, a tumour more frequent in young women (shown in Fig. 3). The reverse situation, also seen in about 4–5% of breast cancers, is a special histological type of breast cancer that is characterized by a slow growth and frequent metastasis—invasive lobular carcinoma (shown in Fig. 4). A third special type of breast cancer should be mentioned because it both has a slow growth rate and rarely metastasizes—the pure tubular and related invasive cribriform carcinomas. Currently, only histology is capable of recognizing the special nature of these tumour types; however, no more than 25–30% of breast carcinomas in any series are made up of these special types of cancers. As several excellent monographs exist detailing the diagnostic criteria for specific types of infiltrating mammary carcinoma (McDivitt *et al*, 1968; Azzopardi, 1979; Page and Anderson, 1987), we focus on our recent efforts to develop methods to characterize premalignant and malignant breast disease, together with and building from the link to histopathological classification.

APPLICATION AND INTEGRATION OF MOLECULAR METHODS OF BREAST CANCER CHARACTERIZATION

Molecular biology provides powerful approaches for analysis of gene expression and gene function and consequently has enormous potential as a tool to study breast cancer in humans. Genetic engineering strategies can rapidly provide countless gene probes that can be evaluated as diagnostic, prognostic or mechanistic markers. The large number of potential gene probes that can be studied forces investigators to focus and characterize only those gene probes that are "useful". A useful probe is one that provides additional information for

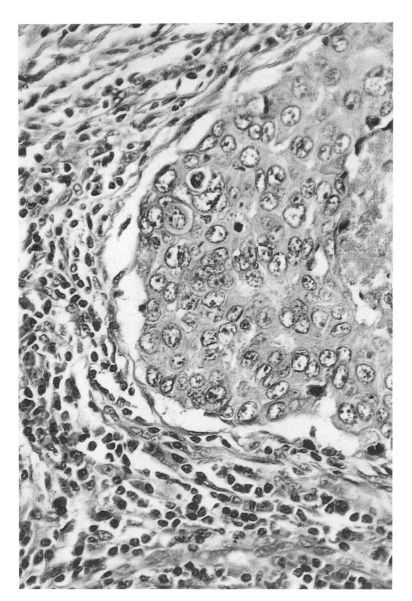

Fig. 3. An island of medullary carcinoma showing an irregularly placed large vesicular nuclei surrounded by a lymphoplasmacyctic infiltrate. The cell density is high and greater nuclear atypia is evident. From Page and Anderson (1987) (used with permission)

use in diagnosis or determination of prognosis or one that contributes to understanding the molecular mechanisms involved in the induction or progression of breast cancer.

Molecular Probes in Invasive Breast Cancer

Cancer can be diagnosed by histopathological means because this method allows us to see the biology of the disease in action and enables the evaluation of

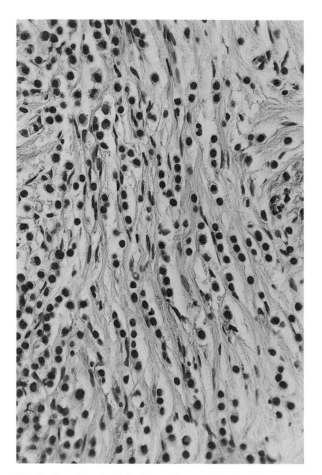

Fig. 4. Pure invasive lobular carcinoma showing individual lines of cells with a regular nuclear pattern of infiltrating between collagen bundles. From Page and Anderson (1987) (used with permission)

nuclear changes or architectural findings such as stromal invasion. Because genes determine function, the histopathological criteria for diagnosis of cancer are simultaneously evaluating a large number of composite genetic changes. It cannot be overemphasized that the use of a single molecular marker is unlikely to provide as much information as a histopathological assessment. The goal of using molecular probes for diagnosis is therefore to provide a companion tool with histopathology and not to develop a simple "stain for cancer". There may often be no advantage in using an RNA or DNA probe if an immuno-histochemical probe (antibody) is available. In fact, it has been determined that there are increasing numbers of genes that are translationally regulated such that an RNA probe would suggest that a gene was being expressed even though the protein was not actually being made. Nucleic acid probes have the advantage that specificity is generally predictable based on knowledge of the DNA sequence and the exquisite specificity of hybridization. By contrast, antibodies may cross react with other proteins in a manner that cannot be predicted. It is also generally easier to assess the specificity of a hybridization reaction by appropriate use of restriction enzymes, DNA sequencing, etc.

Molecular probes will probably be more valuable as prognostic indicators than as diagnostic indicators since present methods of diagnosis are acceptable but prognosis can rarely be predicted with certainty. Although initial studies of a molecular probe will generally test its predictive power as an isolated test, what really matters is whether this probe provides additional information beyond what is already known from pathological grading and clinical staging. Thus, multivariate analysis of probes in combination with known contributing factors is extremely important for determining whether a probe contributes useful prognostic information. Other chapters in this book provide examples of molecular probes that show some potential as prognostic indicators, such as *neu/erbB2* and *TP53*.

In addition to providing information about prognosis or diagnosis, molecular probes whose expression is highly associated with a given stage of breast cancer may contribute important information about the mechanisms of breast cancer induction or repression. The cloning of novel genes whose expression is associated with a certain stage of breast cancer progression by the assumption free methods described below (differential screening, differential display, etc.) may provide insights into disease mechanisms. For example, considerable information can often be gleaned simply by an examination of a gene's sequence or an analysis of its pattern of regulation. If a novel gene is shown to be a member of the steroid hormone receptor family or an intercellular adhesion molecule, then one can readily formulate testable hypotheses to explain why expression of this gene is associated with breast cancer.

Several strategies can be employed to identify molecular probes that are useful as diagnostic, prognostic or mechanistic markers of breast cancer. These include the candidate gene approach, positional cloning or cloning of regulated genes. Each of these methods has its advantages and pitfalls and will be briefly described.

The candidate gene approach has been commonly used as a method for identifying the causes of human genetic diseases and has led to some successes. This method involves testing known genes that are likely to contribute to a disease in rigorous population genetic tests (evaluating a series of patients with known survival for expression of the particular gene probe) and has been used to demonstrate that genes such as *neu/erbB2, TP53* and *nm23* are putative prognostic indicators for breast cancer. Candidate genes for breast cancer could come from several categories: amplified oncogenes (*neu/erbB2, EGF receptor, bcl2/cyclin D1*), known tumour suppressor genes (*TP53, RB, FAP*), and genes with interesting functions (cathepsin D, stromelysins, collagenases). This approach suggests a large number of candidate genes and can be potentially biased: investigators can readily rationalize why the gene that they study is a candidate gene for breast cancer induction or repression.

Positional cloning provides a means for cloning genes from chromosomal regions that are known to be deleted or altered in breast cancer. Human gene mapping approaches have identified a region of chromosome 17 that is linked to some cases of familial breast cancer, and positional cloning methods are presently being used to map precisely the location of this gene. Once this gene is identified, it will be important to determine whether it is altered in a significant number of cases of non-familial (sporadic breast cancer). This is by no means assured, as studies of sporadic Wilms' tumours suggest that the predominant Wilms' tumour gene *WT1* is mutated in less than 10% of sporadic cases. In addition to the mapping of germline familial genes, several chromosomal regions have been shown to exhibit a loss of heterozygosity in breast cancer, using either restriction fragment polymorphisms or the arbitrarily primed polymerase chain reaction (Peinado *et al*, 1992). Genes from these regions may be tested to determine if alterations in their expression serve as useful prognostic indicators.

Molecular methods for identifying genes that are differentially expressed may be used to obtain gene probes that may serve as diagnostic, prognostic or mechanistic markers of breast cancer. Differential cDNA cloning methods (Kulesh *et al*, 1987) or differential display (Liang and Pardee, 1992) have been used to identify genes that are expressed at different (either higher or lower) levels in breast cancer than in non-malignant epithelial cells. These methods have the tremendous advantage that they are assumption free and should not be biased towards the identification of "popular genes" or genes that support present concepts of tumour progression. An example is the stromelysin 3 gene, which was cloned by differential cDNA cloning and is expressed at higher levels in breast cancer than in normal breast (Basset *et al*, 1993). This marker illustrates one of the potential problems in this type of study. Because breast cancers have abundant stroma, it is possible to clone genes from non-malignant stromal cells that are not derived from the tumour. Although this may be useful in some instances, it will be important to develop methods for cloning genes that are differentially expressed in malignant versus benign epithelial cells. In an attempt to avoid this problem, some investigators have used cell lines to perform differential display or differential cDNA cloning. This provides a purer population of epithelial cells, but it is of concern that cultured cells may express genes differently in culture than in vivo.

Molecular Probes in Preinvasive Breast Cancer

Although the morbidity and mortality of breast cancer clearly result from invasion and metastasis, it is important to understand the development of breast cancer in its early stages for two basic reasons: (a) the molecular changes will presumably be simpler in early lesions than in later lesions, which may have acquired numerous non-contributory mutations or "hits", and (b) successful prevention strategies may require "attacking" cancer before it develops the capacity to invade or metastasize.

Non-comedo DCIS may be the best lesion for study because it is the earliest determinant premalignant change. Although comedo DCIS would be technically easier to study because of its generally larger size, its aggressiveness and the presence of numerous genetic alterations (such as *TP53* and *neu/erbB2*) suggest that it may have advanced beyond the earliest stages of carcinogenesis. Although many studies have searched for oncogene mutations, gene amplification and loss of heterozygosity in invasive breast cancer (Lippman *et al*, 1990; Ben *et al*, 1992; Callahan *et al*, 1992; Chen *et al*, 1992), few studies have analysed gene mutations and/or altered gene expression in DCIS. Investigators have demonstrated high levels of TP53 protein in 13–40% of DCIS lesions using a monoclonal antibody to *TP53*, and subsequent sequencing demonstrated a mutation in one case (Poller *et al*, 1993). Studies from our own laboratory on DCIS lesions are in agreement with these findings. In our own series, we examined 39 cases of DCIS and found immunostaining for *TP53* in 4 of 12 cases of comedo DCIS. No immunostaining was identified in any case of non-comedo DCIS. Single-stranded conformational polymorphism analysis and direct sequencing of selected cases demonstrated a mutation in only one case. This result, in conjunction with earlier studies (Thor *et al*, 1992), would suggest that TP53 protein accumulation in DCIS is essentially limited to high grade lesions and that *TP53* positivity by immunohistochemistry does not correlate in all cases with specific mutations in the most conserved regions of the gene (O'Malley *et al*, 1993). The *neu/erbB2* gene also appears to be amplified in a portion of DCIS lesions (Allred *et al*, 1992; Maguire *et al*, 1992). However, histological analysis of these cases suggest that these mutations and altered gene expression events occur predominantly in comedo DCIS (as do changes in chromatin and DNA content), which has a high rate of progression to invasion and metastasis (Komitowski and Janson, 1990; Killeen and Namiki, 1991; Böcker *et al*, 1992).

Molecular methods may be used to determine whether specific molecular probes can serve as diagnostic, prognostic or mechanistic markers for progression of premalignant breast disease. Because these lesions are small, most of the approaches to date have employed immunohistochemistry to determine whether candidate genes are differentially expressed in DCIS versus benign or malignant breast tissue. The candidate genes used have included those that are important in breast cancer progression at later stages such as *TP53* and *nm23* (Poller *et al*, 1993; Royds *et al*, 1993; Simpson *et al*, 1993).

We have developed methods for isolating RNA from small preinvasive breast cancers such as non-comedo DCIS in order to identify genes that may participate in breast cancer progression. We have identified and banked frozen tissue from several patients with extensive microscopic non-comedo DCIS. After frozen section confirmation of the diagnosis, we then use a 2 mm punch to obtain tissue samples that only contain DCIS. Figure 5 shows "before and after" tissue sections that demonstrate that tissue obtained by punch contains a single area of non-comedo DCIS.

This approach was used to obtain RNA from a patient with multifocal non-

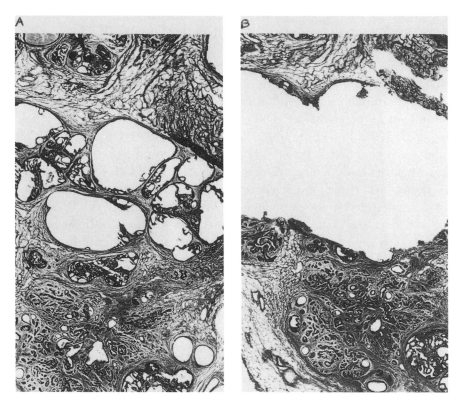

Fig. 5. Non-comedo ductal carcinoma in situ showing (A) before and (B) after tissue sections that demonstrate that tissue obtained by punch dissection of the frozen tissue block contains a single area of DCIS. Original magnification (5x)

comedo DCIS. The tissue sample was minced with a razor blade, lysed and sonicated in guanidinium thiocyanate/phenol, and then chloroform extracted and precipitated with ethanol. Because this DCIS sample was so cellular, we were able to obtain 70 μg of RNA (for comparison, we obtained less than 10 μg of RNA from a similar quantity of normal breast tissue). Polyadenylated RNA was prepared by oligo(dT) chromatography resulting in 7 μg of poly(A)$^+$ RNA; 5 μg of poly(A)$^+$ RNA was then used for construction of a cDNA library in Lambda Zap II (the remaining 2 μg of poly(A)$^+$ RNA was saved for later studies). A similar amount of poly(A)$^+$ RNA was isolated from primary human breast epithelial cells (HMEC) (Hammond *et al*, 1984). We decided to use primary breast epithelial cells for the initial differential screen because normal breast tissue would contain a number of cell types in addition to ductal epithelial cells, unlike the DCIS samples that lack fibroblasts or even myoepithelial cells (Abendroth *et al*, 1991; Schnitt *et al*, 1992). Polyadenylated RNA from both RNA samples was used to synthesize cDNA and was then appropriately linkered and cloned into Lambda Zap. The unamplified HMEC cDNA library contained 7 x 10^5 recombinants and the unamplified cDNA library constructed from DCIS tissue from one patient (X19–12) contained 1.5

x 10^6 recombinants. Characterization of each library demonstrated that in both, greater than 80% of their phage contain inserts. The average insert size of the DCIS library was 1.1–2 kb, and the average insert size of the HMEC library was 2 kb. Phage from the DCIS cDNA library were then differentially screened with two probes: one derived from the DCIS library and the other derived from the HMEC library. We have already screened 200 000 recombinants and have initially identified 24 cDNAs that are differentially expressed. Ten of these showed marked differences in hybridization to the two probes and have been plaque purified through tertiary screening. The plaque purified phage were grown in 20 ml media, and DNA was isolated, slot-blotted and then interrogated with probes derived from either the DCIS library or the HMEC library to confirm that they are expressed at higher levels in the DCIS library than in the normal breast epithelial cell library. We should be able to use these libraries and this screening method to obtain cDNAs that are either increased in DCIS or decreased in DCIS, depending on which library is employed for screening.

We are presently analysing plaque purified cDNAs that appear to be increased in DCIS samples. The following criteria will be used initially to demonstrate that a gene has increased expression in DCIS.

Criteria for DCIS increased cDNAs: (a) present at higher levels in the DCIS library than in the HMEC library, (b) expressed at high levels in DCIS libraries prepared from other patients, (c) expressed at higher levels in mRNA from DCIS tissue samples than in HMEC mRNA (employing RNase protection or quantitative-PCR), (d) not expressed at high levels in fibroblast mRNA (employing our 3T3 cDNA libraries), and (e) in situ hybridization demonstrating higher mRNA levels in DCIS lesions than in areas of normal breast.

Once the cDNAs have been initially screened by these methods, we will confirm that there is differential expression of the mRNAs by analysing the saved samples of mRNAs from patient and HMEC cells. This is an important step in case library amplification, or some other step in the cloning creates an artificial differential expression that is not actually reflected in the mRNA samples obtained from the tissue and/or cell samples. Finally, we will use in situ hybridization with our T7 derived probes to confirm that the DCIS increased cDNAs are expressed at higher levels in DCIS tissue than in adjacent normal breast tissue. We can also identify genes whose expression is decreased in DCIS by screening the HMEC phage library and identifying clones that show significantly stronger hybridization to the HMEC probe than to the probe derived from the patient library. The following criteria will be used initially to demonstrate that a gene has decreased expression in DCIS.

Criteria for DCIS decreased cDNAs: (a) present at higher levels in the HMEC library than in the DCIS library, (b) expressed at low levels in DCIS libraries prepared from other patients, (c) expressed at lower levels in mRNA from DCIS tissue samples than in HMEC mRNA (employing RNase protection or quantitative polymerase chain reaction), (d) not expressed at high levels in fibroblast mRNA (employing 3T3 cDNA libraries), and (e) in situ hybridization demonstrating lower mRNA levels in DCIS lesions than in areas of normal breast.

An important goal of this study is to identify genes whose expression is altered in carcinoma in situ as a probe to investigate the mechanism of progression from benign to preinvasive disease. Once genes have been sequenced and characterized, their functions can be compared to known phenomena that are thought to contribute to tumour progression. For example, oncogenes appear to stimulate cell growth and might induce neoplasia at least in part by increasing cellularity of the preinvasive lesions. Similarly, proteases that are thought to contribute to tumour invasion may be induced in those preinvasive lesions that readily progress to cancer. The identification of genes that are differentially regulated in preinvasive breast cancer will facilitate studies of gene regulation. Once target genes are available, studies may begin to determine the factors responsible for differential gene regulation such as alterations in transcription factor expression or phosphorylation. In addition to these predictable consequences of the identification, it is hoped that the identification of novel genes by these assumption free methods will lead to unexpected ideas about mechanisms of tumour induction or progression. This is the real advantage of an assumption free approach: genes can be identified that have functions which are not presently thought to be related to tumour progression, but may actually be important contributors to the early stages of premalignancy.

SUMMARY

Histopathology remains the benchmark and the only reliable means for diagnosing breast cancer in either invasive or preinvasive stages and for classifying morphologically distinct special types of breast cancer that exhibit different prognoses. Careful epidemiological research performed in tandem with histopathology has demonstrated that certain preinvasive lesions progress to invasive cancer at high frequency, and the detection of these lesions seems certain to increase with increased mammographic screening. Comedo and non-comedo DCIS represent examples of distinct preinvasive lesions in which differing histopathology reflects altered biological behaviour. Certain morphological varieties of invasive cancer are also associated with different biological outcomes, notably the special histological types such as tubular, lobular and medullary. Distinguishing these heterogeneous forms of breast cancer is crucial for diagnosis, prognostic prediction and the acquisition of research material for clinically relevant molecular epidemiological studies.

Acknowledgements

This work was supported by the Molecular Toxicology Program and by the A B Hancock, Jr Memorial Laboratory of the Vanderbilt University Medical Center.

References

Abendroth CS, Wang HH and Ducatman BS (1991) Comparative features of carcinoma in situ and atypical ductal hyperplasia of the breast on fine-needle aspiration biopsy specimens. *American Journal of Clinical Pathology* **96** 654–659

Allred DC, Clark GM, Molina R *et al* (1992) Overexpression of HER-2/neu and its relationship with other prognostic factors change during the progression of in situ to invasive breast cancer. *Human Pathology* **23** 974–979

Azzopardi, J (1979) *Problems in Breast Pathology,* Saunders, Philadelphia

Basset P, Wolf C and Chambon P (1993) Expression of the stromelysin-3 gene in fibroblastic cells of invasive carcinomas of the breast and other human tissues: a review. *Breast Cancer Research and Treatment* **24** 185–193

Ben CM, Rouanet P, Louason G, Jeanteur P and Theillet C (1992) An attempt to define sets of cooperating genetic alterations in human breast cancer. *International Journal of Cancer* **51** 542–547

Betsill WL, Rosen PP, Lieberman PH and Robbins GF (1978) Intraductal carcinoma: long-term follow-up after treatment by biopsy alone. *Journal of the American Medical Association* **239** 1863–1867

Böcker W, Bier B, Freytag G *et al* (1992) An immunohistochemical study of the breast using antibodies to basal and luminal keratins, alpha-smooth muscle actin, vimentin, collagen IV and laminin. Part II: Epitheliosis and ductal carcinoma in situ. *Virchows Archives [A]* **421** 323–330

Bussolati G, Botta G and Gugliotta P (1980) Actin-rich (myoepithelial) cells in ductal carcinoma in situ of the breast. *Virchows Archives [B]* **34** 251–259

Callahan R, Cropp CS, Merlo GR, Liscia DS, Cappa A and Lidereau R (1992) Somatic mutations and human breast cancer: a status report. *Cancer* **69** 1582–1588

Carter D and Smith RRL (1977) Carcinoma in situ of the breast. *Cancer* **40** 1189–1193

Chen L, Kurisu W, Ljung BM, Goldman ES, Moore DI and Smith HS (1992) Heterogeneity for allelic loss in human breast cancer. *Journal of the National Cancer Institute* **84** 506–510

Dupont WD and Page DL (1985) Risk factors for breast cancer in women with proliferative breast disease. *New England Journal of Medicine* **312** 146–151

Dupont WD, Page DL, Rogers LW and Parl FF (1989) Influence of exogenous estrogens, proliferative breast disease and other variables on breast cancer risk. *Cancer* **63** 948–957

Fentiman IS (1992) Ductal carcinoma in situ. *British Medical Journal* **304** 1261–1262

Foulds L (1957) Tumor progression. *Cancer Research* **17** 355–356

Guerry D, Synnestvedt M, Elder DE and Schultz D (1993) Lessons from tumor progression: the invasive radial growth phase of melanoma is common, incapable of metastasis, and indolent. *Journal of Investigative Dermatology* **100** 342s–345s

Hammond SL, Ham RG and Stampfer MR (1984) Serum-free growth of human mammary epithelial cells: rapid clonal growth in defined medium and extended serial passage with pituitary extract. *Proceedings of the National Academy of Sciences of the USA* **81** 5435–5439

Killeen JL and Namiki H (1991) DNA analysis of ductal carcinoma in situ of the breast: a comparison with histologic features. *Cancer* **68** 2602–2607

Komitowski D and Janson C (1990) Quantitative features of chromatin structure in the prognosis of breast cancer. *Cancer* **65** 2725–2730

Kulesh DA, Clive DR, Zarlenga DS and Greene JJ (1987) Indentification of interferon-modulated proliferation-related cDNA sequences. *Proceedings of the National Academy of Sciences of the USA* **84** 8453–8457

Lawrence G (1991) Evaluation of treatment options for ductal carcinoma in situ of the breast. *Archives of Surgery* **126** 1541

Liang P and Pardee AB (1992) Differential display of eukaryotic messenger RNA by means of the polymerase chain reaction. *Science* **257** 967–971

Lippman SM, Lee JS, Lotan R, Hittelman W, Wargovich MJ and Hong WK (1990) Commentary: biomarkers as intermediate endpoints in chemoprevention trials. *Journal of the National Cancer Institute* **82** 555–560

London SJ, Connolly JL, Schnitt SJ and Colditz GA (1992) A prospective study of benign breast disease and risk of breast cancer. *Journal of the American Medical Association* **267** 941–944

Maguire HJ, Hellman ME, Greene MI and Yeh I (1992) Expression of c-erbB-2 in in situ and in adjacent invasive ductal adenocarcinomas of the female breast. *Pathobiology* **60** 117–121

McDivitt RW, Stewart FW and Berg JW (1968) Tumors of the breast. *Atlas of Tumor Pathology*, pp 133-137, Armed Forces Institute of Pathology, Washington, DC

O'Malley FP, Vnencak-Jones CL, Dupont WD, Parl FF, Manning S and Page DL (1993) p53 Mutations in ductal carcinoma in situ of the breast: immunohistochemical and sequencing data. *Laboratory Investigation* **68** 18A

Ottesen GL, Graversen HP, Blichert TM, Zedeler K and Andersen JA (1992) Ductal carcinoma in situ of the female breast: short-term results of a prospective nationwide study. *American Journal of Surgical Pathology* **16** 1183–1196

Page DL (1991) Prognosis and breast cancer—recognition of lethal and favorable prognostic types. *American Journal of Surgical Pathology* **15** 334–349

Page DL and Anderson TJ (eds) (1987) *Diagnostic Histopathology of the Breast,* Churchill Livingstone, Edinburgh

Page DL and Dupont WD (1991) Histologic indicators of breast cancer risk. *Bulletin of the American College of Surgeons* **76** 16–23

Page DL, Dupont WD, Rogers LW and Landenberger M (1982) Intraductal carcinoma of the breast: follow-up after biopsy. *Cancer* **49** 751–758

Page DL, Dupont WD, Rogers LW and Rados MS (1985) Atypical hyperplastic lesions of the female breast: a long term follow-up study. *Cancer* **55** 2698–2708

Page DL, Kidd TE, Dupont WD, Simpson JF and Rogers LW (1991) Lobular neoplasia of the breast: higher risk for subsequent invasive cancer predicted by more extensive disease. *Human Pathology* **22** 1232–1239

Page DL and Dupont WD (1992) Indicators of increased breast cancer risk in humans. *Journal of Cellular Biochemistry* **Supplement 16G** 175–182

Page DL and Rogers LW (1992) Combined histologic and cytologic criteria for the diagnosis of mammary atypical ductal hyperplasia. *Human Pathology* **23** 1095–1097

Page DL, Vander Zwagg R, Rogers LW, Williams LT, Walker WE and Hartmann WH (1978) Relation between component parts of fibrocystic disease complex and breast cancer: A follow-up study. *Journal of the National Cancer Institute* **61** 1055–1063

Peinado MA, Malkhosyan S, Velazquez A and Perucho M (1992) Isolation and characterization of allelic losses and gains in colorectal tumors by arbitrarily primed polymerase chain reaction. *Proceedings of the National Academy of Sciences of the USA* **89** 10065–10069

Pierce SM, Schnitt SJ and Harris JR (1992) What to do about mammographically detected ductal carcinoma in situ? *Cancer* **70** 2576–2578

Poller DN, Roberts EC, Bell JA, Elston CW, Blamey RW and Ellis IO (1993) p53 protein expression in mammary ductal carcinoma in situ: relationship to immunohistochemical expression of estrogen receptor and c-erbB-2 protein. *Human Pathology* **24** 463–468

Posner MC and Wolmark N (1992) Non-invasive breast carcinoma. *Breast Cancer Research and Treatment* **21** 155–164

Royds JA, Stephenson TJ, Rees RC, Shorthouse AJ and Silcocks PB (1993) nm23 protein expression in ductal in situ and invasive human breast carcinoma. *Journal of the National Cancer Institute* **85** 727–731

Schnitt SJ, Connolly JL, Tavassoli FA *et al* (1992) Interobserver reproducibility in the diagnosis of ductal proliferative breast lesions using standardized criteria. *American Journal of Surgical Pathology* **16** 1133–1143

Schwartz GF, Finkel GC, Garcia JC and Patchefsky AS (1992) Subclinical ductal carcinoma in situ of the breast: treatment by local excision and surveillance alone. *Cancer* **70** 2468–2474

Simpson JF and Page DL (1992) Altered expression of a structual protein (fodrin) within epithelial proliferative disease of the breast. *American Journal of Pathology* **141** 285–289

Simpson JF, O'Malley FP, Dupont WD and Page DL (1993) Differential expression of nm23 in non-invasive breast carcinoma. *Laboratory Investigation* **68** 20A

Solin LJ, Recht A, Fourquet A *et al* (1991) Ten-year results of breast-conserving surgery and definitive irradiation for intraductal carcinoma (ductal carcinoma in situ) of the breast. *Cancer* **68** 2337–2344

Swain SM (1992) Ductal carcinoma in situ. *Cancer Investigation* **10** 443–454

Thor AD, Moore DH, Edgerton SM *et al* (1992) Accumulation of p53 tumor suppressor gene protein: an independent marker of prognosis in breast cancers. *Journal of the National Cancer Institute* **84** 845–855

Ward BA, McKhann CF and Ravikumar TS (1992) Ten-year follow-up of breast carcinoma in situ in Connecticut. *Archives of Surgery* **127** 1392–1395

Weed DL, Greenwald P and Cullen JW (1990) The future of cancer prevention and control. *Seminars in Oncology* **17** 504–509

Wellings SR, Jensen HM and Marcum RG (1975) An atlas of subgross pathology of the human breast with special reference to possible precancerous lesions. *Journal of the National Cancer Institute* **55** 231–273

The authors are responsible for the accuracy of the references.

Active Specific Immunotherapy: PEM as a Potential Target Molecule

JOY BURCHELL • ROSALIND GRAHAM • JOYCE TAYLOR-PAPADIMITRIOU

Imperial Cancer Research Fund, PO Box 123, 44 Lincoln's Inn Fields, London WC2A 3PX

INTRODUCTION

The possibility of using active specific immunotherapy (ASI) in the management of cancer is now becoming a feasible proposition. This has been facilitated by the identification of potential target antigens and by the considerable advances now being made in understanding the mechanisms involved in tumour rejection and in antigen presentation and recognition. It now appears that many tumours, including breast cancer, express tumour associated antigens (TAA) that can be recognized by T cells and in this sense they are antigenic. They are not, however, immunogenic since they fail to induce an effective immune response. There is a need therefore not only to identify the TAA, but also to find a way of presenting them to the immune system that generates a response that is effective in rejecting the tumour. Carcinoma cells seem to be particularly ineffective in antigen presentation, and recent data suggest that one important reason for this is their lack of expression of the costimulatory molecules involved in T cell stimulation (Schwartz, 1992; Lanzavecchia, 1993).

Some of the first trials of ASI have been in the management of melanoma

(McGee, 1991; Mitchell, 1991), and in fact, a human tumour antigen present on melanoma cells has been cloned by its ability to stimulate cytotoxic T lymphocytes (Van der Bruggen *et al*, 1991). However, molecules that are potential targets for ASI are now being identified on other tumours, and in this chapter, we focus on the polymorphic epithelial mucin (PEM), which is expressed by most breast cancers and by many adenocarcinomas. The features that make it a suitable target molecule for ASI are explored and the model systems that are available to investigate its efficacy as an immunogen are discussed. In addition, we briefly discuss ways to improve the immunogenicity of tumour cells.

TUMOUR ASSOCIATED ANTIGENS ON BREAST CANCER CELLS

Many TAA were identified using monoclonal antibody technology. In the case of breast cancer, two surface antigens, c-erbB2 and a polymorphic epithelial mucin (PEM), were found to be the target antigen for many antibodies raised against breast epithelial tumours. Overexpression of the proto-oncogene c-*erbB2* has been found to be associated with a poor prognosis (Slamon *et al*, 1987), although there is some indirect evidence that the p185 gene product may be immunogenic in some patients (Menard S, personal communication). Use of the p185 glycoprotein as an immunogen, however, has not been explored, and efforts have been directed largely to targeting antibody and antibody conjugates to tumours.

An advantage of an immunotherapeutic approach based on antigen presentation rather than antibody delivery is that internal antigens may be considered since these can be presented as peptides by the histocompatibility antigens. In this context, a possible candidate as an immunogen is the TP53 protein found to be mutated and upregulated in more than 50% of breast cancers (Bartek *et al*, 1990). Mutations in the *ras* genes, which are frequently seen in other cancers, are not found in breast cancer, although increased levels of Ha-*ras* have been observed (Rochlitz *et al*, 1989).

Planning vaccine formulations based on presentation of peptides through HLA presents certain problems since many cancers lose HLA, and even if the molecules are still expressed, only certain alleles can present a specific peptide, that is, presentation is HLA restricted. As discussed below, these problems may be circumvented in the case of PEM, since there is evidence to suggest that presentation of PEM is not HLA restricted. For this and other reasons, we have focused our efforts on evaluating the potential of PEM based antigens in immunotherapy of breast cancer.

THE POLYMORPHIC EPITHELIAL MUCIN (PEM)

The PEM is a high molecular weight protein that contains a large amount of O-linked sugar. It is expressed on the luminal surface of many simple epi-

A. Diagram of MUC1 gene

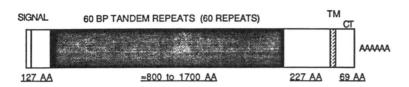

CORE PROTEIN ESTIMATED MOL WT 125,000 TO 225,000 Da

B. Tandem repeat sequence

Immunodominant domain

HGVTSAPDTRPAPGSTAPPA

SM3

HMFG-2

* Probable glycosylation sites

Fig. 1. (A) Diagram of *MUC1* gene. (B) Tandem repeat sequence showing the epitopes recognized by the monoclonal antibodies HMFG-2 and SM3. AA = aminoacids

thelial cells (Zotter *et al*, 1988) and is upregulated by breast epithelium during pregnancy and lactation. Its potential as a target molecule for active specific immunotherapy stems from the fact that in many carcinomas, PEM is both upregulated and aberrantly glycosylated, making it antigenically distinct from the mucin expressed by normal epithelium (Burchell *et al*, 1987). The gene (known as *MUC1*) coding for PEM has been cloned (Siddiqui *et al*, 1988; Gendler *et al*, 1990; Ligtenberg *et al*, 1990; Wreschner *et al*, 1990), and its product has been shown to be a transmembrane protein with a cytoplasmic tail consisting of 69 aminoacids (see Fig. 1). The extracellular domain consists mainly of tandem repeats of 20 aminoacids that are rich in serine, threonine and proline and serve as a scaffold for the large amount of carbohydrate. This structure results in an extended rod like molecule (Jentoff, 1990) that extends far above the glycocalyx of the cell (Hilkens *et al*, 1992). Individual alleles vary in the number of tandem repeats they contain, making this molecule highly polymorphic. The presence of a large number of tandem repeats, ranging between 30 and 90, results in there being many antigenic epitopes per molecule, which is probably one reason why PEM is so highly immunogenic.

Several other genes coding for mucins of the gastrointestinal tract (Gum *et al*, 1989, 1990) and the lung (Porchet *et al*, 1991) have been cloned, as well as mucin genes from species other than human (Hoffman, 1988; Timpte *et al*, 1988). All these genes contain a tandem repeat domain, rich in threonine, serine and proline which allow the attachment of large amounts of carbohydrate. However, in each mucin, the sequence and length of the tandem repeat vary. Moreover, although full length cDNAs for the lung and gastrointestinal mucins are not available, present data suggest that these mucins are not transmembrane proteins. They also contain cysteine rich domains (Gum *et al*, 1992), which are thought to be responsible for intermolecular bonds allowing the molecules to form extremely large aggregates after being released from the cell. Thus, its transmembrane nature and lack of cysteine rich regions make PEM unique among the mucins. The transmembrane and cytoplasmic domain of PEM must have an important function since the sequence is highly conserved in the mouse homologue (*MUC1*), even though the sequence of the tandem repeat is not (Spicer *et al*, 1991).

ABERRANT GLYCOSYLATION OF PEM

Within each tandem repeat of PEM, there are five potential O-glycosylation sites (see Fig. 1). However, statistically, it has been found that only two sites per tandem repeat are glycosylated (Hanisch FG, personal communication). Recent data from Hollingsworth and colleagues (Nishimori *et al*, 1993) using in vitro glycosylation of peptides suggest that in breast carcinoma cell lines, at least, only the two threonines flanking the sequence SAPDTRPAPGS are glycosylated (see Fig. 1 for 20 aminoacid sequence). Interestingly, many of the epitopes recognized by monoclonal antibodies to the core protein have been mapped to within this region (Burchell *et al*, 1989; Taylor-Papadimitriou, 1991). One such antibody, SM3, reacts well with the mucin expressed by breast and other cancer cells but shows little or no reactivity with the normally processed mucin found in the resting breast and many other epithelial tissues (Girling *et al*, 1989). Its epitope has been mapped to PDTRP (Burchell *et al*, 1989), which appears to be masked by carbohydrate on the normal mucin but exposed on tumour associated PEM. Direct analysis of the sugar side chains of PEM derived from milk (Hanisch *et al*, 1989) and from a breast cancer cell line (Hull *et al*, 1989) shows that the chains are longer and form a repeating polylactosamine structure on the normal mucin, whereas the side chains on the tumour associated mucin are much simpler and shorter (see Fig. 2).

IN VITRO MODEL SYSTEMS FOR STUDYING THE ABERRANT GLYCOSYLATION OF PEM

The exposure of epitopes on the mucin expressed by tumour cells which are masked on the normally expressed mucin makes this molecule an excellent

NORMAL

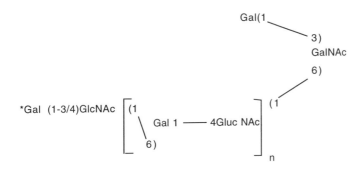

TUMOUR

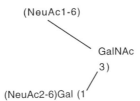

Fig. 2. Major carbohydrate side chains on PEM. n, the sequence Gal 1–4 GlucNAc can be repeated 0–3 times. *The side chains of the normal mucin may be neutral or terminate with sialic acid or sometimes fucose. The side chains of the tumour associated mucin may or may not contain one or two sialic acid molecules

candidate for a target molecule in ASI. Pragmatically, the aberrant glycosylation can start to be exploited by developing immunogens based on the cancer associated mucin or antibodies directed to it. In addition, however, an investigation leading to an understanding of the mechanisms involved in the aberrant glycosylation could help in planning future strategies. To study these underlying mechanisms, it is necessary to have cell lines that glycosylate the PEM normally and those that show aberrant glycosylation. We have developed a cell line (MTSV1-7) from human milk epithelial cells (Bartek *et al*, 1991) that shows many characteristics of normal mammary epithelial cells (Berdichevsky *et al*, 1992). The PEM produced by this cell line does not express the SM3 epitope, but after inhibiting O-glycosylation, the epitope is exposed (see Fig. 3) (Burchell and Taylor-Papadimitriou, 1993). Furthermore, analysis of PEM immunoprecipitates of ^{3}H glucosamine labelled cells suggests in fact that the PEM produced by MTSV1-7 may contain polylactosamine chains (Lloyd K,

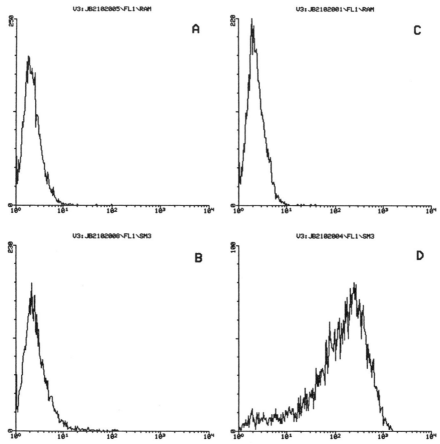

Fig. 3. Expression of the SM3 epitope by MTSV1-7 cells after the inhibition of O-linked glycosylation. Cells were incubated for 48 hr with 2 mM benzyl-n-acetylgalactosamine and then analysed for SM3 binding by fluorescent activated cell sorting. The binding of second antibody control (A, C); SM3 monoclonal antibody (B, D); with (C, D) or without (A, B) prior incubation with benzyl-n-acetylgalactosamine

Burchell J, Taylor-Papadimitriou J, unpublished). This cell line, in comparison with breast carcinoma cell lines, can be used to study the mechanisms responsible for the aberrant glycosylation of PEM.

EVIDENCE FOR IMMUNE RECOGNITION OF PEM IN CANCER PATIENTS

Evidence for immune recognition of the MUC1 product was first noted by Finn and colleagues who isolated cytotoxic T cells from breast and pancreatic cancer patients that killed cancer cell lines expressing PEM (Barnd *et al*, 1989; Jerome *et al*, 1991). The mechanism involved is unclear, although the data show that it is not HLA restricted. The classical model for the presentation of antigen to and recognition of antigen by CD8+ cytotoxic T cells (CTL) involves the interaction of the variable domain of the T cell receptor with an endogenously processed peptide held in the groove of the HLA class I molecule expressed on the tumour cell. The non-HLA restricted killing seen with the PEM activated T cells may arise from the interaction of multiple PEM epitopes with the T cell receptor (not involving the peptide binding groove of the HLA molecule), resulting in signal transduction and activation of the T cell. This mechanism may be similar to that observed when bivalent antibodies bind to the receptor. Interestingly, the use of a vaccinia vector carrying *MUC1* to elicit a mucin specific CTL resulted in HLA restricted killing (Bu D, Domenech N, Lewis J, Taylor-Papadimitriou J and Finn O, unpublished). Sequencing of *MUC1* in the virus showed that recombination had taken place and that all of the vaccinia clones had deleted the perfect tandem repeat region. This lack of tandem repeats and lack of HLA unrestricted killing add further weight to the idea that the tandem repeats are responsible for the phenomena of unrestricted killing. The SM3 antibody has been found to block the unrestricted killing of breast cancer cells expressing PEM, suggesting that core protein epitopes in the vicinity of the PDTRP sequence may be involved in T cell recognition.

Recently, it has been possible to demonstrate that patients can produce antibodies to PEM, both by detecting their presence in serum (Hilgers J, personal communication) and by isolating and immortalizing B cells producing such antibodies from tumour infiltrating lymphocytes of ovarian cancer patients (Rughetti *et al*, 1993).

RODENT MODELS FOR STUDYING TUMOUR REJECTION AND IMMUNE RESPONSES TO PEM

The range of possible PEM based immunogens is wide, including cells, recombinant viruses, peptides, carbohydrates and DNA based formulations. To evaluate the efficacy of the various immunogens and to optimize antigen presentation, model systems are required.

TA3-Ha Tumour Model for Analysis of Carbohydrate Antigens

The shorter carbohydrate side chains that are carried on the core protein of the polymorphic epithelial mucin in many carcinomas are also found on other mucin core proteins in the mouse as well as in humans. The mucin expressed by an extremely aggressive mouse mammary adenocarcinoma TA3-Ha also carries these side chains, and this mouse model has been used effectively to analyse the efficacy of synthetic carbohydrates as immunogens (Fung *et al*, 1990; Singhal *et al*, 1991). Antibody responses to T (Galβ1-3 GalNAc) coupled to KLH have been seen in immunized mice, and inhibition of tumour growth was seen even when the immunogen was administered after the tumour cells were injected (Fung *et al*, 1990). Ovine submaxillary mucin (carrying multiple sialylated Tn, ie NeuAc2-6 GalNAc, epitopes) and also its desialylated product have also been found to be effective in both stimulating an immune response and inhibiting tumour growth in this system (Singhal *et al*, 1991). Although cellular responses to carbohydrates are not well studied, they have been shown to induce delayed type hypersensitivity responses and T cell proliferation in immunized mice.

On the basis of studies in this model, clinical trials have begun to evaluate the therapeutic use of conjugated synthetic carbohydrates in breast and ovarian cancer patients (McLean *et al*, 1992). One advantage of the immunotherapy trials is that important information and possible response data can be obtained by in vitro assessment of immune parameters and responses. This means, however, that the infrastructure to carry out these assessments has to be in place.

Syngeneic Model System Using a Mouse Mammary Tumour Cell Line Transfected with the *MUC1* Gene

A syngeneic model based on PEM was developed by introducing the *MUC1* gene into the mouse mammary epithelial tumour cell line 410.4 (Lalani *et al*, 1991). Expression of the *MUC1* gene did reduce the efficiency of tumour formation in syngeneic Balb/c mice, but tumours developed when sufficient cells were inoculated. To date, we have shown that inhibition of tumour growth can be achieved by preimmunization with transfected cells (Lalani *et al*, 1991), with peptides based on the tandem repeat (Ding *et al*, in press) and with a recombinant vaccinia virus carrying the *MUC1* gene (Lewis J, Stauss H, Lalani EL and Taylor-Papadimitriou J, unpublished).

An examination of proliferative responses to the tandem repeat peptide in vitro of lymphocytes from immunized mice has shown that the responses can be strain dependent (Taylor-Papadimitriou *et al*, 1993). To see whether this relates to tumour rejection, transfectants expressing *MUC1* have been developed from H_2b cell lines in addition to the 410.4 transfectants, which are H_2d.

Transgenic Mice Expressing the Human *MUC1* Gene

To look at immune responses in a host where the human PEM is expressed as a self antigen with the same tissue distribution as in humans, a transgenic mouse has been developed. Such a model can only be developed when the gene coding for a tumour antigen has been cloned and 5′ flanking regulatory sequences have been isolated and analysed (Kovarik *et al*, 1993). The *MUC1* gene is compact, being closely flanked 3′ by the thrombospondin 3 gene (Vos *et al*, 1992) and 5′ by a gene giving a large transcript (13 kb) in most tissues (Gendler SJ and Duhig T, personal communication). It is perhaps not surprising therefore that we have been able to obtain accurate tissue specific expression in a transgenic mouse using a 10.6 kb fragment of genomic DNA containing only 1.6 kb of 5′ sequence and 2.3 kb of 3′ sequence (Peat *et al*, 1992). In humans, the *MUC1* gene is expressed largely by simple epithelial cells, and the

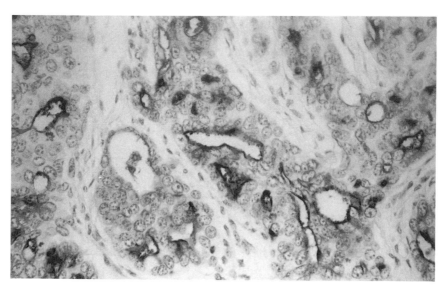

Fig. 4. Staining of MMTV induced tumours in transgenic mice with an antibody to PEM. Methacarn fixed tumours were incubated with HMFG-1 (an antibody to the PEM peptide core) and the binding was visualized using peroxidase conjugated rabbit anti-mouse antibody

same distribution (as determined by staining with antibodies specific for the human PEM) is seen in the transgenic mouse. These mice therefore are an appropriate model for toxicity testing of antibodies or antigens related to the human PEM. It is also possible to look at humoral responses to PEM based immunogens and to examine T cell proliferative responses and non-H_2 restricted cytotoxic T cell responses in vitro. Since the mice are hybrid, they are being backcrossed on to a single strain in order to be able to analyse H_2 restricted cytotoxic T cell responses. Transplantable mouse tumours expressing human PEM can then be used to examine the efficacy of different PEM based antigens in tumour rejection where PEM is expressed as a self antigen.

To extend the transgenic model, we are attempting to develop strains that spontaneously develop carcinomas expressing PEM. To date, we have been able to induce mammary tumours expressing PEM by fostering the *MUC1* transgenics on an MMTV-producing mouse strain (see Fig. 4). Other approaches are to cross the *MUC1* transgenics with a c-*erbB2* transgenic and to make double transgenics by expressing an oncogene from the *MUC1* promoter. The *MUC1* gene is expressed in many epithelial tissues, and it may be possible to produce mouse strains developing spontaneous tumours in the ovary, stomach, lung and colon as well as in the breast.

The *MUC1* transgenic mouse is an extremely important model, since it will allow the possibility not only of examining the efficacy of immunogens, but also of assessing any autoimmune responses that would be expected to be the major side effect of PEM based immunogens where PEM is expressed as a self antigen. We believe such side effects are unlikely, primarily because of the apical location of PEM on normal epithelial tissues (a location less accessible to the effector cells of the immune system), and also because of the higher levels and antigenic differences of the cancer associated mucin.

ENHANCING THE IMMUNE RESPONSE

Although tumours may express TAA, clearly they are not rejected by the immune system and often go on to kill the host. To elicit an immune response, as well as the T cell receptor binding to antigen (conventionally in association with class I molecules), an additional co-stimulatory signal is required. The co-stimulation results from an interaction of CD28 on the T cell surface with its ligand B7 found on the surface of antigen presenting cells (Schwartz, 1992). This leads to the production of IL2 and its receptor and subsequently other cytokines. Most epithelial cells do not express B7, and thus carcinomas do not elicit an effective anti-tumour T cell response. Thus, one avenue that is being extensively explored is the delivery of cytokines to the tumour site. Fearon *et al* (1990) have engineered a mouse colonic tumour cell line to secrete IL2. The transfected, but not the parental, cell line induced a tumour specific CTL response that was mediated by CD8+ cells. More recently, Dranoff *et al* (1993) have introduced a variety of cytokines into B16 melanoma cells using retroviruses. They have found that irradiated cells expressing granulocyte-macrophage colony stimulating factor (GM-CSF) stimulated potent and specific anti-tumour immunity dependent on CD4+ and CD8+ T cells. An extremely interesting approach used by Tao and Levy (1993) is to deliver antigen and cytokine (GM-CSF) as a fusion protein. In the light of recent data showing that in vivo expression of proteins from DNA injected into tumours or tissue can occur (Vile *et al*, 1993), the possibility of vaccines based on DNA formulations is a possibility. Such formulations are, of course, only possible where the gene coding for antigen has been cloned.

Another application of the new molecular understanding of co-stimulation is the transfection of the *B7* gene into tumour cells. Expression of B7 on murine melanoma cells was found to induce the regression of melanoma tumours in vivo (Chen *et al*, 1992; Townsend and Allison, 1993). Experiments are now under way to see whether transfection of the mouse *B7* into mouse mammary tumours expressing PEM increases the immunogenicity of PEM.

ANTIBODIES AND THE ANTI-IDIOTYPIC RESPONSE

In discussing antigen presentation, we have considered possible antigen formulations based on the mucin molecule itself or the gene coding for the core protein. Another possibility, which has been considered in the case of other antigens, is the use of an antibody to the antigen to evoke an anti-idiotypic response, where the binding site of the second antibody, Ab_2, is equivalent antigenically to the epitope on the antigen recognized by the original antibody

(Ab_1). Small doses of antibodies have been given to a large number of patients for tumour imaging and data are emerging—albeit anecdotal, but from several groups—that the prognosis of patients receiving antibody is improved. In the case of antibody 171A, a correlation between survival of colon cancer patients and anti-idiotypic response has been claimed (Frodin et al, 1991). This antibody, unconjugated, has been used in a multicentre trial of colon cancer patients who received several injections after surgery and chemotherapy (Reithmuller W, personal communication). This trial is now completing 8 years, and the survival curves are showing a separation, with antibody treatment being clearly beneficial. This effect may be operating, at least in part, through the anti-idiotype network.

A similar possibility has been raised following the very striking effect of administering yttrium labelled HMFG-1 antibody (directed to PEM) intraperitoneally to ovarian cancer patients. This study by Epenetos and colleagues showed a more than 90% survival in ovarian cancer patients who had minimal residual disease after surgery and chemotherapy and were subsequently treated with antibody (Hird et al, 1993). The dose of yttrium in this study was quite low, and it may be that, again, an anti-idiotype response is involved in the therapeutic effect.

The disadvantage of the anti-idiotype approach is that only one epitope of the antigen is expressed, compared to presenting the antigen itself with multiple epitopes. However, the presentation on an antibody may be very important in inducing a good immune response. With this in mind, other investigators have engineered sequences coding for an epitope on an antigen into the variable region of an antibody to improve presentation. All of these possible forms of antigen presentation can be tested in the mouse models we have described here.

SUMMARY

An understanding of the mechanisms involved in a biological phenomenon increases its potential for clinical exploitation. Thus, the simultaneous identification of TAA and the molecular mechanisms involved in antigen presentation and recognition by the immune system make the use of ASI a real possibility. The polymorphic epithelial mucin is expressed on most carcinomas and is highly immunogenic. Furthermore, it has many characteristics that make it potentially an ideal target molecule for ASI: (a) not only is it expressed, but it is upregulated by most carcinomas; (b) it is aberrantly glycosylated by carcinomas, resulting in the exposure of cryptic epitopes; (c) its tandem repeat structure results in there being many epitopes per molecule; (d) its extended structure at the surface means it is one of the first molecules the cells of the immune system encounter; and (e) its apparent ability to elicit HLA unrestricted killing already demonstrated in cancer patients makes it applicable to all individuals.

To move from the initial concept to preclinical testing, and eventually to clinical trial, is a long journey down an untravelled road, no doubt full of obstacles. Because the gene coding for PEM has been cloned, it has been possible to develop good preclinical models that we believe will allow rapid progress in evaluating the best form of antigen presentation. While these studies are going on, a start has been made in the clinic with the synthetic carbohydrate components of mucins. Some of us are optimistic that immunotherapy could quite soon become part of the repertoire of therapeutic modalities offered to breast and ovarian cancer patients, and indeed may even begin to be considered in prophylaxis of these diseases. As with any therapy in a disease as heterogeneous in its prognosis as breast cancer, evaluation of immunotherapy in the clinic will take time and commitment from the clinician and the patient as well as the laboratory research workers.

References

Barnd DL, Lan MS, Metzgar RS and Finn OJ (1989) Specific, major histocompatibility complex-unrestricted recognition of tumor-associated mucins by human cytotoxic T cells. *Proceedings of the National Academy of Sciences of the USA* **86** 7159–7164

Bartek J, Bartkova B and Vojtessek B (1990) Patterns of expression of the p53 tumor suppressor in human breast tissues and tumors in situ and in vitro. *International Journal of Cancer* **46** 839–844

Bartek J, Bartkova J, Kyprianou N *et al* (1991) Efficient immortalisation of luminal epithelial cells from the human mammary gland by the introduction of SV40 large T antigen using recombinant retrovirus. *Proceedings of the National Academy of Science of the USA* **88** 3520–3524

Berdichevsky F, Gilbert C, Shearer M and Taylor- Papadimitriou J (1992) Collagen-induced rapid morphogenesis of human mammary epithelial cells: the role of the α2β1 integrin. *Journal of Cell Science* **102** 437–446

Burchell J and Taylor-Papadimitriou J 1993 Effect of modification of carbohydrate side chains on the reactivity of antibodies with core-protein epitopes of the MUC1 gene product. *Epithelial Cell Biology* **2** 155–162

Burchell J, Gendler SJ, Taylor-Papadimitriou J *et al* (1987) Development and characterization of breast cancer reactive monoclonal antibodies directed to the core protein of the human milk mucin. *Cancer Research* **47** 5476–5482

Burchell J, Taylor-Papadimitriou J, Boshell M, Gender SJ and Duhig T (1989) A short sequence within the amino acid tandem repeat of a cancer associated mucin, contains immunodominant epitopes. *International Journal of Cancer* **44** 691–696

Chen L, Ashe S, Brady W *et al* (1992) Costimulation of antitumor immunity by the B7 counter-receptor for the T lymphocyte molecules CD28 and CTLA-4. *Cell* **71** 1093–1102

Ding L, Lalani E-N, Reddish M *et al* Immunogenicity of synthetic peptides related to the core peptide sequence encloded by the human MUC1 mucin gene: effect of immunization on the growth of murine mammary adenocarcinoma cells transfected with the human MUC1 gene. *Journal of Cancer Immunology and Immunotherapy* (in press)

Dranoff G, Jaffee E, Lazenby A *et al* (1993) Vaccination with irradiated tumor cells engineered to secrete murine GM-CSF stimulates potent, specific and long lasting antitumor immunity. *Proceedings of the National Academy of Sciences of the USA* **90** 3539–3543

Fearon ER, Pardoll DM, Itaya T *et al* (1990) Interleukin and production by tumor cells bypasses T helper function in the generation of an antitumor response. *Cell* **60** 397–403

Frodin JE, Faxas ME, Hagstrom B *et al* (1991) Induction of anti-idiotypic (ab$_2$) and anti-anti-idiotypic (ab$_3$) antibodies in patients treated with the mouse monoclonal antibody 17-1A

(ab_1): relation to the clinical outcome—an important antitumoral effector function? *Hybridoma* **10** 421–431

Fung PYS, Madej M, Koganty R and Longnecker BM (1990) Active specific immunotherapy of a murine mammary adenocarcinoma using a synthetic tumor-associated glycoconjugate. *Cancer Research* **50** 4308

Gendler SJ, Lancaster CA, Taylor-Papadimitriou J *et al* (1990) Molecular cloning and expression of the human tumor-associated polymorphic epithelial mucin. *Journal of Biological Chemistry* **265** 15286–15293

Girling JR, Bartkova J, Burchell J, Gendler S, Gillett C and Taylor-Papadimitriou J (1989) A core protein epitope of the polymorphic epithelial mucin detected by the monoclonal antibody SM-3 is selectively exposed in a range of primary carcinomas. *International Journal of Cancer* **43** 1072–1076

Gum JR, Byrd J, Hicks J, Toribara N, Lamport D and Kim Y (1989) Molecular cloning of human intestinal mucin cDNAs. *Journal of Biological Chemistry* **264** 6480–6487

Gum JR, Hicks J, Swallow D *et al* (1990) Molecular cloning of cDNAs derived from a novel human intestinal mucin gene. *Biochemical and Biophysical Research Communications* **171** 407–415

Gum JR, Hicks JW, Toribara NW, Rothe EM, Lagace RE and Kim YS (1992) The human MUC2 intestinal mucin has cysteine-rich subdomains located both upstream and downstream of its central repetitive region. *Journal of Biological Chemistry* **267** 21375–21383

Hanisch FG, Uhlenbruck G, Peter-Katalinic J, Egge H, Dabrowski J and Dabrowski U (1989) Structures of neutral O-linked polylactosaminoglycans on human skim milk mucins: a novel type of linearly extended poly-N-acetyl-lactosamine backbones with Galβ(1-4) GlcNAcβ(1-6) repeating units. *Journal of Biological Chemistry* **265** 872–883

Hilkens J, Ligtenberg MJ, Vos H and Litvinov SV (1992) Cell membrane-associated mucins and their adhesion-modulating property. *Trends in Biochemical Science* **17** 359–363

Hird V, Snook D, Dhokia B *et al* (1993) Adjuvant therapy of ovarian cancer with radioactive monoclonal antibody. *British Journal of Cancer* **68** 403–406

Hoffman W (1988) A new repetitive protein from *Xenopus laevis* skin highly homologous to pancreatic spasmolytic polypeptide. *Journal of Biological Chemistry* **263** 7686–7690

Hull SR, Bright A, Carraway KL, Abe M, Hayes DF and Kufe DW (1989) Oligosaccharide differences in the DF3 sialomucin antigen from normal human milk and the BT-20 human breast carcinoma cell line. *Cancer Communications* **1** 261–267

Jentoff N (1990) Why are proteins o-glycosylated? *Trends in Biochemistry* **15** 291–294

Jerome KR, Barnd KL, Bendt KM *et al* (1991) Cytotoxic T-lymphocytes derived from patients with breast adenocarcinoma recognize an epitope present on the protein core of a mucin molecule preferentially expressed by malignant cells. *Cancer Research* **51** 2908–2916

Kovarik A, Peat N, Wilson D, Gendler SJ and Taylor-Papadimitriou J (1993) Analysis of the tissue specific promoter of the MUC1 gene. *Journal of Biological Chemistry* **268** 9917–9926

Lalani EN, Berdichevsky F, Boshell M *et al* (1991) Expression of the gene coding for a human mucin in mouse mammary tumor cells can affect their tumorigenicity. *Journal of Biological Chemistry* **266** 15420–15426

Lanzavecchia A (1993) Identifying strategies for immune intervention. *Science* **260** 937–944

Ligtenberg M, Vos H, Gennissen A and Hilkens J (1990) Episialin, a carcinoma-associated mucin, is generated by a polymorphic gene encoding splice variants with alternative amino termini. *Journal of Biological Chemistry* **265** 5573–5578

McGee JM (1991) Immunotherapy for malignant melanoma: a review and update. *Seminars in Surgical Oncology* **7** 217–220

McLean GD, Howen-Yacyshyn MB, Samuel J *et al* (1992) Active immunization of human ovarian cancer patients against a common carcinoma (Thomsen-Friedenreich) determinant using a synthetic carbohydrate antigen. *Journal of Immunotherapy* **11** 292–305

Mitchell MS (1991) Attempts to optimize active specific immunotherapy for melanoma. *Inter-*

national Review of Immunology **7** 331–347

Nishimori I, Perini F, Mountjoy K, Caffray T and Hollingworth A (1993) Identification of o-glycosylation sites on MUC1 tandem repeat peptides glycosylated by pancreatic and breast adenocarcinoma cell lines. *Journal of Cellular Biochemistry* **Supplement 17A** 374

Peat N, Gendler SJ, Lalani E-N, Duhig T and Taylor-Papadimitriou J (1992) Tissue-specific expression of a human polymorphic epithelial mucin (MUC1) in transgenic mice. *Cancer Research* **52** 1954–1960

Porchet N, Van Cong N, Dufosse J *et al* (1991) Molecular cloning and chromosomal localization of a novel human tracheo-bronchial mucin cDNA containing tandemly repeated sequences of 48 base pairs. *Biochemical and Biophysical Research Communications* **175** 414–422

Rochlitz CF, Scott GK, Dodson JM *et al* (1989) The incidence of activating ras oncogene mutations associated with primary and metastatic human breast cancer. *Cancer Research* **15** 357–360

Rughetti A, Turchi V, Ghetti CA *et al* 1993) Human B-cell immune response to the polymorphic epithelial mucin. *Cancer Research* **53** 2457–2459

Schwartz RM (1992) Costimulation of T lymphocytes: the role of CD28, CTLA-4 and B7/BB1 in interleukin-2 production and immunotherapy. *Cell* **71** 1065–1068

Siddiqui J, Abe M, Hayes D, Shani E, Yunis E and Kufe D (1988) Isolation and sequencing of a cDNA coding for the human DF3 breast carcinoma-associated antigen. *Proceedings of the National Academy of Sciences of the USA* **85** 2320–2323

Singhal A, Fohn M and Hakomori S (1991) Induction of α-N-acetylgalactosamine-O-serine/threonine (Tn) antigen-mediated cellular immune response for active immunotherapy in mice. *Cancer Research* **51** 1406–1414

Slamon DJ, Clark GM, Wong WJ *et al* (1987) Human breast cancer: correlation of relapse and survival with amplification of the HER-2/neu oncogene. *Science* **235** 177–182

Spicer AP, Parry G, Patton S and Gendler SJ (1991) Molecular cloning and analysis of the mouse homologue of the tumor-associated mucin, MUC1, reveals conservation of potential O-glycosylation sites, transmembrane and cytoplasmic domains and a loss of minisatellite-like polymorphism. *Journal of Biological Chemistry* **266** 15099–15109

Tao MH and Levy R (1993) Idiotype/granulocyte-macrophage colony-stimulating factor fusion protein as a vaccine for B-cell lymphoma. *Nature* **362** 756–758

Taylor-Papadimitriou J (1991) Report on the First International Workshop on Carcinoma-associated Mucins. *International Journal of Cancer* **49** 1–5

Taylor-Papadimitriou J, Stewart L, Burchell J and Beverley P (1993) The polymorphic epithelial mucin as a target for immunotherapy. *Cancer Vaccines* **3** (1347) 73–93

Timpte C, Eckhardt A, Abernethy J and Hill R (1988) Porcine submaxillary gland apomucin contains tandemly repeated, identical sequences of 81 residues. *Journal of Biological Chemistry* **263** 1081–1088

Townsend S and Allison J (1993) Tumor rejection after direct costimulation of CD8+ cells by B7-transfected melanoma cells. *Science* **259** 368–370

Van der Bruggen P, Travewari C, Chomez P *et al* (1991) A gene encoding an antigen recognized by cytolytic T lymphocytes on a human melanoma. *Science* **254** 1643–1647

Vile RG, Goss M and Hart I (1993) In vitro and in vivo targeting of gene-expression to melanoma cells. *Journal of Cellular Biochemistry* **(Supplement 17E)** 209

Vos HL, Devarayalu Y, de Vries and Bornstein P (1992) Thrombospondin 3 (Thbs3), a new member of the thrombospondin gene family. *Journal of Biological Chemistry* **267** 12192–12196

Wreschner DH, Hareuveni M, Tsarfaty I *et al* (1990) Human epithelial tumor antigen cDNA sequences. *European Journal of Biochemistry* **189** 463–473

Zotter S, Hageman PC, Lossnitzer A, Mooi WJ and Hilgers J (1988) Tissue and tumor distribution of human polymorphic epithelial mucin. *Cancer Reviews* **11-12** 55–107

The authors are responsible for the accuracy of the references.

The Hormonal Milieu and Prognosis in Operable Breast Cancer

IAN S FENTIMAN • WALTER M GREGORY

ICRF Clinical Oncology Unit, Guy's Hospital, London SE1 9RT

Introduction
Menstrual cycle changes
The unopposed oestrogen hypothesis
Supportive and contradictory data
Meta-analysis of published studies
Direct endocrine measurements
Why are the results so heterogeneous?
Summary

INTRODUCTION

The outcome of treatment for operable breast cancer is in part dependent on characteristics of the primary tumour. Thus, patients with poorly differentiated lesions tend to have a worse prognosis and those with axillary nodal metastases have an increased risk of relapse that is arithmetically related to the number of nodes involved (Nemoto *et al*, 1980). However, the characteristics of the patient herself may also have an impact on survival. Postmenopausal women who are obese have a worse 5 year survival than thinner patients after controlling for tumour size and nodal involvement (Boyd *et al*, 1981).

The heterogeneous behaviour of breast cancer is a result of differences not only between tumours and patients, but also in primary treatment. There is evidence of shedding of malignant cell clumps at the time of surgery, and these may be detected by immunocytochemistry of bone marrow aspirates (Mansi *et al*, 1987; Cote *et al*, 1988). Further evidence of perioperative dissemination of malignant cells is suggested by the study that showed that a 6 day course of postoperative cyclophosphamide achieved a significant reduction in recurrence and mortality from breast cancer compared with untreated control cases (Nissen-Meyer *et al*, 1978).

MENSTRUAL CYCLE CHANGES

Hormonal fluctuations within the normal menstrual cycle produce multiple functional changes in breast tissue, the most noticeable being premenstrual fullness, sometimes amounting to discomfort and occasionally to pain for which treatment is required (Fentiman, 1992). At a cellular level within the normal breast, it has been shown that the thymidine labelling index of lobules is higher during the second half (luteal phase) of the menstrual cycle (Goring *et al*, 1988).

Ratajczak *et al* (1988) postulated that the menstrual cycle could influence the behaviour of breast tumours and investigated this using the C3HeB/FeJ mouse model. The animals were implanted in the left hind leg with a transplantable mammary carcinoma from an inbred C3H mouse. The leg and tumour were resected 14–17 days later and the animals still alive were sacrificed 28–42 days later. The menstrual phase was determined by cytological evaluation of vaginal washings.

The menstrual phase at the time of tumour inoculation had no effect on metastatic spread, whereas the timing of tumour resection had a significant impact. Thus, of the mice who had postoestrus resection, 16% showed no evidence of disease 1 month later compared with 40% of those who underwent surgery during the near oestrus phase. Similarly at 5 months, of those whose tumours were amputated in the postoestrus phase, 12% were disease free against 27% of the preoestrus surgery group.

As a result of this work, a review was conducted of 41 premenopausal women who had undergone surgery in Los Angeles for breast cancer and were having regular menstrual cycles and not taking oral contraception. The date of last menstrual period (LMP) was known for all cases and they were divided into two groups, mid-cycle (days 7–20) and perimenstrual (days 0–6 and 21–36). All were followed up for 7–14 years. There were 22 women in the mid-cycle group of whom one (5%) developed local relapse. In the perimenstrual group, there were 19 cases and 5 (26%) of these developed local relapse. Distant recurrence occurred in two (9%) of the mid-cycle cases and six (32%) of the perimenstrual cases. There was one (5%) death in the former group and four (21%) in the latter. Both overall recurrence and local recurrence occurred with significantly increased frequency in those undergoing surgery in the perimenstrual phase.

Subsequent analyses by other groups using similar criteria to divide the menstrual cycle, however, were not able to confirm these findings (Gelber and Goldhirsch, 1989; Powles *et al*, 1989). In another attempt to study this question, for a consecutive series of 21 premenopausal patients who had a mastectomy in the University of Minnesota Hospitals, menstrual information was available for only one (Gruber *et al*, 1989). It was suggested that an accurate menstrual history should be an essential part of preoperative evaluation of women with breast cancer. This prompted another analysis of 279 premenopausal women treated at Centre René Huguenin (Ville *et al*, 1990). There were 136 women who underwent surgery in the perimenstrual phase and 143 whose operations were performed mid-cycle. After a median follow-up of 5 years, the mortality rate was 20% in the mid-cycle group and 21% in the premenstrual group. Thus, examined in this way, timing of surgery within the menstrual cycle did not appear to have any significant impact on prognosis.

THE UNOPPOSED OESTROGEN HYPOTHESIS

Several lines of evidence suggest that oestrogens exert an effect on established breast cancers. Firstly, castration can induce regression of lesions in patients with advanced breast cancer, and this was first demonstrated by Beatson almost a century ago (Beatson, 1896). Subsequent work has indicated that the responsiveness of tumours depends on the presence of functional oestrogen receptors (Jensen *et al*, 1967). This is related to the differentiation of the primary carcinoma. Thus, grade I infiltrating ductal carcinomas are more likely to have oestrogen receptors and respond to oestrogen withdrawal or blockade than grade III carcinomas (Millis, 1987). Furthermore, studies of breast carcinoma cells in vitro have shown that the addition of oestrogens can lead to cell proliferation and the induction of proteases, which might play a part in invasion and metastasis (Lippman *et al*, 1986; Rochefort *et al*, 1988; Manni *et al*, 1990).

This being so, the hormonal milieu at the time of surgery might have an impact on the cohesion of the primary tumour and the possibility for dissemination during resection of the tumour. It was postulated that unopposed oestrogens might be responsible for loss of tumour cohesion and thus the patient who had surgery between days 3 and 12 of the menstrual cycle would be at increased risk of dissemination of malignant cells as a result of tumour handling during the operative procedure.

To test this hypothesis, a review was conducted of all premenopausal patients with operable breast cancer treated at Guy's Hospital between 1975 and 1985 (Badwe *et al*, 1991a). A total of 560 cases were identified from the database. No information was available for LMP in 151 of these and a further 96 had irregular periods so that their menstrual phase could not be calculated. In addition, there were 24 patients who had a prior hysterectomy with presentation of at least one ovary, 22 taking oral contraceptives and 18 excluded for miscellaneous reasons including pregnancy, lactation and hormone replacement therapy. Thus, there was a residue of 249 cases who formed the basis of the analysis. A comparison of the overall survival of those for whom LMP data were available and the 151 with unknown LMP showed that there was no significant difference.

The study group was divided into two subgroups: those who underwent surgery between days 3 and 12 of the cycle (n=75) and those who had an operation on days 0–2 and 13–32 (n=174). In terms of conventional prognostic factors including tumour size, type, nodal involvement, receptor status or use of adjuvant therapy, there were no significant differences between the two subgroups. As Fig. 1 shows, there was a highly significant difference in terms of overall survival. At 10 years, there was an actuarial survival of 54% in those treated between days 3 and 12, and 84% among the subgroup treated at other times of the cycle. There was a small difference between the two subgroups in terms of local relapse free survival, which was worse in the group treated between days 3 and 12 (p<0.04), and a highly significant difference in terms of recurrence free survival (p<0.001) and distant metastases free survival

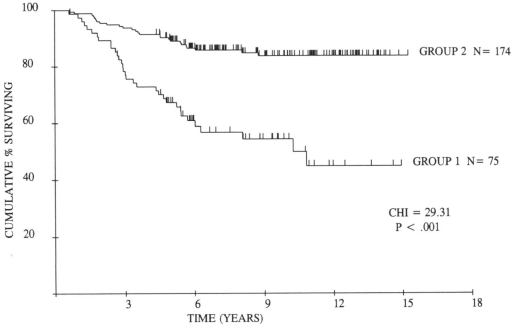

Fig. 1. Overall survival by timing of surgery. Group 1 = patients with late menstrual period (LMP) 3–12 days before surgery. Group 2 = patients with LMP 0–2 and 13–33 days before surgery. CHI = χ square value

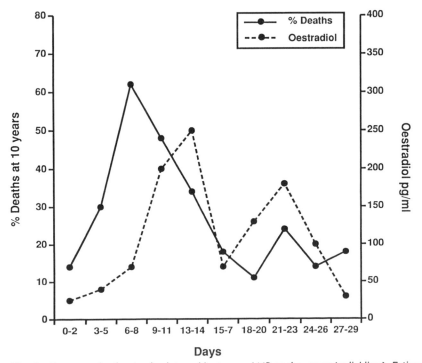

Fig. 2. Ten year death rates by interval between LMP and surgery (solid line). Estimated oestradiol levels at same intervals (broken line)

TABLE 1. Significance of prognostic factors for survival and recurrence free survival

Factor	Univariate χ^2	p	Multivariate χ^2	p
Survival				
number of nodes	33.3	<0.0001	39.7	<0.0001
LMP day	25.1	<0.0001	33.1	<0.0001
tumour type/grade	20.9	<0.0001	23.5	<0.0001
age	3.1	0.8	4.6	0.03
Recurrence free survival				
number of nodes	33.0	<0.0001	45.4	<0.0001
LMP day	22.6	<0.0001	25.2	<0.0001
tumour type/grade	16.4	0.0001	19.5	<0.0001
adjuvant therapy	0.2	0.69	5.6	0.02
age	3.4	0.07	4.3	0.04

(p<0.0001), all favouring the group who had surgery during either the immediate postmenstrual or luteal phases. Percentage death rates were calculated for 3 day intervals within the menstrual cycle, and these are shown in Fig. 2, together with expected oestradiol levels at those times. There is a close congruence between death rates and oestradiol levels.

A multivariate analysis of survival was performed using Cox's proportional hazards model (Cox, 1972). A comparison of univariate and multivariate analyses of prognostic factors is given in Table 1. For overall survival, the number of involved axillary nodes, LMP day and tumour type/grade were significant on both univariate and multivariate analyses. Similar results were obtained in terms of prognosis factors for relapse free survival.

Finally, the original data presented by Hrushesky et al (1989) were recalculated using the Guy's timing intervals, and it was found that the relapse free survival was 62% for those who had surgery between days 3 and 12 and 79% in those who had tumours excised at other times. Because of the small numbers, the difference did not achieve statistical significance, but it was similar in both magnitude and direction to the difference found in the Guy's study.

The overall survival within the various prognostic subgroups was calculated for those operated upon in the two different menstrual phases, as shown in Table 2. The same magnitude of difference was found in all subgroups, except for axillary node metastasis. For patients operated upon between days 3 and 12, who were node negative, the 10 year survival was 82% compared with 89% for those who had surgery at other times (p=0.24). However, among node positive cases, the survival for the former group was 33% compared with 78% in the latter group. Thus, the menstrual phase was of particular prognostic importance for node positive patients.

Interestingly, the oestrogen receptor (ER) status did not seem to have a significant role, with a similar magnitude of effect occurring in both ER positive and ER negative cases. This suggests that the predominant effect might be

TABLE 2. Survival within LMP and prognostic subgroups

| | Ten year actuarial survival | | |
	group 1[a] no. (%)	group 2[b] no. (%)	p
Tumour size			
<2 cm	30 (55)	75 (93)	<0.001
2–4 cm	35 (59)	80 (80)	<0.02
>4 cm	10 (44)	19 (63)	0.32
Lymph node metastasis			
negative	33 (82)	91 (89)	0.24
1–3 nodes positive	27 (39)	55 (85)	<0.001
4–9 nodes positive	9 (30)	16 (81)	<0.001
≥10 nodes positive	7	12 (42)	0.19
Oestrogen receptors (ER)			
ER negative	19 (42)	46 (83)	<0.001
ER positive	43 (57)	102 (81)	<0.001
Histopathology			
grade I/II	36 (64)	91 (90)	<0.001
grade III	21 (43)	49 (70)	<0.01
Primary treatment			
breast conservation	15 (70)	39 (84)	0.44
mastectomy	60 (52)	135 (85)	<0.001
Adjuvant systemic therapy			
no treatment	26 (33)	35 (65)	<0.002
melphalan	8 (14)	19 (89)	<0.001
cyclophosphamide			
methotrexate 5 fluorouracil	7 (71)	27 (85)	0.42

[a]Group 1: surgery days 0–2, 3–12
[b]Group 2: surgery days 13–32

on normal (ER containing) tissue around the tumour rather than a direct effect on the tumour cells.

Because of the size of the observed effect and the potential implications in terms of rescheduling surgery, a second review was performed of patients treated at Guy's Hospital after 1985 (Badwe *et al,* 1991b). There were 150 patients for whom data were available on LMP; 95 underwent tumour excision between days 0–2 and 13–33, with 55 women whose surgery was conducted between days 3 and 12. Relapse free survival of the two groups is shown in Fig. 3. As in the previous study, the survival of those undergoing surgery between days 3 and 12 was significantly worse than that of patients treated at other times of the menstrual cycle ($\chi^2 = 13$; p<0.001). However, the magnitude of the difference was less than that observed in the previous study.

Further analysis suggested that the reduction in the effect of LMP might result from the different method of making the histological diagnosis in patients treated after 1985. Whereas previously the majority of patients had an

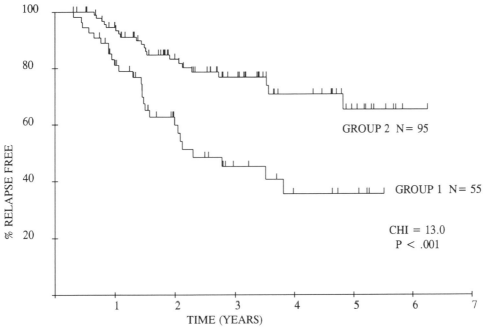

Fig. 3. Relapse free survival of patients treated after 1985. Group 1 = patients with LMP 3–12 days before surgery. Group 2 = patients with LMP 0–2 and 13–33 days before surgery. CHI = χ square value

excision of the carcinoma for histological confirmation of malignancy, many of the later patients had a trucut needle biopsy performed under a local anaesthetic when first seen in the clinic (Fentiman *et al*, 1986). Thus, some patients had a trucut needle biopsy performed between days 3 and 12 but subsequent tumour excision/mastectomy between days 0–2 and 13–33. The comparative relapse free survival for patients who had surgery performed at a "favourable" time is shown in Fig. 4, which shows three subgroups: needle biopsy at a favourable time, no needle biopsy and needle biopsy at an unfavourable time. The latter group fared very badly, suggesting that a needle biopsy between days 3 and 12 could lead to a high risk of development of metastatic disease. That tumour handling at this time could be dangerous was also suggested by analysis of timing of mammography and outcome. In a univariate analysis, this had a prognostic effect if performed in the first half of the menstrual cycle, although the effect was lost on multivariate analysis.

SUPPORTIVE AND CONTRADICTORY DATA

At almost the same time, supportive data were published from Memorial Sloan-Kettering Cancer Center, New York (Senie *et al*, 1991). The study group comprised 283 premenopausal women with breast cancer treated by mastectomy and axillary clearance. Patients were divided into two groups, those un-

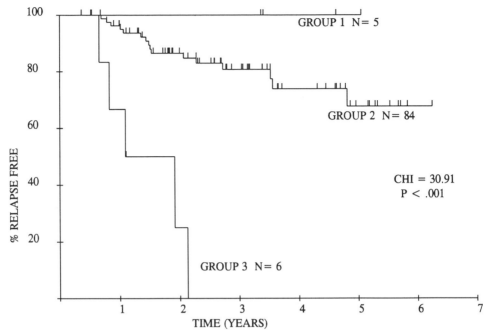

Fig. 4. Relapse free survival of patients who underwent surgery between days 0–2 and 13–33. Group 1 = needle biopsy at favourable time. Group 2 = no needle biopsy. Group 3 = needle biopsy at unfavourable time. CHI = χ square value

dergoing surgery in the follicular phase (1–14) and in the luteal phase (15–28). The group who underwent follicular phase surgery had a significantly worse 10 year survival (29% v. 43%). Further analysis showed that, as in the Guy's studies, the risk was carried predominantly by women with positive axillary lymph nodes with a hazard rate of 1.97 for node positive cases operated on during the follicular phase and 1.07 for node negative patients.

In an accompanying editorial to the Senie paper, McGuire (1991) expressed scepticism about the relation between timing of surgery and outcome. McGuire's major argument was that the findings could be the result of chance, since if the menstrual cycle were divided up arbitrarily into enough subgroups there was a high probability of finding a difference in at least one of these by chance. It was suggested that other negative studies backed the assertion that the positive results were statistical artefacts.

This was disputed by the Guy's group, who pointed out that results were obtained as a result of a prior hypothesis and not from data manipulation to obtain the best fit (Gregory, 1992). In addition, the Guy's data were split into random subgroups to test McGuire's hypothesis. Using a p value of 0.05 as the definition of positivity, there were 28% positive results in 100 such random assignments. However, with the p value of 6×10^{-8}, which was the actual Guy's result, no positive results occurred in 10 000 further random assignments.

Furthermore, a meta-analysis was conducted of data from ten published studies. This showed a significant overall effect for timing of surgery (p=0.003). The χ square for heterogeneity was 18.9 (9 degrees of freedom), suggesting that the differences between the studies could not be explained by random chance. Since the original meta-analysis, several new studies have been published, both supporting and contradicting the hypothesis that timing of surgery influences survival, and therefore a new overview has been conducted.

META-ANALYSIS OF PUBLISHED STUDIES

Each survival curve was carefully measured to establish a 5 year survival figure. In a few cases, survival curves were not shown, but 5 year survival figures were reported. In cases where survival data were not given, 5 year progression free data were used instead. Nearly all the studies had a minimum follow-up of more than 5 years. For the few exceptions, it was necessary to make an approximation of the numbers followed up at 5 years and the likely censoring times of patients censored before this time. This was then used to estimate an effective sample size at 5 years, using the method described by Simon (1986). It was then usually a straightforward calculation to establish the number of deaths that must have occurred up to this time. Having estimated the number of deaths in the different arms of the trial at 5 years, the expected number of deaths, given no difference between the treatments, could be calculated. Thus, the overview methodology described in detail by Peto (1987) could be applied to these figures. In brief, the difference between the number of observed and number of expected deaths is derived for each trial. These O–E figures are then summed over the whole set of trials to form a grand total. The variance of the individual estimates is also derived and summed, giving a variance and thus a standard deviation (SD) for the grand total. The number of standard deviations (z) by which the grand total differs from zero gives an estimate of the significance of any effect. The O–Es can also be tested for heterogeneity to see whether the scatter of results is unexpected (the quantity [C–DD/V] where C is the sum of $[O-E]^2$/variance, D is the sum of [O–E] and V is the sum of variances, should be distributed as χ square with n – 1 degrees of freedom if the scatter is random, where n is the number of studies).

The size of any treatment effect, specifically the typical odds ratio (TOR), is simply estimated as exp(z/SD), with approximate 95% confidence limits exp(z/SD +/- 1.96/SD). Confidence limits for the individual trials can be calculated in the same fashion. The TORs and their confidence limits for each trial, along with the grand total, can then be displayed as in Fig. 5. The sizes of the solid squares are chosen to be directly proportional to the amount of information each trial contains. Since many individual trials are displayed, 99% confidence limits are shown for the individual trials. For the single overall result, 95% confidence limits are given (these are represented by the unshaded diamond in Fig. 5).

OVERVIEW OF PUBLISHED LMP STUDIES (5 YEAR SURVIVAL RESULTS)

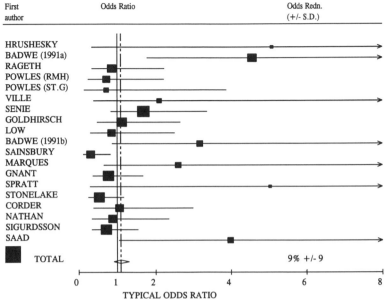

Fig. 5. Meta-analysis of published LMP studies (5 year survival results)

The TORs for all the trials, along with 99% confidence intervals, are shown in Fig. 7, ordered (approximately) by time of publication. The grand total of summed O–Es is 10.7 (implying the possible avoidance of 21 deaths by treating in the luteal phase of the cycle), with SD equal to 10.9, and thus z = grand total/SD = 0.98, which is not statistically significant (p=0.33). This initially suggests that there is no difference in survival by treatment in different phases of the menstrual cycle. However, three trials showed anomalous results (in different directions), with 99% confidence limits that did not include a TOR of 1 (equivalent to no effect). Furthermore, the test for heterogeneity of the O–Es was significant (χ^2_{18} = 57.9, p=0.000004) confirming that the scatter of results is unexpected and not normally distributed. Thus, differences are apparent between centres that cannot be explained as chance findings.

DIRECT ENDOCRINE MEASUREMENTS

It could be argued that information on the phase of the menstrual cycle that had been gathered retrospectively from hospital notes might not be reliable. Direct endocrine measurements on blood taken at the time of surgery would provide a more accurate estimate of the phase of the menstrual cycle, certainly insofar as whether patients were in the luteal phase.

Between 1975 and 1985, blood had been collected from the majority of patients with operable breast cancer treated at Guy's Hospital. The original intention was to examine both prospectively and retrospectively a variety of

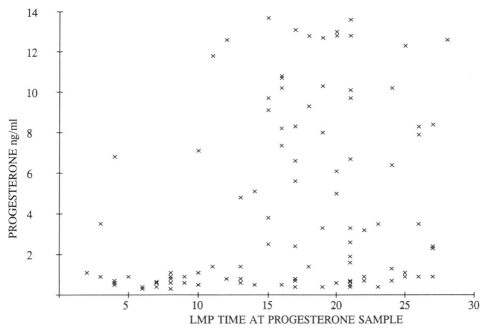

Fig. 6. Relation between last menstrual period and serum progesterone levels

putative prognostic markers. Blood had been taken and serum stored at −20°C from 271 premenopausal patients, usually 1 day before or 2 days after excision of the primary tumour. Among the 271 patients, blood was taken within 3 days of tumour excision in 210 (77%).

Data on LMP and regular cycle were available for 121 patients (45%). Levels of both oestradiol and progesterone were measured using radioimmunoassay (Badwe *et al*, in press). When oestradiol levels were plotted against time since last LMP, no relation was observed, nor was there any relation between oestradiol levels and survival. However, as Fig. 6 shows, there was a close relation between time elapsed since LMP and serum progesterone levels. This indicates that the majority of women who had blood samples taken during the first 12 days of the cycle had progesterone levels of less than 1.5 ng/ml. Some of the patients sampled in the second half of the cycle may have had anovulatory cycles and therefore low progesterone levels, but these data in general validate the accuracy of LMP derived from clinical notes.

Using a cutoff point of 1.5 ng/ml, the patients were divided into two groups (<1.5 and >1.5). Among the node negative cases, there was no difference in the survival of the two groups. However, as Fig. 7 shows, stratification of node positive cases based on serum progesterone levels demonstrated a better survival among the group with progesterone levels greater than 1.5 ng/ml, who underwent surgery during the luteal phase.

A multivariate analysis indicated that the time of LMP gave significant prognostic information for node positive patients, but when this was taken into account, progesterone levels no longer had prognostic significance. Among

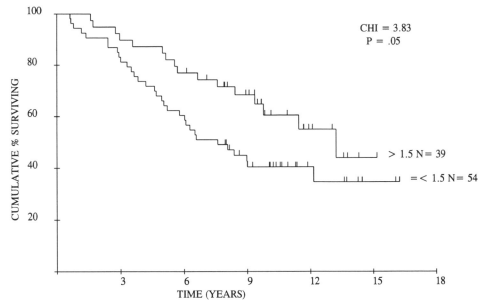

Fig. 7. Survival of node positive patients with serum progesterone levels <1.5 ng/ml and >1.5 ng/ml. CHI = chi square value

patients with progesterone levels less than 1.5 ng/ml, the relative risk of dying was twice that for those with levels greater than 1.5 ng/ml. Thus, this third study provided further evidence that the endocrine milieu at the time of tumour excision had a major effect on patient outcome. Taking all these lines of evidence into account has convinced those working on the ICRF Clinical Oncology Unit that this is an important phenomenon deserving further study and has meant that surgical procedures have been rescheduled for the luteal phase in women aged 30 years or more who have a lesion that might be malignant.

WHY ARE THE RESULTS SO HETEROGENEOUS?

As shown in the meta-analysis, although there is no overall significant effect, there is great heterogeneity among the results of studies examining the relation between timing of surgery and prognosis. The distribution of results is not normal. Why should this be? Firstly, it is important that the date of LMP before surgery is correct. This depends on checking primary records, not computer files, and ascertaining those individuals with regular cycles where menstrual phase could then be calculated.

Secondly, it is not just the time at which tumour excision or mastectomy occurs that is important. The timing of needle biopsy and possibly fine needle aspiration cytology and mammography may also be responsible for predisposing to shedding of viable micrometastases in susceptible individuals (those with axillary nodal involvement). One reason why the results were so clear cut in the first Guy's study may have been the structured way in which patients were managed, with biopsies being performed at definite times and with an almost constant interval between primary biopsy and definitive surgery.

Finally, the primary treatment may also be important. At Guy's, patients were treated either by modified radical mastectomy or by breast conservation comprising tumour excision, axillary clearance, iridium implant and external radiotherapy. Both regimens have been compared in a prospective randomized trial of over 900 patients that showed that both were equally effective in terms of local control and overall survival (van Dongen *et al*, 1992). Those using less adequate primary treatment such as simple mastectomy or axillary sampling may fail to achieve maximal local control which might mask the effect of timing of surgery (Axelsson *et al*, 1992).

Although the Guy's group are convinced that the finding is real, it is accepted that others do not. For the sceptics, it is important that they should keep accurate records of LMP and cycle length as a minimum. Others may wish to ask their patients to take part in a prospective randomized trial so that the important question of timing of surgery can be answered definitively.

SUMMARY

Evidence is presented from those studies which have shown that the timing of surgery affects the prognosis of premenopausal women with operable breast cancer. Those undergoing surgery at a time of unopposed oestrogen (days 3–12) had a significantly worse prognosis than those who had operations at other phases of the menstrual cycle.

This was also borne out by another study that indicated that progesterone levels at the time of surgery had prognostic significance, with node positive patients in the luteal phase (progesterone >1.5 ng/ml) having a significantly better outcome.

A meta-analysis has shown a highly significant heterogeneity of results, which do not overall show an effect. Possible reasons for this heterogeneity are discussed together with the need for prospective studies.

References

Axelsson CK, Mouridsen HT, Zedeler K *et al* (1992) Axillary dissection of level I and II lymph nodes is important in breast cancer classification. *European Journal of Cancer* **28A** 1415–1418

Badwe RA, Richards MA, Fentiman IS *et al* (1991a) Surgical procedures, menstrual cycle phase and prognosis in operable breast cancer. *Lancet* **338** 815–816

Badwe RA, Gregory WM, Chaudary MA *et al* (1991b) Timing of surgery during menstrual cycle and survival of premenopausal women with operable breast cancer. *Lancet* **i** 1261–1264

Badwe RA, Wang DY, Gregory WM *et al* Serum progesterone at the time of surgery and survival in women with premenopausal operable breast cancer. *European Journal of Cancer* (in press)

Beatson CT (1896) On treatment of inoperable cases of carcinoma of the mamma: suggestions for a new method of treatment with illustrative cases. *Lancet* **2** 104–107

Boyd NF, Campbell JE, Germanson T *et al* (1981) Body weight and prognosis in breast cancer. *Journal of the National Cancer Institute* **67** 785–789

Corder AP, Cross M, Julions SA, Mullee MA and Taylor I The timing of breast cancer surgery within the menstrual cycle. *British Journal of Surgery* (in press)

Cote RJ, Rosen PP, Hakes TB *et al* (1988) Monoclonal antibodies detect occult breast carcinoma metastases in the bone marrow of patients with early stage disease. *American Journal of Surgical Pathology* **12** 333–340

Cox DR (1972) Regression models and life tables. *Journal of the Royal Statistical Society* **34** 187–220

Fentiman IS (1992) Mastalgia mostly merits masterly inactivity. *British Journal of Clinical Practice* **46** 158

Fentiman IS, Millis RR, Chaudary MA *et al* (1986) The effect of the method of biopsy on the prognosis and reliability of receptor assays in patients with operable breast cancer. *British Journal of Surgery* **73** 610–612

Gelber RD and Goldhirsch A (1989) Menstrual effect on surgical cure of breast cancer. *Lancet* **ii** 1344

Gnant FX, Seifert M, Jakesz R, Adler A, Mittlboeck M and Sevelda P (1992) Breast cancer and timing of surgery during menstrual cycle. A 5-year analysis of 385 premenopausal women. *International Journal of Cancer* **52** 707–712

Goldhirsch A, Gelber RD, Forbes J *et al* (1991) Timing breast cancer surgery. *Lancet* **338** 692 (letter)

Goring JJ. Anderson TJ, Battersby S and MacIntyre CCA (1988) Proliferative and secretory activity in human breast during natural and artificial menstrual cycles. *American Journal of Pathology* **130** 193–204

Gregory WM, Richards MA and Fentiman IS (1992) Optimal timing of initial breast cancer surgery. *Annals of Internal Medicine* **116** 268–269

Gruber SA, Nichol KC, Sothern RB *et al* (1989) Menstrual history and breast cancer surgery. *Breast Cancer Research and Treatment* **13** 278

Hrushesky WJM, Bluming AZ, Gruber SA and Sothern RB (1989) Menstrual influence on surgical cure of breast cancer. *Lancet* **ii** 949–952

Jensen EV, De Sombre ER and Jungblut PW (1967) Estrogen receptors in hormone-responsive tissues and tumors, In: Wissler RW, Dao TL and Wood S Jr (eds). *Endogenous Factors Influencing Host-Tumor Balance*, pp 15–30, University of Chicago, Chicago

Lippman ME, Dickson RB, Bates S *et al* (1986) Autocrine and paracrine growth regulation of human breast cancer. *Breast Cancer Research and Treatment* **7** 59–70

Low SC, Galea MH and Blamey RW (1991) Timing breast cancer surgery. *Lancet* **338** 691 (letter)

McGuire WL (1991) The optimal timing of mastectomy: low tide or high tide? *Annals of Internal Medicine* **115** 401–403

Manni A, Wright C, Badger B *et al* (1990) Role of transforming growth factor alpha-related peptides in the autocrine/paracrine control of experimental breast cancer growth by estradiol, prolactin and progesterone. *Breast Cancer Research and Treatment* **15** 73–83

Mansi JL, Berger U, Easton D *et al* (1987) Micrometastases in bone marrow in patients with primary breast cancer: evaluation as an early predictor of bone metastases. *British Medical Journal* **295** 1093–1096

Marques LA and Franco EL (1993) Association between timing of surgery during menstrual cycle and prognosis in premenopausal breast cancer. *International Journal of Cancer* **53** 707–708 (letter)

Millis RR (1987) The relationship between the pathology of breast cancer and hormone sensitivity. *Reviews on Endocrine-Related Cancer* **20** 13–18

Nathan B, Bates T, Anbazhagan R and Norman AR (1993) Timing of surgery for breast cancer in relation to the menstrual cycle and survival of premenopausal women. *British Journal of*

Surgery **80** 43

Nemoto T, Vana J, Bedwani R *et al* (1980) Management and survival of female breast cancer: results of a national survey by the American College of Surgeons. *Cancer* **45** 2917–2924

Nissen-Meyer R, Kjellgren K, Malmio K, Mansson B and Norin T (1978) Surgical adjuvant chemotherapy. *Cancer* **41** 2088–2098

Peto R (1987) Why do we need systematic overviews of randomised trials. *Statistics in Medicine* **6** 233–240

Powles TJ, Jones AL, Ashley S and Tidy A (1989) Menstrual effect on surgical cure of breast cancer. *Lancet* **ii** 1343–1344

Powles TJ, Ashley SE, Nash AG, Tidy A, Gazet J-C and Ford HT (1991) Timing of surgery for breast cancer. *Lancet* **337** 1604 (letter)

Rageth JC, Wyss P, Unger C and Hochuli E (1991) Timing of breast cancer surgery within the menstrual cycle: influence on lymph node involvement receptor status, postoperative metastatic spread and local recurrence. *Annals of Oncology* **2** 269–272

Ratajczak HV, Sothern RB and Hruschesky WJM (1988) Estrous influence on surgical cure of a mouse breast cancer. *Journal of Experimental Medicine* **168** 73–83

Rochefort H, Angereau P, Briozzo P *et al* (1988) Structure, function, regulation and clinical significance of the 52K pro-cathepsin D secretion by breast cancer cells. *Biochimie* **70** 943–949

Saad Z, Bramwell V, Duff J *et al* Timing of surgery in relation to menstrual cycle in premenopausal women with operable breast cancer. *British Journal of Surgery* (in press)

Sainsbury R, Jones M, Parker D, Hall R and Close H (1991) Timing of surgery for breast cancer. *Lancet* **338** 392 (letter)

Senie RT, Rosen PP, Rhodes P *et al* (1991) Timing of breast cancer excision during the menstrual cycle influences duration of disease-free survival. *Annals of Internal Medicine* **115** 337–342

Siggurdson H, Baldetorp B, Borg A *et al* (1992) Timing of surgery in the menstrual cycle does not appear to be a significant determinant of outcome in primary breast cancer. *Proceedings of the American Society of Clinical Oncology* **11** 62

Simon RJ (1986) Confidence intervals for reporting results of clinical trials. *Annals of Internal Medicine* **105** 429–435

Spratt JS, Zirnheld J and Yancey JM (1993) Breast cancer detection demonstration project data can determine whether the prognosis of breast cancer is affected by the time of surgery during the menstrual cycle. *Journal of Surgery and Oncology* **53** 4–9

Stonelake PS, Baker PR and Morrison JM (1993) Timing of surgery during menstrual cycle for premenopausal women with breast cancer. Cancer UK Meeting, Sheffield [Abstract]

van Dongen JA, Bartelink H, Fentiman IS *et al* (1992) Factors influencing local relapse and survival and results of salvage treatment after breast conserving therapy in operable breast cancer: EORTC 10801 trial comparing breast conservation with mastectomy in TNM Stage I and II breast cancer. *European Journal of Cancer* **28** 801–804

Ville Y, Lasry S, Spyratos F *et al* (1990) Menstrual status and breast cancer surgery. *Breast Cancer Research and Treatment* **16** 119

The authors are responsible for the accuracy of the references.

Prognostic Factors and Response to Therapy in Breast Cancer

JAN G M KLIJN • ELS M J J BERNS • JOHN A FOEKENS

Division of Endocrine Oncology, Department of Medical Oncology, Rotterdam Cancer Institute (Daniel den Hoed Kliniek), Groene Hilledijk 301, 3075 EA Rotterdam, The Netherlands

INTRODUCTION

Since about 1985, a large number of modern cell biological parameters such as oncogenes/suppressor genes, growth factors and secretory proteins appear to influence strongly the behaviour of a tumour with respect to metastatic pat-

TABLE 1. Classification of prognostic factors in breast cancer (modified from review of Klijn and Foekens, 1990)

A. Patient characteristics:
    race
    age
    menopausal status
    performance status
    metabolic diseases

B. Variables determined in blood:
    tumour marker levels (carcinoembryonic antigen, CA15-3)
    haemoglobin, alkaline phsophatase, liver function tests
    fragment c receptor for Igτ (immunoglubulin τ) on mononuclear cells
    hormone levels
    growth factor levels

C. Tumour characteristics:
    1. histological features: type, grade, number of blood vessels, vascular invasion, necrosis
    2. stage (tumour, node, metastasis), bone marrow micrometastases
    3. cytoplasmic and nuclear steroid receptors: ER, PGR, AR, vitamin-D-receptor
    4. membrane receptors for hormones and growth factors:
        LHRHR
        Prolactin receptor
        IGF1R
        EGFR
        TGFBR
        SSR
    5. enzymes, proteins and other cytoplasmic factors:
        plasminogen activator expression
        plasminogen activator inhibitors (PAI1, PAI2)
        cathepsin D
        PS2 protein
        growth factor content (EGF, TGFA and B, IGF1)
        tyrosine kinase activities
        heat shock proteins
        aromatase activity
        haptoglobin-related protein (Hpr) epitope expression
        adhesion factors
        glutathione S transferase 3
        human milk fat globule antigens (HMFG-1)
        prostaglandin levels
    6. chromosomal abnormalities:
        cytogenetic
        ploidy
        amplification, (over)expression of oncogenes (*c-myc*, *HER2/neu/c-erbB2*, *int2*, *ras*)
        deletion or mutation of suppressor genes (*TP53*, *RB*, *nm23*)
    7. cell proliferation indices:
        labelling index
        S-phase fraction
        Ki-67 antigen
    8. clonogenicity
    9. immunological phenotypes

D. Response to treatment

UICC = International Union Against Cancer

TABLE 2. Clinical application of modern cell biological parameters in patients with breast cancer

1. For estimation of prognosis in patients with primary or metastatic breast cancer
2. For selection of high and low risk patients with respect to treating or not treating
3. For selection of type of therapy depending on tumour and patient characteristics
4. As target for new treatment modalities

tern, extent of cellular differentiation, growth rate and the development of resistance to therapy. Oncogenes may encode for growth factors, growth factor receptors, protein kinases, signal transducers, nuclear proteins and transcription factors. Most of these parameters have been tested as prognostic factors in order to refine risk assessment as routinely done by classical prognostic factors such as stage, grade and steroid receptor status. This is important in view of the discussion on overtreatment of a significant proportion of patients with early breast cancer and on cost effectiveness of adjuvant systemic therapy (McGuire, 1989). Accurate identification of high risk and low risk patients is therefore important. Consequently, at present, a large series of classical and modern prognostic factors has been reported (Table 1). Most of these factors have been evaluated with respect to relapse free survival and overall survival, but very few with respect to response to hormonal or chemotherapy in primary or metastatic disease (Klijn and Foekens, 1990; Foekens *et al*, 1991; Elledge *et al*, 1992; Klijn *et al*, 1993a,b, in press a). However, for patients with recurrent disease (macrometastases), prognostic factors and predictors of response to treatment are also clinically important for reaching decisions on type of therapy. Finally, a number of cell biological parameters such as growth factor receptors and proteases might be used in future studies as possible targets for new treatment modalities (Table 2). Therefore, the characterization of individual tumours is increasingly relevant. In this paper, we update and review the clinical significance of the most relevant cell biological parameters especially with respect to their predictive value for response to systemic therapy, focusing on our own results.

GENETIC ALTERATIONS

Apart from genetic modulation of the oestrogen receptor (ER) system (Fuqua, 1992), other genetic alterations may be related to the development of resistance for systemic endocrine therapy and chemotherapy. Amplification and overexpression of several oncogenes have been detected in breast cancers and have been found to be frequently related to more aggressive breast tumours, to poor prognosis and either negatively or positively to steroid receptor status (Klijn *et al*, 1993a, in press a). In human primary breast cancer, changes in three oncogenes—*HER2/neu*, *c-myc* and *int2*—occur relatively frequently. Changes in some suppressor genes (*nm23*, *TP53* and *RB*) might also be important for prognosis and prediction of response to treatment.

HER2/neu/c-erbB2

In a recent review of 11 408 breast tumours, we calculated a mean *HER2/neu* positivity of 20% without finding any significant difference between the incidence of amplification (20.6%) and overexpression (19.2%) (Klijn *et al*, 1992c). In our own large series of 1000 human primary breast tumours, we found an incidence of *HER2/neu* amplification of 18.7% (Berns *et al*, 1992a). Recent reviews indicate that there is no association between elevated *HER2/neu* and patient age, only a tentative relationship with tumour grade, size or node involvement, and an inverse association with steroid hormone receptor status (Gullick, 1990; Perren, 1991). There are increasing number of data on the predictive value of *HER2/neu* for response to endocrine therapy and chemotherapy. These data indicate quite uniformly that *HER2/neu* positive tumours show a poor response to endocrine therapy, but the data on the relation between *HER2/neu* and response to chemotherapy are conflicting.

In a preclinical study, MCF7 breast cancer cells transfected with *HER2* cDNA (MCF/HER2-18 cells) showed a 45-fold increase of *HER2/neu* expression compared with the parental cells (Benz *et al*, 1992). In contrast to the parental MCF7 cells, these MCF/HER2-18 cells appeared to be tamoxifen resistant both in vitro and in vivo in nude mice. In our clinical study (Berns *et al*, 1991; Klijn *et al*, 1992a), in 126 patients with metastatic breast cancer, *HER2/neu* amplified tumours showed a poor response to endocrine therapy with tamoxifen (Table 3), but a good response to subsequent chemotherapy resulting in no difference in overall postrelapse survival. Tumour growth inhibition as measured by complete remission, partial remission and stabilization of disease occurred in 53% of *HER2/neu* negative tumours and in only 21% of *HER2/neu* positive tumours ($p < 0.05$). Patients with *HER2/neu* positive tumours showed a shorter progression free survival (Fig. 1). A similar negative association between *HER2/neu* and response to tamoxifen treatment has been described by Nicholson *et al* (1990) and Wright *et al* (1992a). Measuring *HER2/neu* expression instead of amplification, they also found a low response rate (1 out of 14) to tamoxifen in tumours overexpressing *HER2/neu*. The extracellular domain of the HER2/neu oncogene product may circulate in human plasma. High levels of this neu related protein (≥ 2000 U/ml) were found in 36% of 242 patients with metastatic breast cancer (Hayes *et al*, 1993). Patients with high levels of neu related protein appeared to respond poorly to megestrol acetate compared with patients with low levels, although the efficacy of chemotherapy was not different between these subgroups of patients. However, in 33 patients with locally advanced disease, Quéenel *et al* (1993) did not observe a significant correlation between c-*erbB2* RNA levels (measured by dot blot hybridization from drill biopsy) and clinical response to neo-adjuvant therapy with tamoxifen.

With respect to chemotherapy, the results of studies on the relation between *HER2/neu* and response to therapy are conflicting and more difficult to interpret. Benz *et al* (1992) previously showed that MCF/HER2-18 cells had acquired resistance to cisplatin. In addition, in the in vitro studies of Pegram *et*

TABLE 3. Response rates (CR, PR, SD) by first line endocrine therapy (n=126) and second line chemotherapy (n=63) in patients with metastatic breast cancer in relation to oncogene amplification

Oncogene	Endocrine therapy (%)	Chemotherapy (%)
HER2/neu⁺	21	75
	p<0.05	
HER2/neu⁻	53	45
C-myc⁺	44	29
		p<0.02
C-myc⁻	47	64
int2⁺	40	58
int2⁻	46	50

+ = amplified; − = not amplified; CR = complete remission; PR = partial remission; SD = stabilization of disease

al (1993), using human breast and ovarian cancer cell lines, transfection of the *erbB2* gene caused no increase in drug sensitivity to doxorubicin, carboplatin, etoposide, 5-fluorouracil and thiotepa. However, the c-*erbB2* expressing MCF7 breast cancer cells were 2.5-fold less sensitive to carboplatin and 5-fluorouracil in their study than the maternal cell line without *erbB2* gene expression (Pegram *et al*, 1993). However, after transplantation of the transfected MCF7 cells into a nude mouse, increased chemosensitivity was observed in vivo (Pegram *et al*, 1993). In patients with metastatic disease, *HER2/neu* positive tumours were also related to a high sensitivity to chemo-

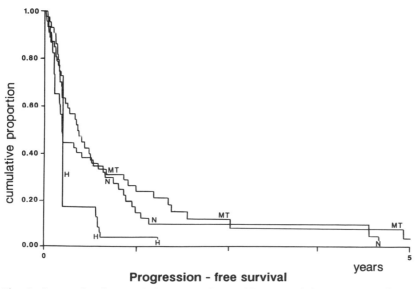

Progression - free survival

Fig. 1. Progression free survival in 126 patients with metastatic breast cancer after start of first line endocrine therapy according to type of oncogene amplified. H = patients with *HER2/neu* amplification; MT = patients with c-*myc* or *int2* amplification; N = patients with no amplification of any of the three oncogenes in their primary breast tumours

therapy. Seventy five percent of our patients with a *HER2/neu* positive tumours showed a response to chemotherapy (mainly CMF) in contrast to 45% of *HER2/neu* negative tumours (see Table 3). The median length of progression-free and overall survival from start of chemotherapy was 6 months longer in our patients whose tumours exhibited *HER2/neu* amplification as compared to patients with normal *HER2/neu* gene copy number. However, Wright *et al* (1992b), studying the relation between c-*erbB2* expression and response to mitoxanthrone in 68 patients with advanced breast cancer, reported opposite results as compared to our data. In contrast to our findings (Berns *et al,* 1991; Klijn *et al,* 1992a), that is, a positive relation between *HER2/neu* amplification and response to chemotherapy (mainly CMF), they found that tumours overexpressing c-*erbB2* showed a lower response rate (50% v. 58%) and shorter duration of response to chemotherapy (mitoxanthrone), compared with c-*erbB2* negative tumours. These associations, however, were not statistically significant, but survival after starting chemotherapy was indeed significantly shorter in the c-*erbB2* positive group. In a third study concerning metastatic disease, as mentioned above, Hayes *et al* (1993) found no difference in chemosensitivity between patients with metastatic breast cancer with high or low circulating levels of neu related protein. With respect to the adjuvant role, two studies reported on a negative association between *HER2/neu* expression and response to adjuvant chemotherapy (Allred *et al,* 1992; Gusterson *et al,* 1992), and a third reported on a positive association (Muss *et al,* 1993). Allred *et al* (1992) and Gusterson *et al* (1992) reported that overexpression of *HER2/neu* was associated with resistance to chemotherapy in patients with either node negative or node positive breast cancer. This is puzzling because *HER2/neu* expression has been associated with high S phase fraction (O'Reilly *et al,* 1991; Perren, 1991) and poor differentiation (Perren, 1991), indicating more rapid tumour proliferation; consequently, a higher sensitivity of *HER2/neu* positive tumours for chemotherapy might be expected. However, from both a methodological (Levine and Andrulis, 1992) and endocrine (Klijn *et al,* in press a) point of view, criticism on the conclusions of these studies is warranted. Their relatively good results with adjuvant chemotherapy in patients with *HER2/neu* negative tumours can be partly explained by an indirect endocrine action, since both our group (Berns *et al,* 1991) and Nicholson *et al* (1990) reported a higher efficacy of endocrine treatment in *HER2/neu* negative tumours than in *HER2/neu* positive tumours. In this respect, it is also important to stress that a longer relapse free survival has been significantly correlated with the occurrence of amenorrhoea in four of six studies (Trudeau and Pritchard, 1992) (including the Ludwig trial studied by Gusterson *et al,* 1992) and with tumour progesterone receptor (PGR) levels (Padmanabhan *et al,* 1986; Raemaekers *et al,* 1987). Furthermore, oophorectomy appeared to be just as effective as adjuvant CMF according to both an indirect (Early Breast Cancer Trialists' Collaborative Group, 1992) and direct (Scottish Cancer Trials Breast Group and ICRF Breast Unit, 1993) comparison. In addition, in the study of Gusterson *et al* (1992), low dose prednisone plus tamoxifen was added to chemotherapy. Also in the study of Allred *et al* (1992), an endocrine treatment component (ie prednisone) has been used, and this combined chemoendocrine treatment appeared to be twice as effective in ER positive tumours than in ER negative tumours (Mansour *et al*, 1989). All these data suggest that in the treatment regimens used by Allred *et al* (1992) and Gusterson *et al* (1992), the endocrine components were dominant over the chemotherapeutic components with respect to treatment efficacy. In the third study (Muss *et al*, 1993) no endocrine component was included in the treatment regimen consisting of cyclophosphamide, doxorubicin and fluorouracil (CAF). In this CALGB 8869 study, *erbB2* expression was measured immunohistochemically in the tumours of 461 randomly selected patients from 1572 patients included in trial CALBG 8541. C-*erbB* positivity was found in 29% of the tumours. Patients randomized to higher doses of CAF had a significantly better relapse free survival and overall survival when *erbB2* was overexpressed in their tumours, in contrast to patients without *erbB2* expression. Thus, evidence of a CAF dose effect was found mainly in patients with *erbB2* positive tumours. Since the lowest doses of chemotherapy used in this trial might actually be at the threshold of chemotherapy effectiveness, the authors concluded that *erbB2* overexpression may be useful in identifying patients who are unlikely to derive benefit from low or moderate doses of adjuvant chemotherapy, in contrast to patients with *erbB2* positive tumours treated with high dose chemotherapy who will benefit from chemotherapy.

In conclusion, most evidence indicates that *HER2/neu* positive tumours respond poorly to endocrine therapy, but there is no consensus on response to chemotherapy. This might be explained by differences in techniques used (amplification v. expression), differences in patient age (pre- v. postmenopausal) and populations (patients with primary v. metastatic disease), differences in dose and type of cytotoxic agents used, the absence or presence of endocrine components in the treatment regimen and in potential differences in sequences of various treatment modalities used (first or second line).

C-*myc*

In a series of 1000 primary breast cancers, we found an incidence of c-*myc* amplification in 17.1% (Berns *et al*, 1992a), but the incidence was higher (33%) in tumours of patients developing metastases later on (Berns *et al*, 1992a,d). C-*myc* amplification was more prevalent in the PGR negative subpopulation (p<0.05). Reviewing the literature (Berns *et al*, 1992d), we calculated the incidence of c-*myc* amplification in 20% of 2493 breast cancers, including our series. Recently, we reported on the strong prognostic value of c-*myc* amplification as a marker for survival (Berns *et al*, 1992c). C-*myc* amplification appeared to be highly predictive for short term relapse free and overall survival, especially among patients with node negative or steroid receptor positive tumours.

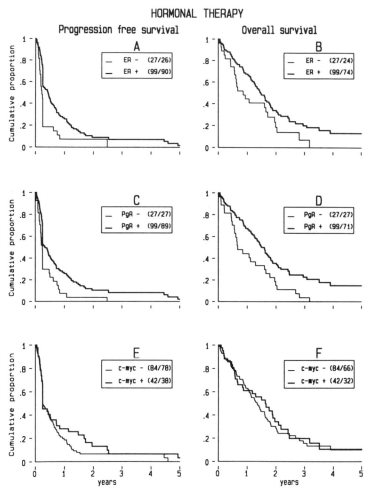

Fig. 2. Progression free and overall survival in 126 patients with metastatic breast cancer from start of first line endocrine therapy according to steroid receptor (ER, PGR) status and c-*myc* amplification. Bold lines indicate patients with receptor positive (ER⁺, PGR⁺) or c-*myc* amplified (c-*myc*⁺) tumours. The numbers in parentheses are number of patients/number of failures

To our knowledge, only our group has so far reported on the relation between c-*myc* and response to systemic therapy. In our experience, patients with c-*myc* amplified tumours tend to respond to treatment in a manner opposite to that of patients with *HER2/neu* amplification (Berns *et al*, 1991; Klijn *et al*, 1992a). With respect to the efficacy of endocrine therapy, we found no significant difference in response to endocrine therapy between patients with or without c-*myc* amplification (see Table 3), but the progression free survival from first line endocrine treatment tended to be better in patients with c-*myc* amplified tumours than in those with no c-*myc* amplification (Fig. 2E). With respect to chemotherapy, 64% of patients with no c-*myc* amplification responded to CMF in contrast to only 29% of patients with c-*myc* amplified tumours (Table 3, p<0.02). This group of patients with c-*myc* amplification

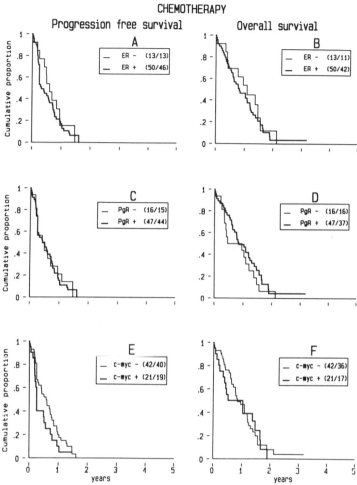

Fig. 3. Progression free and overall survival in 63 patients with metastatic breast cancer from start of first chemotherapeutic regimen at tumour progression after first line endocrine therapy according to steroid receptor (ER, PGR) status and c-*myc* amplification. Bold lines indicate patients with receptor positive (ER$^+$, PGR$^+$) or c-*myc* amplified (c-*myc*$^+$) tumours. The numbers in parentheses are number of patients/number of failures

tended to have a shorter progression free survival (Fig. 3E), but the difference was not significant. The opposite effects of endocrine and chemotherapy on progression free survival resulted in the absence of a relation between c-*myc* amplification and total survival after relapse (Fig. 2F). The poor response of our patients with c-*myc* amplified tumours to chemotherapy may be in agreement with preclinical experimental findings in erythroleukaemia cells showing that the degree of cis-platinum resistance correlated directly with the level of c-*myc* expression (Sklar and Prochownik, 1991). These findings suggest that c-*myc* levels may influence the efficacy of therapy in some tumours and may regulate specific processes by which cells cope with DNA damage caused by chemotherapy.

Int2/bcl1

The *int2* gene, which encodes a protein homologous to fibroblast growth factor, is located on chromosome 11q13. In a series of 1000 breast cancers, we found *int2/bcl1* amplification in 14.1% (Berns *et al*, 1992a). In this large series, a significant positive association with ER was found. Reviewing the literature, we calculated the incidence of *int2/bcl1* amplification as 13% in more than 1500 breast cancers (Klijn *et al*, 1993a). However, there is little evidence of overexpression of *int2*. A few reports indicate that *int2* amplification might predict a poor prognosis (Tsuda *et al*, 1989; Borg *et al*, 1991), but not all indicate this (Roux-Dosseto *et al*, 1992). In a series of 263 patients with primary breast cancer, we recently noted that patients with *int2* amplified tumours did indeed show a poorer relapse free survival (unpublished).

To our knowledge, no data are available regarding the relation between *int2/bcl1* amplification and response to systemic treatment. In a small series of 126 patients with metastatic breast cancer, we found no significant association between *int2/bcl1* amplification and response to endocrine or chemotherapy (Table 3) (Klijn *et al*, 1992a). However, after 12 months of endocrine therapy, a higher rate of progression free survival was found in patients with *int2* positive tumours than in patients with *int2* negative tumours (59% v. 32%). This might be caused by the weak positive association between *int2/bcl1* amplification and ER.

TP53

The gene encoding the nuclear phosphoprotein TP53 is the most commonly mutated gene yet identified in human (breast) cancer (Elledge *et al*, 1992; Harris, 1992; Thor and Yandell, 1993; Thorlacius *et al*, 1993; Klijn *et al*, in press a). Loss of heterozygosity or (over)expression of (mutated) TP53 protein occurs in about 30–55% of human breast cancers. A negative association with ER and prognosis has been found. In our experience, using polymerase chain reaction–single strand conformation polymorphism analysis of exon 5–8 of the *TP53* suppressor gene, changes indicative of mutations have been found thus far in 35 of 61 tumours (57%). Abnormalities of the *TP53* gene were more prevalent in the ER negative subgroup and in about half of the cases accompanied by amplification of the c-*myc*, HER2/*neu* and/or *int2/bcl1* oncogenes. As yet, no clear clinical data on a possible association between *TP53* gene alterations and response to systemic treatment have been reported. However, in view of the observed negative association with ER levels, it might be expected that *TP53* gene alterations may predict a poor response to endocrine therapy. Both endocrine and many chemotherapeutic agents induce apoptosis. Tumour cells may become resistant to chemotherapeutic drugs by turning on genes such as *bcl2* that block apoptosis or, conversely, by turning off genes such as *TP53* that may induce apoptosis (Marx, 1993). Therefore, it can be expected that *TP53* mutation might also be related to a poor response to chemotherapy.

Retinoblastoma (*RB*) Gene

Loss of heterozygosity of the *RB* gene occurs in about 25% and decreased expression in 10–20% of primary breast cancer patients (Varley *et al*, 1989; Borg *et al*, 1992; Klijn *et al*, in press a). In a collaborative study with Bootsma *et al* (1993), genetic alterations (deletion or rearrangement) of the *RB* gene occurred in 24% of 95 breast cancers (23 of 95). In six of these 23 tumours, the genetic alterations were accompanied by amplification of one of the three oncogenes (unpublished). We found no significant correlation with relapse free or overall survival. There are no data available on the relation between loss of heterozygosity of the *RB* gene and response to treatment.

Nm23

Expression of *nm23*, a putative metastasis suppressor gene, mapped to chromosome 17q21, has been detected in human breast cancers (Royds *et al*, 1993; Steeg *et al*, 1993). Reduced *nm23* expression has been found to be correlated with comedo-type ductal carcinoma in situ and with high histological grade (poor differentiation), lymph node metastasis and poor survival in patients with invasive ductal carcinoma. In a series of 58 invasive ductal carcinomas, 26 (45%) were *nm23* negative (Royds *et al*, 1993). Although in human breast cancer, five studies have demonstrated a significant association between reduced *nm23* expression and aggressive tumour behaviour (Steeg *et al*, 1993), so far no data are available on the relation between *nm23* expression and response to systemic therapy.

RECEPTORS FOR GROWTH FACTORS AND PEPTIDE HORMONES

Several growth factors and peptide hormones are directly or indirectly involved in the growth regulation of breast cancer (Klijn *et al*, 1992c). The relation between the receptors for some of these factors and response to therapy will be described.

Epidermal Growth Factor Receptor (EGFR)

Epidermal growth factors, as well as transforming growth factor alpha (TGFA), both of which can activate EGF receptors, are probably produced locally in many normal and malignant tissues as local growth factors rather than as systemic hormones. Malignant tumours frequently contain higher EGFR levels than normal tissues. Recently, we reviewed extensively the clinical significance of EGFR in breast cancer (Klijn *et al*, 1992b, in press b). EGFR positivity was shown to be present in 2500 (48%) of 5232 breast tumours in 40 different series of patients. The mean of the percentages of EGFR positivity in individual series reported by these 40 different groups is 45% (range 14–91%). Overall, there are generally no clear differences between results obtained by radioligand binding assays, immunological methods, autoradiography and measurement of EGFR transcripts, although the mean percentage of EGFR positive tumours determined by immunological methods tends to be somewhat lower. Also in a recent update of over 8000 patients (Klijn *et al*, in press b), nearly all studies indicate a negative relation between EGFR and steroid receptor status (35 of 38 studies for ER, 14 of 21 for PGR), showing that EGFR positivity is twice as high in ER or PGR negative tumours than in ER or PGR positive tumours (50–60% v. 30%). With regard to other prognostic factors, the majority of investigators (12 of 21) also reported a significant (positive) correlation with tumour grade, but only a minority found a significant relation between EGFR status and patient age (3 of 11), menopausal status (2 of 9), histological type (3 of 8), tumour size (3 of 21), nodal status (6–11 of 26), ploidy (1 of 7) or proliferation indices (5 of 11). No relation was observed with tumour insulin like growth factor 1 receptor, prolactin receptor and LHRH receptor status, but an inverse relation between EGFR and somatostatin receptor may be present. We calculated the presence of EGFR positivity overall in 35% of 253 aneuploid tumours v. only 15% of 114 diploid tumours ($p < 0.0001$). In addition, most studies reported a trend, if no significant correlation, between higher EGFR levels in tumours with the highest percentages of S phase or Ki-67 expression. Finally, three of nine studies showed a relation between EGFR and *HER2/neu* expression, and two of two studies with *TP53* mutation.

There is no agreement on the prognostic value of EGFR. Of 15 different studies, 9 showed in some way a significant negative association between EGFR and relapse free survival by univariate analysis, whereas two others showed a tendency ($0.05 < p < 0.10$) to such a relation (Klijn *et al*, in press b). Of seven studies using multivariate analysis, two demonstrated an independent prognostic value of EGFR for relapse free survival and two others showed a tendency to a significant correlation, whereas three did not. There is no agreement on the subgroups of patients in which EGFR may have had a discriminative prognostic effect (Foekens *et al*, 1989c; Klijn *et al*, 1992b).

As yet, only a few data are available on the relation between EGFR and response to systemic treatment. In common with our data (Berns *et al*, 1991; Klijn *et al*, 1992a) and Nicholson *et al's* (1990) data on *HER2/neu*, an EGFR related protein, Nicholson *et al* (1989, 1990) found that expression of EGFR is associated with a lack of response to endocrine therapy in recurrent breast cancer. Only 8% of EGFR positive tumours showed an objective response to first line treatment with tamoxifen in metastatic breast cancer, whereas 30% of EGFR negative tumours responded ($p < 0.05$). In addition, only 1 of 28 EGFR positive/ER negative tumours showed an objective response. Furthermore, EGFR and c-erbB2 protein also appeared to have additive effects in reducing the likelihood of responses; none of eight patients with EGFR positive/c-*erbB2* positive tumours derived benefit from endocrine therapy (Wright *et al*, 1992a). Patients with EGFR positive primary tumours showed more rapid disease progression after first line endocrine therapy than those with EGFR negative tumours. Interestingly, Van Agthoven *et al* (1992) showed that transfection of EGFR in human hormone dependent breast cancer cells induced progression of these cells to hormone independence. Long *et al* (1992) also found that acquired tamoxifen resistance was associated with an increase in EGFR numbers accompanied by loss of ER and PGR. Furthermore, reciprocal modulation of the genes for EGFR and ER by butyrate suggests that the expression of ER and EGFR may be co-regulated (De Fazio *et al*, 1992).

With respect to response to chemotherapy, in a preliminary study in 25 patients who received first line single therapy with mitoxanthrone, there was no correlation between EGFR status and response to therapy, time to tumour progression or survival (Harris, 1990a). In another small study, Cantwell *et al* (1991) investigated the relation between EGFR status and response to doxorubicin plus ifosfamide in recurrent breast cancer. Nine of ten patients with EGFR positive tumours and three of five with EGFR negative tumours showed an objective response, but the numbers are too small to prove a significant difference. Growth inhibitory concentrations of doxorubicin, 5-fluorouracil and 4-hydroperoxycyclophosphamide had no effect on EGF binding to MCF7 human breast cancer cells in vitro, but cisplatin and vinblastine reduced EGF binding affinity (Hanauske *et al*, 1987). On the other hand, EGF treatment, accompanied by increased EGFR expression, enhanced cisplatin cytotoxicity for cervical carcinoma cells (Nishikawa *et al*, 1992). Epidermal growth factor also increased sensitivity to doxorubicin of human squamous cell lines, especially the doxorubicin resistant sublines (A131/A5 and A431/A10) containing higher EGFR levels (Kwok and Sutherland, 1991). The enhanced drug responsiveness was considered not to be directly related to EGF effects on growth. Interestingly, in human large cell lung cancer, reduced EGFR expression has been associated with non-P-glycoprotein mediated multidrug resistance (MDR) (Reeve *et al*, 1990). With respect to the development of MDR, both high and low EGFR levels may be involved (Meyers *et al*, 1986; Reeve *et al*, 1990). In breast cancer, overexpression of the *MDR1* gene may be associated with decreased expression of steroid hormone receptors and oestrogen inducible PS2 protein, and increased EGFR expression, but there is no agreement that *MDR1* gene overexpression results in cross resistance to anti-oestrogens (Clarke *et al*, 1992b).

Receptors for Insulin Like Growth Factors (IGFRs)

Insulin like growth factors (IGF1 and IGF2) are potent mitogens for breast cancer cells (Osborne *et al*, 1990; Clarke *et al*, 1992a). Apart from oestrogens, they are the most powerful growth stimulating factors in vitro. The growth effects of both are mediated predominantly via IGF1 receptors, which have been demonstrated in 67–93% of primary human breast cancers (Klijn *et al*, 1992c, 1993a, in press a).

At present, there is no agreement on the prognostic value of IGF1R. Possibly both very low (Bonneterre *et al*, 1990; Peyrat *et al*, 1990) and very high levels (Berns *et al*, 1992b) may predict poor survival. Little is known about the possible relation between tumour IGF1 or IGF1R levels and response to sys-

temic treatment. In human primary breast cancer, we found a negative association between tumour IGF1 like activity and ER or PGR levels with higher
cytosolic IGF1 like activity in ER negative tumours (Foekens *et al*, 1989b).
Some endocrine agents such as anti-oestrogens and somatostatin analogues
might affect tumour IGF1 secretion, but no data are available on the in vivo
effects of these treatment modalities on the autocrine/paracrine regulation of
IGF1 secretion or IGF1R production in patients with metastatic breast cancer.
On the other hand, with respect to the endocrine effects, both tamoxifen
(Coletti *et al*, 1989; Pollak *et al*, 1990; Bontenbal *et al*, 1992; Kiang *et al*, 1992)
and somatostatin analogues (Lamberts *et al*, 1990; Peyrat *et al*, 1990; Santen *et
al*, 1990) can decrease plasma IGF1 levels by 25–80%. Increased plasma IGF1
concentrations have been found in patients with breast cancer (Peyrat *et al*,
1993). Interestingly, Kiang *et al* (1992) recently showed in patients with
metastatic breast cancer that, in contrast to megestrol acetate and oophorectomy, tamoxifen and high dose oestrogens diethylstilbestrol decreased plasma
IGF1 levels and that the degree of IGF1 suppression correlated with tumour
response to tamoxifen. The mean IGF1 nadir was 21.9 ng/ml for eight
responders against 48.0 ng/ml for nine non-responders ($p<0.01$). Thus, insufficient suppression of plasma IGF1 levels may predict an absence of response to
tamoxifen. Of clinical importance also might be the observation that hydrox-
ytamoxifen can prevent growth factor mitogenic activity through a marked
(60%) decrease in high affinity IGF1 binding sites apart from a strong impair-
ment of EGFR signal transduction (Freiss *et al*, 1992). Progestins also appear
to downregulate IGF1R, possibly due to an increased biosynthesis of the lig-
and IGF2 (Goldfine *et al*, 1992). To date, no data are available on the relation
between tumour IGF1R levels and response to therapy in patients with breast
cancer.

With respect to IGF2, Cullen *et al* (1992) showed that IGF2 overexpression may be capable of mediating malignant progression in human breast cancer. Recently, Brünner *et al* (1993) reported that growth inhibiting endocrine
treatment with tamoxifen or oestrogens strongly reduced IGF2 mRNA and
protein expression in ER positive T61 human breast cancer xenografts. This
downregulation was found to be specific for IGF2, since analyses on the expression of IGF1 mRNA, 36B4 mRNA, TGFA mRNA and EGFR mRNA in
these T61 tumours did not reveal any downregulation. Blockade by monoclonal antibodies of IGF1R and downregulation of IGF2 by tamoxifen or
oestrogens resulted in growth inhibition, suggesting that IGF2 expression is
correlated to breast tumour growth. Furthermore, both IGF2 and IGF1 may
be involved in hormone independence (Brünner *et al*, 1992). For more extensive data on IGF2, we refer to the excellent review of Clarke *et al* (1992a).

Transforming Growth Factor Beta (TGFB)

Short term treatment with tamoxifen during a few weeks may increase TGFB
expression in the stroma of primary breast cancers (Butta *et al*, 1992) and may

increase plasma TGFB levels (Knabbe, 1993). So far, it is unclear whether TGFB might be involved in drug resistance. Hypothetically, loss of this TGFB inducing property of tamoxifen during long term treatment may lead to tamoxifen resistance. On the other hand, the presence of TGFB transcripts in 53 of 104 breast carcinomas showed no relation with survival and other clinical features (Coombes *et al*, 1990)

Fibroblast Growth Factors (FGFs)

Very few data are available on the role of FGFs and drug resistance. Interestingly, McLeskey *et al* (1993) recently showed that transfection of FGF4 into MCF7 cells resulted in cell lines that form progressively growing and metastatic tumours in ovariectomized or tamoxifen treated athymic nude mice. The growth of these transfected cells appeared to be stimulated by tamoxifen and inhibited by oestrogen treatment. These data suggest a possible role for FGFs in the progression of breast cancer to an oestrogen independent anti-oestrogen resistant, metastatic phenotype.

In human primary breast cancer, high affinity (Kd <1 nM) and low affinity (Kd >2 nM) binding sites for basic FGF (bFGF) were found in 19 and 29 of 36 cases, respectively (Peyrat *et al*, 1992). No association between bFGF binding sites and node involvement or grade was found, but a negative correlation with ER and PGR was demonstrated. This suggests that high bFGF receptor levels in primary breast cancer may indicate a poor response to endocrine therapy

Somatostatin Receptor (SSTR)

Receptors for SSTR have been found in 36–67% of primary breast cancers (Fekete *et al*, 1989; Reubi *et al*, 1990; Klijn *et al*, 1992c; Bootsma *et al*, 1993). The incidence increased even to 77% (38 of 49) when SSTR was measured by receptor scintigraphy in vivo in patients with primary breast cancer (in vivo imaging) (Lamberts *et al*, 1992). A negative association of SSTR with EGFR and a positive association with ER and PGR status have been reported (Reubi *et al*, 1990). In agreement with these findings, we observed that patients with SSTR positive primary tumours had a significantly longer 5 year relapse free survival than those with SSTR negative tumours (Foekens *et al*, 1989c, 1990b).

Less is known about the relation between SSTR and response to endocrine therapy. Treatment with somatostatin analogues may have both indirect endocrine inhibitory effects on tumour growth (through a decrease of growth hormone and IGFI secretion) and a direct growth inhibitory effect via tumour SSTR (Lamberts *et al*, 1990). Indeed, we (Setyono-Han *et al*, 1987; Klijn *et al*, 1990) and later others have demonstrated in vitro direct growth inhibitory effects of somatostatin analogues on human breast cancer cells containing SSTR. However, thus far only a few clinical results have been published showing a low response rate (16%) in heavily pretreated patients with metastatic breast cancer (Santen *et al*, 1990; Klijn *et al*, 1992c). Studies on the efficacy of somatostatin analogues in previously untreated patients are warranted, especially with combination therapies designed to block other growth stimulatory pathways. In a preliminary clinical randomized study using octreotide in combination with a new anti-prolactin and tamoxifen, we observed interesting endocrine and anti-tumour effects (11% non-responders), although octreotide did not add to the plasma *IGF1* lowering effect of tamoxifen (Bontenbal *et al*, 1992). In endocrine gastroenteropancreatic tumours and carcinoids, response appeared to be related to tumour SSTR levels (Kvols and Reubi, 1990). Tumours with high SSTR levels showed a better response. Therefore, it might be expected that somatostatin analogue treatment may have (additive) growth inhibitory effects in patients with breast tumours containing the highest SSTR levels. From experiences in other tumour types (Lamberts *et al*, 1990), it may be concluded that the absence of SSTR predicts a low chance of response to endocrine therapy with somatostatin analogues.

Luteinizing Hormone Releasing Hormone Receptors (LHRHR)

In two different large series of patients, receptors for LHRH have been found in 52% of primary breast cancers (Fekete *et al*, 1989; Baumann *et al*, 1993). No correlation was found with steroid receptor status, *EGFR*, lymph node status and S phase index. Treatment with LHRH analogues has been shown to be active especially in premenopausal patients (Klijn and De Jong, 1982; Klijn, 1992). The main mechanism of action of LHRH agonist treatment is medical castration, but direct tumour growth inhibitory effects through LHRHR as observed in vitro (reviewed in Foekens and Klijn, 1992) cannot be excluded. Kiesel *et al* (1993) have recently shown that patients with LHRHR positive primary tumours have a worse prognosis than patients with LHRHR negative tumours. So far, no data have been reported on a possible association between LHRHR levels and response to endocrine therapy, especially with LHRH analogues, in patients with metastatic breast cancer.

STEROID RECEPTORS AND OESTROGEN REGULATED PROTEINS

Steroid hormones are an important category of hormones involved in the growth regulation of breast cancer. Oestradiol is one of the most potent tumour growth stimulatory factors. The mechanism of action of oestrogens on breast cancer and the development of hormone independence or resistance are not completely understood. Nevertheless, oestrogens induce many effects on the expression of various genes, on growth factor secretion, on growth factor receptor expression and on the production of a number of oestrogen regulated proteins such as PGR, PS2, cathepsin D and plasminogen activators. Together with ER (Foekens *et al*, 1989a), all these proteins are positively or negatively associated with metastasis and prognosis, but so far there are few data on the predictive value of these proteins for response to therapy, with the exception of PGR.

Steroid Receptors (ER, PGR, AR)

Patients with high tumour levels of ER and PGR receive more benefit from adjuvant endocrine therapy than patients with ER/PGR negative tumours (Early Breast Cancer Trialists' Collaborative Group, 1992). In patients with metastatic disease, the response rate to endocrine therapy is highly dependent on the steroid receptor status of the tumours (Horwitz et al, 1985; Santen et al, 1990; Muss, 1992; Ravdin et al, 1992), being about 10% in ER negative tumours, 50% in ER positive tumours and 75% in ER and PGR positive tumours. In a large prospective trial, multivariate analysis including 13 variables seemed to show that PGR is also an independent predictive factor for response to tamoxifen, time to progression and overall survival (Ravdin et al, 1992). Response rates in subgroups ranged from 24% to 86% (postmenopausal patients with ER >38 and PGR >329 fmol/mg). The predictability of response by PGR can even be increased to 90% by measuring in vivo induction of PGR as a result of the partial oestrogen agonist activity of tamoxifen, indeed reflecting an intact ER machinery. Of 21 patients (90%) showing an increase of PGR in a second biopsy after an average of 13 days' treatment with tamoxifen, 19 responded objectively to continued endocrine therapy in contrast to only a 35% response in 31 patients with no increase in PGR levels (Howell et al, 1987). However, in clinical practice, this approach is not feasible because most patients refuse a second biopsy or have no accessible metastases. Finally, the PGR might be especially predictive for response to treatment with anti-progestins (Bakker et al, 1989; Klijn et al, 1989; Horwitz, 1992). Also, the presence of the androgen receptor (AR) is a good indicator of response to endocrine therapy, especially high dose progestins (Teulings et al, 1980). Metastases in liver and brain are more frequently ER negative than soft tissue metastases (Alexieva-Figusch et al, 1988). Resistance to endocrine therapy can be present from the beginning, even in ER/PGR positive tumours, or can develop later during the disease (Klijn, 1991). Patients developing detectable recurrences during or shortly after adjuvant therapy show a low response rate to subsequent endocrine therapy for metastatic disease (Fornander et al, 1987; Rubens, 1993). On the other hand, patients with a long disease free interval generally have higher tumour ER levels and respond better to endocrine therapy for metastatic disease (Muss, 1992).

The majority of papers do not show an association between steroid receptor status and response to chemotherapy (Henderson, 1987). We also observed the lack of an association (see Fig. 3).

PS2 Protein

Several investigators have observed a positive association among ER, PGR and PS2 levels (Rio and Chambon, 1990). Recently, we (Foekens et al, 1990a,b, 1993a) and other investigators (Predine et al, 1992; Thor et al, 1992) have reported on the prognostic value of PS2 protein. In our initial study in 205 patients with breast cancer (Foekens *et al*, 1990a), the death rate for patients with PS2 positive tumours was one tenth that for patients with PS2 and ER negative tumours.

The discriminatory effect of PS2 was present especially in the subgroup of patients with ER+/PGR+ tumours. Recently, we confirmed our data on the prognostic value of quantitatively assessed PS2 in a larger second series of 710 patients (Foekens *et al*, 1993a). Other investigators using immunohistochemical techniques found that PS2 had less or no prognostic value for relapse free and overall survival (Henry *et al*, 1991; Thor *et al*, 1992). In our large series, node negative patients with tumours containing low PS2 levels (≤2 ng/mg protein) and high cathepsin D values (>70 pmol/mg protein) experienced a 4.5-fold increase in relapse rate compared with those with high PS2 levels (>2 ng/mg protein) and low cathepsin D values (≤30 pmol/mg protein) (Foekens *et al*, 1993a).

Less is known about the relation between PS2 and response to systemic therapy. Henry *et al* (1991), in a small series of 55 patients, and in 21 patients analysing mRNA expression (Henry *et al*, 1989), and Schwarz *et al* (1991), in a series of 72 patients, have shown that immunohistochemically assessed PS2 positivity is predictive of response to endocrine therapy for recurrent disease. Patients with PS2 (or *pNR2*) positive tumours responded in 67% and 52% of cases and patients with PS2 negative tumours responded in 26% and 27% of the cases reported in both these series. Unexpected findings in these studies were the absence of a relation between PS2 positivity and duration of response to first line hormonal therapy (Schwartz *et al*, 1991) and the absence of a predictive value of immunohistochemically assessed ER (Henry *et al*, 1991; Schwartz *et al*, 1991) and PGR (Schwartz *et al*, 1991) with respect to response, which is in sharp contrast to the generally accepted view regarding quantitatively determined ER and PGR status (Horwitz *et al*, 1985; Muss, 1992; Ravdin *et al*, 1992). In a third preliminary study in only 21 patients with recurrent breast cancer, expression of Md2 protein (found to be homologous to PS2) correlated with response to endocrine therapy and was of similar predictive value as ER status (Skilton *et al*, 1989). We recently found in a series of 289 patients with metastatic breast cancer that PS2 does indeed identify patients in the ER+/PGR+ subgroup, which is likely to benefit from hormonal therapy due to the intactness of the ER pathway (Foekens *et al*, 1992a; Klijn *et al*, 1992a). Quantitatively assessed PS2 negativity predicted a higher failure rate, a shorter duration of response and a faster death rate after the start of endocrine therapy.

With respect to adjuvant therapy, Predine *et al* (1992) reported that in a series of 98 patients treated with adjuvant tamoxifen therapy, the PS2 concentration was shown in a multivariate analysis to be the most potent prognostic factor for predicting clinical outcome, preceding even the well established ER determination. The difference in 5 year overall survival between PS2 positive and PS2 negative patients (receiving adjuvant hormone therapy) was about 40%.

Cathepsin D (CTSD)

A large number of studies have shown that CTSD is a valuable prognostic marker, with high tumour levels related to poor prognosis (Rochefort, 1992). In the largest series of patients published, we found a continuous positive association between the level of CTSD and relapse rate (Foekens *et al*, 1993a). In our experience, CTSD and PS2 appear to be independent and additive prognostic factors in primary breast cancer.

There are, however, very few data on the possible association between CTSD and response to systemic therapy. In a recent study (Foekens *et al*, 1992a; Klijn *et al*, 1992a) in 289 patients with metastatic breast cancer, we found no relation between quantitatively assessed CTSD levels in the primary tumour and type of response, duration of response or length of postrelapse survival following first line hormonal therapy for recurrent disease, suggesting that CTSD is a marker of metastasis rather than of hormone responsiveness. Also, using immunocytochemical staining for the Mr 52 000 precursor of CTSD in tumours in a series of 89 patients, Damstrup *et al* (1992) showed that Mr 52 000 is not of value in predicting response to endocrine therapy in advanced or recurrent disease. The observation that patients with node positive tumours with low CTSD levels treated with adjuvant chemotherapy had a significantly prolonged survival compared with treated patients with high CTSD levels, although CTSD levels did not modify the outcome of node negative and untreated node positive patients (Namer *et al*, 1991), may nevertheless indicate the possible importance of CTSD measurement for therapeutic decision making, for example patients with high tumour CTSD levels may gain less or no benefit from adjuvant chemotherapy.

Plasminogen Activators and Inhibitors

Among other proteases such as cathepsins and collagenases, plasminogen activators are involved in the process of cancer invasion and metastasis (Markus, 1988). The expression of tissue type plasminogen activator (t-PA) seems to be regulated in vitro by ER and/or PGR, whereas urokinase type plasminogen activator (u-PA) may not be regulated by steroid hormones. An inverse correlation between u-PA and t-PA has been found in breast cancer tissue (Jänicke *et al*, 1991). High t-PA tumour levels are associated with ER positivity and good prognosis, whereas high u-PA tumour levels are associated with ER negativity and poor prognosis. Recently, in a large series of 671 patients with breast cancer, we found significantly higher u-PA levels in ER and PGR negative tumours ($p < 0.02$) but no significant correlation between u-PA and ER or PGR levels (Foekens *et al*, 1992b). In our study, u-PA appeared to be an independent prognostic factor associated with increased rates of relapse and death, especially in the subgroups of node negative ($p = 0.002$), node positive ($p < 0.0001$), postmenopausal ($p < 0.0001$) and steroid receptor positive patients ($p < 0.0001$). Apart from the u-PA receptor, two plasminogen activator inhibitors (PAI1 and PAI2) are involved in the plasminogen activator system. In a study on 657 patients (Foekens *et al*, 1993b), we found that PAI1 levels were strongly positively correlated with the rates of relapse (p<0.0001) and death (p<0.001). A positive association was observed between PAI1 and both u-PA and CTSD levels, and, in contrast, a negative association was found between PAI1 and both steroid hormone receptors and PS2 levels. Of these six cytosolic parameters, PAI1 was the strongest prognostic factor for early relapse, in both node negative and node positive breast cancer.

There are, to date, no reports on the relation between u-PA or t-PA levels and response to systemic therapy. However, in a series of 240 patients, we recently found that high tumour u-PA levels (>1.6 ng/mg protein) were associated with a low rate of response to endocrine therapy for metastatic disease, especially in the subgroup of patients with ER negative tumours (Klijn *et al*, 1992a), but the numbers are small. In our study on 671 patients (Foekens *et al*, 1992b), the beneficial effect of adjuvant therapy (in node positive patients) was present most strongly in the u-PA positive group (relative relapse rate in comparison to no treatment group 0.42; p<0.001) but less pronounced in the u-PA negative group (relative relapse rate 0.71; p=0.13). Although this difference in relative relapse rates did not reach significance (p=0.07), this observation suggests that tumours with high cytosolic u-PA levels are more sensitive to adjuvant therapy. Thus, u-PA is probably not only a prognostic factor, but also a predictive factor for the efficacy of adjuvant systemic therapy. No data are available on the possible relation between the levels of the plasminogen activator inhibitors and response to therapy. In our study concerning a multivariate analysis (including u-PA) for relapse free survival in 373 node positive patients (Foekens *et al*, 1993b), adjuvant systemic therapy caused a lower relative relapse rate in PAI1 positive patients (0.59 compared with no treatment) than in PAI1 negative patients (0.86), suggesting a higher efficacy of adjuvant therapy in PAI1 positive patients. However, these data must be interpreted with caution due to the strong association between application of systemic adjuvant therapy and some patient and tumour characteristics.

Other Oestrogen Regulated Proteins

A significant correlation between Mr 24 000 protein and the presence of ER in breast cancers has been established. However, despite such association, Mr 24 000 protein appeared not to correlate with response to endocrine therapy in a small series of 103 patients (Damstrup *et al*, 1992).

Heat shock proteins are also correlated with ER status and prognosis. Specific heat shock proteins appear to be associated with doxorubicin resistance in certain human breast cancer cells but independent of the multidrug resistance system (Ciocca *et al*, 1992).

CELL PROLIFERATION INDICES

Proliferation indices, commonly used for predicting tumour aggressiveness and patient prognosis, are [^{3}H]thymidine labelling index, flow cytometric S phase cell fraction, and Ki-67 immunoreactivity. For a review of proliferative variables and their predictive value, we refer to the papers of Silvestrini (Silvestrini, in press; Silvestrini and Daidone, 1993). A high proliferation index clearly appeared to be associated with poor relapse free and overall survival. Little information is available on their relevance as predictors of response to specific treatments. Accumulating evidence from retrospective analyses indicates that slowly proliferating tumours respond better to endocrine therapy and rapidly proliferating tumours respond better to chemotherapy (Silvestrini and Daidone, 1993; Muss *et al,* 1993).

DETOXIFYING ENZYMES

A wide variety of mechanisms have been implicated in the aetiology of resistance to chemotherapeutic agents including expression of the *MDR* gene, enhanced DNA repair, topoisomerases and the action of detoxifying enzymes such as the glutathione S transferases (GST) (Harris and Hochhauser, 1992). Multidrug resistance and GST3 overexpression are associated with the loss of oestrogen receptors in adriamycin resistant MCF7 cells. In the primary breast tumours of 139 node positive, mainly premenopausal patients treated with adjuvant chemotherapy, we found in a collaborative study that GST3 was negatively correlated with ER and PGR and positively correlated with CTSD (Peters *et al,* 1993).

There was no correlation between GST isoenzymes and the length of disease free survival, suggesting that GSTs are not useful as markers to predict response to adjuvant chemotherapy in human breast cancer. However, in node negative patients with primary breast cancer not treated with systemic adjuvant therapy, Gilbert *et al* (1993) found a highly prognostic value of GST3 indicating poor relapse free and overall survival in both ER negative and positive breast cancer patients with high immunohistochemically determined concentrations of GST3 in their tumours. In multivariate analysis (including ER status, PGR status, nuclear grade and tumour size), GST3 expression most accurately predicted shorter relapse free and overall survival in node negative patients. However, in node positive patients, who had received a variety of different adjuvant chemical and hormonal therapies, no association between GST3 expression and survival was found, which is in agreement with our findings (Peters *et al,* 1993). This suggests that adjuvant chemotherapy is especially effective in patients with GST3 positive tumours.

Very few clinical data are available on the relation between GST3 levels and response to systemic therapy in metastatic disease. Wright *et al* (1992b) showed no correlation between GST content and response to mitoxanthrone therapy in 68 patients with advanced breast cancer. Whether or not the GSTs are relevant in patients receiving endocrine therapy needs to be investigated. In a preliminary study in 33 patients with ER positive locally advanced breast cancer, treated with tamoxifen, GST3 levels were significantly (p=0.007) higher in patients with stable or progressive disease than in 13 patients with an objective response (Quénel *et al*, 1993).

CELL BIOLOGICAL FACTORS AND SITES OF RELAPSE

For some of these factors, a relation with site of relapse has been shown. This is important because there is an association between site of relapse and response to endocrine therapy—that is, soft tissue metastases respond more frequently to endocrine therapy (30–60%) than visceral metastases (5–40%) (Muss, 1992). This association is probably related to steroid receptor status in view of our observation that ER and PGR negative tumours relapse more frequently in brain, liver and lung (Alexieva-Figusch *et al*, 1988). Recently, we also found that *HER2/neu* amplified breast cancers tend to relapse relatively frequently in visceral organs (Table 4) perhaps because of the negative correlation between *HER2/neu* status and steroid receptor levels. Patients with liver and lung metastases showed a higher incidence of *HER2/neu* amplification (ie 42% and 33%, respectively) in their primary tumours compared with the total group of patients (19%). Our data on *HER2/neu* are in agreement with those of Kallioniemi *et al* (1991) who also demonstrated a significant association between *HER2/neu* overexpression and increased risk of visceral metastases.

In addition, EGFR positive tumours have been reported to relapse more frequently at visceral sites and less frequently in bone (Nicholson *et al*, 1989). In our experience, c-*myc* amplification is positively correlated with brain (50%) and negatively correlated with bone metastases (p=0.04) compared with the incidence (33%) in the total group of patients with metastases (Table 4).

CRITICAL REMARKS

Over the last decade, molecular biological and immunological techniques have revealed an increasing number of cell biological parameters involved in the development of malignancy and in the regulation of tumour cell function and growth. With respect to these parameters, there appears to be a great heterogeneity either between cells within a certain breast tumour or between individual breast tumours. This explains why there are so many differences in clinical behaviour between breast cancers. Most of these parameters have been investigated with respect to their value as prognosticators for relapse free and overall survival (Klijn and Foekens, 1990; Klijn *et al*, 1993a, in press a). Indeed, many of them appeared to be negatively or positively, dependent or independent, correlated with clinical outcome.

In parallel with this expansion in number of prognostic factors, however, there is increasing criticism by some clinicians. The main questions are (a) how useful are these prognostic factors for daily routine clinical practice and (b) if useful, how to integrate them? At present, there are several practical problems. Firstly, the value of many cell biological parameters as prognostic factors

TABLE 4. Relationship between sites of relapse at start of first line hormonal therapy and *HER2/neu* and c-*myc* status in primary tumours

	Total No. (%)		*HER2/neu* No. (%)		c-*myc* No. (%)	
Total	126	(100)	24	(19)	42	(33)
Single sites	82	(100)	16	(20)	29	(35)
Multi-sites	44	(100)	8	(18)	13	(30)
Locoregional						
breast	6	(100)	0	(0)	3	(50)
nodes	22	(100)	3	(14)	9	(41)
Viceral						
pleura	16	(100)	4	(25)	6	(38)
lung	18	(100)	6	(33)	3	(17)
liver	12	(100)	5	(42)	4	(33)
brain	4	(100)	0	(0)	2	(50)
Skeletal	73	(100)	11	(15)	19	(26)[a]
Skin	24	(100)	6	(25)	9	(38)

[a]$p = 0.04$

needs to be validated in large studies with sufficient sized subgroups of patients using multivariate analysis with inclusion of the classical and relevant new prognostic factors (Clark, 1992). Furthermore, agreement is needed on the optimal laboratory method and cut off levels used. Although it is clear that some prognostic factors or combination of factors (prognostic index) provide a much better discrimination between high and low risk patients than others, there is discussion on how large this discriminative effect must be before applying such factors in clinical practice. It is our opinion that prognostic factors or indices that indicate more than a 20–30% difference between high and low risk patients with node negative primary breast cancer in retrospective studies are valuable for testing in prospective studies if in the low risk group there are recurrences in not more than 10–15% of the patients over 10 years of follow-up and they are not too small subgroup. Otherwise, the costs of measuring these prognostic factors in all patients are not worthwhile. A second problem is, however, that most clinical investigators prefer to investigate the value of a new treatment modality over that of a new prognostic factor. In addition, it is quite complicated to assess adequately in the same trial and study design the value of both a new treatment regimen and a new prognosticator. A third problem is that there are fewer data on the relation of a certain cell biological parameter to type of response to systemic therapy than to prognosis. The question of which patients will benefit from which treatment modality is important. If high risk patients determined by a certain prognostic factor receive no benefit from a specific (adjuvant) therapy, then such a prognostic factor is of low value. Therefore, we have reviewed in this paper (as summarized in Table 5) all available data in this respect. It seems that a valuable prognostic factor can be a worthless predictive factor for response to either endocrine therapy or chemotherapy, and vice versa. For instance, *HER2/neu* is a weak prog-

TABLE 5. Relationship between various predictive factors, steroid receptors and type of response to endocrine therapy (ET) or chemotherapy (CT) in breast cancer

Predictive factor	ER/PR	Relative tumour response ET	CT
ER+	+/+	good[a]	–
PGR+	+/+	good	–
AR+	+/+	good	–
pS2+	+/+	good	–
CTSD+	+/+	no value	no value (m)
u-PA+	–/–	poor (m)	good (adj)
t-PA+	+/+	?	?
PAI1	–/–	?	good (adj)
Mr 24 000+	+/0	no value	?
Heat shock proteins		?	poor[b]
PRLR+	±/±	no value (adj tamoxifen)	
SSR+	+/+	good?	?
EGFR+	–/–	poor	no value? (m) good[b]
TGF-A/EGF+	–/–	poor[b]	good?
IGF1R+	+/+	?	?
IGF1+	–/–	?	?
Plasma IGF1↓		good	?
HER2/neu+	–/–	poor	good (m) poor/good (adj)
c-myc+	0/–	good?	poor
int2+	+/–	good?	no value
TP53+	–/–	?	?
RB	?	?	?
Aneuploidy	–/–	poor	?
High proliferation (LI, S-phase, Ki-67)		poor	good
GTS3+	–/–	poor	no value/good (adj) poor[b]

[a] Good and poor indicate relative response, not value as a marker
[b] In vitro
ER = oestrogen receptor; PGR = progesterone receptor; AR = androgen receptor; LI = labelling index
m = in metastatic disease; adj = in adjuvant setting; + = positively correlated; – = negatively correlated;
0 = not correlated

nosticator but a valuable marker for response to endocrine therapy, whereas CTSD is a valuable marker for early metastasis but of low value for prediction of response to systemic therapy. So, it can be expected in the future that a panel of clinical and cell biological parameters related to tumour differentiation, proliferation and metastatic capacity will be selected to be measured to enable the clinician to select adequately the patients who need not only additional (systemic) therapy, but also the most suitable type of therapy. Finally, new cell biological parameters will be detected, which may further refine our ability to predict prognosis and response to therapy. They will nevertheless improve our insight in to tumour biology, which may lead to the development of better diagnostic tools and new treatment modalities using these cell biological parameters as targets for therapy (Klijn *et al*, 1990; Harris, 1990b; Lippman, 1993).

CONCLUSIONS

(a) There is a large series of cell biological prognostic factors available to estimate prognosis, but because of a lack of hard data, only a few are suitable for the prediction of tumour response to endocrine therapy and/or chemotherapy.

(b) A valuable prognostic factor can be a worthless predictive factor of response to therapy, and vice versa.

(c) Low proliferation indices and high tumour levels of ER, PGR, AR and PS2 predict a relatively good response to endocrine therapy, whereas EGFR positivity, *HER2/neu* positivity, aneuploidy and possibly high u-PA or GST3 levels indicate a high probability of poor response to endocrine therapy.

(d) With respect to chemotherapy, a high proliferation rate and *HER2/neu* amplification predict a good response to chemotherapy, whereas *MDR* gene expression and possibly c-*myc* amplification are related to a worse response.

(e) Patients with high u-PA, PAI1 or GST3 tumour levels may benefit more from adjuvant chemotherapy than patients with low levels.

(f) Results on the relation between a certain cell biological marker and response to chemotherapy could be different in primary and metastatic disease as a consequence of a protracted indirect endocrine effect by chemical oophorectomy in premenopausal women treated with adjuvant chemotherapy.

(g) Cell biological factors can be used as targets for new treatment modalities.

SUMMARY

For the integration of new cell biological prognostic factors in daily clinical practice, we need to know not only their prognostic power with respect to prediction of relapse free and overall survival, but also their possible relation to response to endocrine therapy or chemotherapy in order to select adequate treatment for each patient. A large number of cell biological parameters are currently available to predict the prognosis of patients with breast cancer, but it is still difficult to predict the response to treatment accurately. A valuable prognostic factor can be a worthless predictive factor for endocrine therapy or chemotherapy, and vice versa. High tumour levels of ER, PGR, AR and PS2 protein predict a relatively good response to endocrine therapy, whereas EGFR positivity, *HER2/neu* positivity, aneuploidy, high proliferation indices and possibly high u-PA levels indicate a good chance of a poor response to endocrine therapy in metastatic breast cancer. With respect to chemotherapy, a high proliferation rate and *HER2/neu* amplification predict a good response to therapy in metastatic disease, whereas *MDR* gene expression and possibly c-*myc* amplification are related to a worse response. In conclusion, the newer cell biological parameters can be used to select high and low risk patients and type of systemic treatment and can be used as targets for new treatment modalities.

Acknowledgements

We would like to thank the Dutch Cancer Society for grants RRTI 88-9 and DDHK 92-04, and Ms R Kalkman for typing the manuscript.

References

Alexieva-Figusch J, Van Putten WLJ, Blankenstein MA, Blonk-van der Wijst J and Klijn JGM (1988) The prognostic value and relationships of patient characteristics, progestin receptor, estrogen receptor, and site of relapse in primary and metastatic human breast cancer. *Cancer* **61** 758–768

Allred DC, Clark GM, Tandon AK *et al* (1992) HER-2/neu in node-negative breast cancer: prognostic significance of overexpression influenced by the presence of in situ carcinoma. *Journal of Clinical Oncology* **10** 599–605

Bakker GH, Setyono-Han B, Portengen H, De Jong FH, Foekens JA and Klijn JGM (1989) Endocrine and antitumor effects of combined treatment with an antiprogestin and antiestrogen or luteinizing hormone-releasing hormone agonist in female rats bearing mammary tumors. *Endocrinology* **125** 1593–1598

Baumann KH, Kiesel L, Kaufmann M, Bastert G and Runnebaum B (1993) Characterization of binding sites for a GnRH-agonist (buserelin) in human breast cancer biopsies and their distribution in relation to tumor parameters. *Breast Cancer Research and Treatment* **25** 37–46

Benz CC, Scott GK, Sarup JC *et al* (1992) Estrogen-dependent, tamoxifen-resistant tumorigenic growth of MCF-7 cells transfected with HER2/neu. *Breast Cancer Research and Treatment* **24** 85–95

Berns PMJJ, Foekens JA, Van Staveren IL *et al* (1991) Amplification of the HER2/neu gene and not of c-*myc* is associated with a poor response to endocrine- and good response to chemotherapy in recurrent breast cancer. *Abstracts of 5th EORTC Breast Cancer Working Conference*, Leuven, 3-6 September 1991 [Abstract A 213]

Berns PMJJ, Klijn JGM, Van Staveren IL, Portengen H, Noordegraaf E and Foekens JA (1992a) Prevalence of amplification of the oncogenes c-*myc*, HER2/neu and int-2 in one thousand human breast tumours: correlation with steroid receptors. *European Journal of Cancer* **28** 697–700

Berns PMJJ, Klijn JGM, Van Staveren IL, Portengen H and Foekens JA (1992b) Sporadic amplification of the insulin-like growth factor 1 receptor gene in human breast tumors. *Cancer Research* **52** 1036–1039

Berns PMJJ, Klijn JGM, Van Putten WLJ, Van Staveren IL, Portengen H and Foekens JA (1992c) C-*myc* amplification is a better prognostic factor than HER2/neu amplification in primary breast cancer. *Cancer Research* **52** 1107–1114

Berns PMJJ, Foekens JA, Van Putten WLJ *et al* (1992d) Prognostic factors in human primary breast cancer: comparison of c-*myc* and HER2/neu amplification. *Journal of Steroid Biochemistry and Molecular Biology* **43** 13–19

Bonneterre J, Peyrat JP, Beuscart R and Demaille A (1990) Prognostic significance of IGF-1 receptors in human breast cancer. *Cancer Research* **50** 6931–6935

Bontenbal M, Foekens JA, Klijn JGM and other collaborators from a Dutch South West Oncology Group (1992) Phase II trial of tamoxifen versus tamoxifen plus Sandostatin and CV 205-502 in metastatic breast cancer. *Breast Cancer Research and Treatment* **23** 170 [Abstract 157[3]

Bootsma AH, Van Eijk C, Schouten KK *et al* (1993) Somatostatin receptor-positive primary breast tumors: genetic, patient and tumor characteristics. *International Journal of Cancer* **54** 357–362

Borg A, Sigurdsson H, Clark GM *et al* (1991) Association of int2/hst1 coamplification in primary breast cancer with hormone dependent phenotype and poor prognosis. *British Journal of Cancer* **63** 136–142

Borg A, Zhang Q-X, Alm P, Olsson H and Sellberg G (1992) The retinoblastoma gene in breast cancer: allele loss is not correlated with loss of gene protein expression. *Cancer Research* **52** 2991–2994

Brünner N, Moser C, Clarke R and Cullen K (1992) IGF-I and IGF-II expression in human breast cancer xenografts: relationship to hormone independence. *Breast Cancer Research and Treatment* **22** 69–79

Brünner N, Yee D, Kern FG, Spang-Thomsen M, Lippman ME and Cullen KJ (1993) Effect of endocrine therapy on growth of T61 human breast cancer xenografts is directly correlated to a specific down-regulation of insulin-like growth factor II (IGF-II). *European Journal of Cancer* **29A** 562–569

Butta A, Machennan K, Flanders KC *et al* (1992) Induction of transforming growth factor-β in human breast cancer in vivo following tamoxifen treatment. *Cancer Research* **52** 4261–4264

Cantwell BMJ, Hennessy C, Millward MJ and Lennard TWJ (1991) Epidermal growth factor receptors and doxorubicin plus ifosfamide/mesna in recurrent breast cancer. *Lancet* **337** 1417

Ciocca DR, Fuqua SAW, Lock-Lim S, Toft DO, Welch WJ and McGuire WL (1992) Response of human breast cancer cells to heat shock and chemotherapeutic drugs. *Cancer Research* **52** 3648–3654

Clark GM (1992) Integrating prognostic factors. *Breast Cancer Research and Treatment* **22** 187–191

Clarke R, Dickson RB and Lippman ME (1992a) Hormonal aspects of breast cancer: growth factors, drugs and stromal interactions. *Critical Reviews in Oncology/Hematology* **12** 1–23

Clarke R, Currier S, Kaplan O *et al* (1992b) Effect of P-glycoprotein expression on sensitivity to hormones in MCF-7 human breast cancer cells. *Journal of the National Cancer Institute* **84** 1506–1512

Coletti RB, Roberts JD, Devlin JT and Copeland KC (1989) Effects of tamoxifen on plasma insulin-like growth factor I in patients with breast cancer. *Cancer Research* **49** 1882–1884

Coombes RC, Barrett-Lee P and Luqmani Y (1990) Growth factor expression in breast tissue. *Journal of Steroid Biochemistry and Molecular Biology* **37** 833–837

Cullen KJ, Lippman ME, Chow D, Hill S, Rosen N and Zwiebel JA (1992) Insulin-like growth factor-II expression in MCF-7 cells induces phenotypic changes associated with malignant progression. *Molecular Endocrinology* **6** 91–100

Damstrup L, Andersen J, Kufe DW, Hayes DF and Skovgaard Poulsen H (1992) Immunocytochemical determination of the estrogen regulated proteins Mr 24 000 Mr 52 000 and DF3 breast cancer associated antigen: clinical value in advanced breast cancer and correlation with estrogen receptor. *Annals of Oncology* **3** 71–77

De Fazio A, Chiew YE, Donoghue C, Lee CS and Sutherland RL (1992) Effect of sodium butyrate on estrogen receptor and epidermal growth factor receptor gene expression in human breast cancer cell lines. *Journal of Biological Chemistry* **267** 18008–18012

Early Breast Cancer Trialists' Collaborative Group (1992) Systemic treatment of early breast cancer by hormonal, cytotoxic, or immune therapy. *Lancet* **339** 1–15,

Elledge RM, McGuire WL and Osborne CK (1992) Prognostic factors in breast cancer. *Seminars in Oncology* **19** 244–253

Fekete M, Wittliff JL and Schally AV (1989) Characteristics and distribution of receptors for [D-Trp^6]-luteinizing-hormone-releasing hormone, somatostatin, epidermal growth factor, and sex steroids in 500 biopsy samples of human breast cancer. *Journal of Clinical Laboratory Analysis* **3** 137–141

Foekens JA and Klijn JGM (1992) Direct antitumor effects of LH-RH analogs, In: Höffken K (ed). *Peptides in Oncology I, LHRH Agonist and Antagonist. Recent Results in Cancer Research 124*, pp 7–17, Springer-Verlag, Heidelberg

Foekens JA, Portengen H, Van Putten WLJ *et al* (1989a) Prognostic value of estrogen and progesterone receptors measured by enzyme immunoassays in human breast cancer cytosols. *Cancer Research* **49** 5823–5828

Foekens JA, Portengen H, Janssen M and Klijn JGM (1989b) Insulin-like growth factor-1 receptors and insulin-like growth factor-1-like activity in human primary breast cancer. *Cancer* **63** 2139–2147

Foekens JA, Portengen H, Van Putten WLJ *et al* (1989c) Prognostic value of receptors for insulin-like growth factor 1 somatostatin, and epidermal growth factor in human breast cancer. *Cancer Research* **49** 7002–7009

Foekens JA, Rio M-C, Seguin P *et al* (1990a) Prediction of relapse and survival in breast cancer patients by pS2 protein status. *Cancer Research* **50** 3832–3837

Foekens JA, Van Putten WLJ, Portengen H *et al* (1990b) Prognostic value of pS2 protein and receptors for epidermal growth factor (EGF-R), insulin-like growth factor-1 (IGF-1-R) and somatostatin (SS-R) in patients with breast and ovarian cancer. *Journal of Steroid Biochemistry and Molecular Biology* **37** 815–823

Foekens JA, Peters HA, Portengen H, Noordergraaf E, Berns PMJJ and Klijn JGM (1991) Cell biological prognostic factors in breast cancer: a review. *Journal of Clinical Immunoassay* **14** 184–196

Foekens JA, Van Putten WLJ, Thirion B and Klijn JGM (1992a) PS2 and cathepsin-D as predictors of prognosis in primary breast cancer and of response to first-line hormonal therapy in metastatic disease. *Proceedings of the 83rd Annual Meeting of the American Association for Cancer Research*, San Diego, 20–23 May 1992, vol 33, p 284 [Abstract 1697]

Foekens JA, Schmitt M, Van Putten WLJ, Peters HA, Bontenbal M, Jänicke F and Klijn JGM (1992b) Prognostic value of urokinase-type plasminogen activator (uPA) in 671 primary breast cancer patients. *Cancer Research* **52** 6101–6105

Foekens JA, Van Putten WLJ, Portengen H, De Koning HYWCM, Thirion B, Alexieva-Figusch J and Klijn JGM (1993a) Prognostic value of pS2 and cathepsin D in 710 human primary breast tumors: multivariate analysis. *Journal of Clinical Oncology* **11** 899–909

Foekens JA, Jänicke F, Schmitt M *et al* (1993b) The combined prognostic value of urokinase (uPA) and plasminogen activator inhibitor-1 (PAI-1) in 654 primary breast cancer patients. *Proceedings of the 84th Annual Meeting of the American Association for Cancer Research*, Orlando, 19–22 May 1993, vol 34, p 192 [Abstract 1146]

Fornander T, Rutqvist LE and Glas U (1987) Response to tamoxifen and fluoxymesterone in a group of breast cancer patients with disease recurrence after cessation of adjuvant tamoxifen. *Cancer Treatment Reports* **71** 685–688

Freiss G, Rochefort H and Vignon F (1992) Anti-growth factor action of antiestrogens in breast cancer cells. *Abstracts of the International Symposium on Hormones and Breast Cancer: From Biology to the Clinic*, Nice, 29–30 August 1992 [Abstract 13]

Fuqua SAW (1992) Where is the lesion in hormone-independent breast cancer? An editorial.

Journal of the National Cancer Institute **84** 554–555

Gilbert L, Elwood LJ, Merino M *et al* (1993) A pilot study of pi-class glutathione S-transferase expression in breast cancer: correlation with estrogen receptor expression and prognosis in node-negative breast cancer. *Journal of Clinical Oncology* **11** 49–58

Goldfine ID, Papa V, Vigneri R, Siiteri P and Rosenthal S (1992) Progestin regulation of insulin and insulin-like growth factor I receptors in cultured human breast cancer cells. *Breast Cancer Research and Treatment* **22** 69–79

Gullick WJ (1990) New developments in the molecular biology of breast cancer. *European Journal of Cancer* **26** 509–510

Gusterson BA, Gelber RD, Goldhirsch A *et al* (1992) Prognostic importance of c-erbB-2 expression in breast cancer. *Journal of Clinical Oncology* **10** 1049–1056

Hanauske A-R, Osborne CK, Chamness GC *et al* (1987) Alteration of EGF-receptor binding in human breast cancer cells by antineoplastic agents. *European Journal of Cancer and Clinical Oncology* **23** 545–551

Harris AL (1990a) Epidermal growth factor receptor: a marker of early relapse in breast cancer: interactions with neu. *European Journal of Cancer* **26** 154 [Abstract 29]

Harris AL (1990b) The epidermal growth factor receptor as a target for therapy. *Cancer Cells* **2** 321–323

Harris AL (1992) p53 Expression in human breast cancer. *Advances in Cancer Research* **59** 69–89

Harris AL and Hochhauser D (1992) Mechanisms of multidrug resistance in cancer treatment. *Acta Oncologica* **31** 205–213

Hayes DF, Cirrincione C, Carney W *et al* (1993) Elevated circulating HER-2/neu related protein (NRP) is associated with poor survival in patients with metastatic breast cancer. *Proceedings of the 29th Annual Meeting of the American Society of Clinical Oncology*, Orlando, 16–18 May 1993, vol 12, p 58 [Abstract 35]

Henderson IC (1987) Endocrine therapy in metastatic breast cancer, In: Harris JR, Hellman S Henderson IC, and Kinne DW (eds). *Breast Diseases*, pp 398–428, JB Lippincott, Philadelphia

Henry JA, Nicholson S, Hennessy C, Lennard TWJ, May FEB and Westley BR (1989) Expression of the oestrogen regulated pNR-2 mRNA in human breast cancer: relation to oestrogen receptor mRNA levels and response to tamoxifen therapy. *British Journal of Cancer* **61** 32–38

Henry JA, Piggott NH, Mallick UK *et a l* (1991) pNR-2/pS2 immuno-histochemical staining in breast cancer: correlation with prognostic factors and endocrine response. *British Journal of Cancer* **63** 615–622

Horwitz KB (1992) The molecular biology of RU 486: is there a role for antiprogestins in the treatment of breast cancer? *Endocrine Reviews* **13** 146–163

Horwitz KB, Wei LL, Sedlacek SM and d'Arville CN (1985) Progestin action and progesterone receptor structure in human breast cancer: a review. *Recent Progress in Hormone Research* **41** 249–316

Howell A, Harland RNL, Barnes DM *et al* (1987) Endocrine therapy for advanced carcinoma of the breast: relationship between the effect of tamoxifen upon concentrations of progesterone receptor and subsequent response to treatment. *Cancer Research* **47** 300–304

Jänicke F, Graeff H and Schmitt M (1991) Clinical relevance of the urokinase-type and tissue-type plasminogen activators and of their type 1 inhibitor in breast cancer. *Seminars in Thrombosis and Hemostasis* **17** 303–312

Kallioniemi PO, Holli K, Visakorpi T, Koivula T, Helin HH and Isola JJ (1991) Association of c-erbβ-2 protein over-expression with high rate of cell proliferation, increased risk of visceral metastatis and poor long-term survival in breast cancer. *International Journal of Cancer* **49** 650–655

Kiang DT, Kollander R, Kiang B and Kao PC (1992) Role of plasma IGF-I in endocrine therapy for breast cancer. *Proceedings of the 28th Annual Meeting of the American Society of Clini-*

cal Oncology, San Diego, 17–19 May 1992, vol 11, p 51 [Abstract 31]

Kiesel L, Bentzien F, Baumann KH, Kaufmann M, Runnebaum B and Bastert G (1993) Bindung und direkte wirkung von GnRH-Releasing-Hormone-Analoga in mammakarzinomen. *13th Annual Meeting of the German Society of Senology*, Berlin, 3–5 June 1993

Klijn JGM (1991) Clinical parameters and symptoms for the progression to endocrine independence of breast cancer, In: Berns PMJJ, Romijn JC and Schröder FH (eds). *Mechanisms of Progression to Hormone-independent Growth of Breast and Prostatic Cancer*, pp 11–19, Parthenon, Carnforth

Klijn JGM (1992) LH-RH agonists in the treatment of metastatic breast cancer: ten years' experience, In: Höffken K (ed). *Peptides in Oncology I, LHRH Agonists and Antagonists. Recent Results in Cancer Research 124*, pp 75–90, Springer-Verlag, Heidelberg

Klijn JGM and De Jong FH (1982) Treatment with a luteinizing hormone-releasing-hormone analogue (buserelin) in premenopausal patients with metastatic breast cancer. *Lancet* **i** 1213–1216

Klijn JGM and Foekens JA (1990) Prognostic factors in breast cancer, In: Goldhirsch A (ed). *Endocrine Treatment of Breast Cancer IV. Monograph Series of the European School of Oncology*, pp 17–25, Springer-Verlag, Berlin

Klijn JGM, De Jong FH, Bakker GH et al (1989) Antiprogestins, a new form of endocrine therapy for human breast cancer. *Cancer Research* **49** 2851–2856

Klijn JGM, Setyono-Han B, Bakker GH, Van der Burg MEL, Bontenbal M, Peters HA, Sieuwerts AM, Berns PMJJ and Foekens JA (1990) Growth factor-receptor pathway interfering treatment by somatostatin analogs and suramin: preclinical and clinical studies. *Journal of Steroid Biochemistry and Molecular Biology* **37** 1089–1097

Klijn JGM, Berns PMJJ, Van Putten WLJ et al (1992a) The prognostic value of oncogene amplification and of tumoral secretory proteins with respect to response to endocrine and chemotherapy in metastatic breast cancer. *Proceedings of the 28th Annual Meeting of the American Society of Clinical Oncology*, San Diego, 17–19 May 1992, vol 11, p 53 [Abstract 37]

Klijn JGM, Berns PMJJ, Schmitz PIM and Foekens JA (1992b) The clinical significance of epidermal growth factor receptor (EGF-R) in human breast cancer: a review on 5232 patients. *Endocrine Reviews* **13** 3–18

Klijn JGM, Berns PMJJ, Bontenbal M, Alexieva-Figusch J and Foekens JA (1992c) Clinical breast cancer, new developments in selection and endocrine treatment of patients. *Journal of Steroid Biochemistry and Molecular Biology* **43** 211–221

Klijn JGM, Berns PMJJ, Van Putten WLJ, Bontenbal M, Alexieva-Figusch J and Foekens JA (1993a) Critical review of growth factors as clinical tools in primary and metastatic breast cancer, In: Senn HJ, Goldhirsch A, Gelber RD and Thürlimann B (eds). *Adjuvant Therapy of Breast Cancer IV. Recent Results in Cancer Research 127*, pp 77–89, Springer-Verlag, Heidelberg

Klijn JGM, Berns PMJJ, Bontenbal M and Foekens JA (1993b) Cell biological factors associated with the response of breast cancer to systemic treatment. *Cancer Treatment Reviews* **19** (Supplement B 45–63

Klijn JGM, Berns PMJJ, Dorssers LCJ and Foekens JA Molecular markers of resistance to endocrine treatment of breast cancer, In: Dickson RB and Lippman ME (eds). *Drug and Hormone Resistance in Breast Cancer: Cellular and Molecular Mechanisms*, Ellis Horwood, Chichester (in press a)

Klijn JGM, Berns PMJJ, Schmitz PIM and Foekens JA Epidermal growth factor receptor in clinical breast cancer: update 1993. *Monographs of Endocrine Reviews* (in press b)

Knabbe C (1993) Paracrine regulation of breast cancer cells. *13th Annual Meeting of the German Society of Senology*, Berlin, 3–5 June 1993

Kvols LK and Reubi J-C (1990) Treatment of metastatic carcinoid tumors with somatostatin analogue (Octreotide) and correlation of response with presence of somatostatin receptors, In: Klijn JGM, Foekens JA and Schröder FH (eds). *Abstracts of the Second International*

Symposium on Hormonal Manipulation of Cancer: Peptides, Growth Factors and New (Anti-)Steroidal Agents, Rotterdam, 9–11 April 1990, p 38 [Abstract 64]

Kwok TT and Sutherland RM (1991) Epidermal growth factor reduces resistance to doxorubicin. *International Journal of Cancer* **49** 73–76

Lamberts SWJ, Krenning EP, Klijn JGM and Reubi J-C (1990) Clinical use of somatostatin analogs in the treatment of cancer. *Baillière's Clinical Endocrinology and Metabolism* **3** 29–49

Lamberts SWJ, Reubi J-C and Krenning EP (1992) Somatostatin receptor imaging in the diagnosis and treatment of neuroendocrine tumors. *Journal of Steroid Biochemistry and Molecular Biology* **43** 185–188

Levine MN and Andrulis I (1992) The HER2/neu oncogene in breast cancer: so what is new? An editorial. *Journal of Clinical Oncology* **10** 1034–1036

Lippman ME (1993) The development of biological therapies for breast cancer. *Science* **259** 631–632

Long B, McKibben BM, Lynch M and Van den Berg HW (1992) Changes in epidermal growth factor receptor expression and response to ligand associated with acquired tamoxifen resistance or oestrogen independence in the ZR-75-1 human breast cancer cell line. *British Journal of Cancer* **65** 865–869

Mansour EG, Gray R, Shatila AH *et al* (1989) Efficacy of adjuvant chemotherapy in high-risk node-negative breast cancer. *New England Journal of Medicine* **320** 485–490

Markus C (1988) The relevance of plasminogen activators to neoplastic growth: a review of recent literature. *Enzyme* **40** 158–172

Marx J (1993) Cell death studies yield cancer clues. *Science* **259** 760–762

McGuire WL (1989) Adjuvant treatment of node-negative breast cancer. *New England Journal of Medicine* **320** 525–527

McLeskey SW, Kurebayashi J, Honig SF *et al* (1993) Fibroblast growth factor 4 transfection of MCF-7 cells produces cell lines that are tumorigenic and metastatic in ovariectomized or tamoxifen-treated athymic nude mice. *Cancer Research* **53** 2168–2177

Meyers MB, Merluzzi VJ, Spengler BA and Biedler JL (1986) Epidermal growth factor receptor is increased in multidrug-resistant Chinese hamster and mouse tumor cells. *Proceedings of the National Academy of Sciences of the USA* **83** 5521–5525

Muss HB (1992) Endocrine therapy for advanced breast cancer: a review. *Breast Cancer Research and Treatment* **21** 15–26

Muss H, Thor A, Kute T *et al* for the CALGB (1993) Erbβ-2 (c-erbβ-2, HER-2/neu) and S-phase fraction predict response to adjuvant chemotherapy in patients with node-positive breast cancer: Cancer and Acute Leukemia Group B (CALGB) Trial 8869. *Proceedings of the 29th Annual Meeting of the American Society of Clinical Oncology*, Orlando, 16–18 May 1993, vol 12, p 72 [Abstract 88]

Namer M, Ramaioli A, Fontana X *et al* (1991) Prognostic value of total cathepsin-D in breast tumors. *Breast Cancer Research and Treatment* **19** 85–93

Nicholson S, Sainsbury JRC, Halcrow P, Chambers P, Farndon JR and Harris AL (1989) Expression of epidermal growth factor receptors associated with lack of response to endocrine therapy in recurrent breast cancer. *Lancet* **i** 182–184

Nicholson S, Wright C, Sainsbury JRC *et al* (1990) Epidermal growth factor receptor (EGFr) as a marker for poor prognosis in node-negative breast cancer patients: neu and tamoxifen failure. *Journal of Steroid Biochemistry and Molecular Biology* **37** 811–815

Nishikawa K, Rosenblum MG, Newman RA, Pandita TK, Hittelman WN and Donato NJ (1992) Resistance of human cervical carcinoma cells to tumor necrosis factor correlates with increased sensitivity to cisplatin: evidence of a role for DNA repair and epidermal growth factor receptor. *Cancer Research* **52** 4758–4765

O'Reilly SM, Barnes DM, Camplejohn RS, Bartkoua J, Gregory WM and Richards MA (1991) The relationship between c-erbB-2 expression, S-phase fraction and prognosis in breast cancer. *British Journal of Cancer* **63** 444–446

Osborne CK, Clemmons DR and Arteaga CL (1990) Regulation of breast cancer growth by insulin-like growth factors. *Journal of Steroid Biochemistry and Molecular Biology* **37** 805–809

Padmanabhan N, Howell A and Rubens RD (1986) Mechanism of action of adjuvant chemotherapy in early breast cancer. *Lancet* **ii** 411–415

Pegram MD, Pietras RJ, Chazin VR, Ellis L and Slamon DJ (1993) Effect of erbβ-2 (HER2/neu) overexpression on chemotherapeutic drug sensitivity in human breast and ovarian cancer cells. *Proceedings of the 84th Annual Meeting of the American Association for Cancer Research,* Orlando, 19–22 May 1993, vol 34, p 26 [Abstract 152]

Perren TJ (1991) C-erbB-2 oncogene as a prognostic marker in breast cancer. *British Journal of Cancer* **63** 328–332

Peters WHM, Roelofs HMJ, Van Putten WLJ, Jansen JBBJ, Klijn JGM and Foekens JA (1993) Response to adjuvant chemotherapy in primary breast cancer: no correlation with expression of glutathione S-transferases. *British Journal of Cancer* **68** 86–92

Peyrat JP, Bonneterre J, Vermin PH *et al* (1990) Insulin-like growth factor 1 receptors (IGF-1-R) and IGF-1 in human breast tumors. *Journal of Steroid Biochemistry and Molecular Biology* **37** 823–827

Peyrat JP, Bonneterre J, Hondermarck H *et al* (1992) Basic fibroblast growth factor (bFGF) mitogenic activity and binding sites in human breast cancer. *Journal of Steroid Biochemistry and Molecular Biology* **43** 87–94

Peyrat JP, Bonneterre J, Hecquet B *et al* (1993) Plasma insulin-like growth factor-I (IGF-I) concentrations in human breast cancer. *European Journal of Cancer* **29A** 492–497

Pollak M, Constantino J, Polychronakos C *et al* (1990) Effect of tamoxifen on serum insulin-like growth factor-1 levels in stage I breast cancer patients. *Journal of the National Cancer Institute* **82** 1693–1697

Predine J, Spyratos F, Prud'homme JF *et al* (1992) Enzyme-linked immunosorbent assay of pS2 in breast cancers, benign tumors, and normal breast tissues: correlation with prognosis and adjuvant hormone therapy. *Cancer* **69** 2116–2123

Quénel N, Dorion-Bonnet F, Coindre JM *et al* (1993) Relationship between GSTpi and c-erbβ-2 RNA levels and response to tamoxifen therapy: analysis of 33 primary locally advanced breast carcinomas. *Proceedings of the 29th Annual Meeting of the American Society of Clinical Oncology,* Orlando, 16–18 May 1993, vol 12, p 120 [Abstract 279]

Raemaekers JMM, Beex LVAM, Pieters GFFM, Smals AGH, Benraad ThJ, Kloppenborg PWC and the Breast Study Group (1987) Progesterone receptor activity and relapse-free survival in patients with primary breast cancer: the role of adjuvant chemotherapy. *Breast Cancer Research and Treatment* **9** 191–199

Ravdin PM, Green S, Melink Dorr T *et al* (1992) Prognostic significance of progesterone receptor levels in estrogen receptor-positive patients with metastatic breast cancer treated with tamoxifen: results of a prospective Southwest Oncology Group study. *Journal of Clinical Oncology* **10** 1284–1291

Reeve JG, Rabbitts PH and Twentyman PR (1990) Non-P-glycoprotein-mediated multidrug resistance with reduced EGF receptor expression in a human large cell lung cancer cell line. *British Journal of Cancer* **61** 851–855

Reubi J-C, Waser B, Foekens JA, Klijn JGM, Lamberts SWJ and Laissue J (1990) Somatostatin receptor incidence and distribution in breast cancer using receptor autoradiography: relationship to EGF receptors. *International Journal of Cancer* **46** 416–421

Rio M-C and Chambon P (1990) The pS2 gene, mRNA, and protein: a potential marker for human breast cancer. A review. *Cancer Cells* **2** 269–274

Rochefort H (1992) Cathepsin-D in breast cancer: a tissue marker associated with metastasis. *European Journal of Cancer* **28A** 1780–1783

Roux-Dosseto M, Romain S, Dassault N *et al* (1992) c-*Myc* gene amplification in selected node-negative breast cancer patients correlates with high rate of early relapse. *European Journal of Cancer* **28A** 1600–1604

Royds JA, Stephenson TJ, Rees RC, Shorthouse AJ and Silcocks PB (1993) Nm23 protein expression in ductal in situ and invasive human breast carcinoma. *Journal of the National Cancer Institute* **85** 727–731

Rubens RD (1993) Effect of adjuvant systemic therapy on respone to treatment after relapse. *Cancer Treatment Reviews* **19 (Supplement B)** 3–10

Santen RJ, Manni A, Harvey H and Redmond C (1990) Endocrine treatment of breast cancer in women. *Endocrine Reviews* **11** 221–265

Schwartz LH, Koerner FC, Edgerton SM *et al* (1991) pS2 expression and response to hormonal therapy in patients with advanced breast cancer. *Cancer Research* **51** 624–628

Scottish Cancer Trials Breast Group and ICRF Breast Unit (1993) Adjuvant ovarian ablation versus CMF chemotherapy in premenopausal women with pathological stage II breast carcinoma: the Scottish trial. *Lancet* **341** 1293–1298

Setyono-Han B, Henkelman MS, Foekens JA and Klijn, JGM (1987) Direct inhibitory effects of somatostatin (analogues) on the growth of human breast cancer cells. *Cancer Research* **47** 1566–1570

Silvestrini R Biological markers for designing clinical protocols. *Proceedings of the Pisa Symposium on Breast Cancer: From Biology to Therapy,* Pisa, 19–21 October 1992, New York Academy of Sciences, New York (in press)

Silvestrini R and Daidone MG (1993) Review of proliferative variables and their predictive value, In: Senn H-J, Gelber RD, Goldhirsch A and Thürlimann B (eds). *Adjuvant Therapy of Breast Cancer IV Recent Results in Cancer Research 127,* pp 71–77, Springer-Verlag, Heidelberg

Skilton RA, Luqmani YA, McClelland RA and Coombes RC (1989) Characterization of a messenger RNA selectively expressed in human breast cancer. *British Journal of Cancer* **60** 168–175

Sklar MD and Prochownik EV (1991) Modulation of *cis*-platinum resistance in Friend erythroleukemia cells by c-*myc. Cancer Research* **51** 2118–2123

Steeg PS, De La Rosa A, Flatow U, MacDonald NJ, Benedict M and Leone A (1993) Nm23 and breast cancer metastasis. *Breast Cancer Research and Treatment* **25** 175–187

Teulings FAG, Van Gilse HA, Henkelman MS, Portengen H and Alexieva-Figusch J (1980) Estrogen, androgen, glucocorticoid, and progesterone receptors in progestin-induced regression of human breast cancer. *Cancer Research* **40** 2557–2561

Thor AD and Yandell DW (1993) Prognostic significance of p53 overexpression in node-negative breast carcinoma: preliminary studies support cautious optimism. An editorial. *Journal of the National Cancer Institute* **85** 176–177

Thor AD, Koerner FC, Edgerton SM and Schwartz LM (1992) pS2 expression in primary breast carcinomas: relationship to clinical and histological features and survival. *Breast Cancer Research and Treatment* **21** 111–119

Thorlacius S, Börresen A-L and Eyfjörd JE (1993) Somatic p53 mutations in human breast carcinomas in an Icelandic population: a prognostic factor. *Cancer Research* **53** 1637–1641

Trudeau ME and Pritchard KI (1992) Adjuvant endocrine therapy of breast cancer, In: Henderson IC (ed). *Adjuvant Therapy of Breast Cancer,* pp 69–115, Kluwer Academic, Boston

Tsuda H, Hirohashi S, Shimosato Y *et al* (1989) Correlation between long term survival in breast cancer patients and amplification of two putative oncogene-coamplication units; hst-1/int-2 and c-erbB-2/ear-1. *Cancer Research* **49** 3104–3108

Van Agthoven T, Van Agthoven TLA, Portengen H, Foekens JA and Dorssers LCJ (1992) Ectopic expression of epidermal growth factor receptors induces hormone independence in ZR-75-1 human breast cancer cells. *Cancer Research* **52** 5082–5088

Varley JM, Armour J, Swallow JE *et al* (1989) The retinoblastoma gene is frequently altered leading to loss of expression in primary breast tumors. *Oncogene* **4** 725–729

Wright C, Nicholson S, Angus B *et al* (1992a) Relationship between c-erbβ-2 protein product expression and response to endocrine therapy in advanced breast cancer. *British Journal of Cancer* **65** 118–121

Wright C, Cairns J, Cantwell BJ *et al* (1992b) Response to mitoxantrone in advanced breast cancer: correlation with expression of c-erbB-2 protein and glutathione S-transferases. *British Journal of Cancer* **65** 271–274

The authors are responsible for the accuracy of the references.

Improving Treatment for Advanced Breast Cancer

R D RUBENS

ICRF Clinical Oncology Unit, Guy's Hospital, London SE1 9RT

Introduction
Incidence and prevalence
Selection of treatment
Endocrine treatment
Chemotherapy
Cost effectiveness of treatment
Effects of prior adjuvant treatment
Bone metastases
Appropriate use of investigations
Summary

INTRODUCTION

"... we retard what we cannot repel, ... we palliate what we cannot cure".
Samuel Johnson, 1775

Breast cancer advanced beyond the possibility of radical surgical resection is not usually curable with current treatments and most patients have a severely shortened life expectancy. Nevertheless, important advances have been made in treatment, some of which have been applied to the early disease to extend the survival of patients significantly (Early Breast Cancer Trialists' Collaborative Group, 1992). In advanced disease, prolongation of survival is not usually a primary objective of treatment; rather, the intention is to relieve symptoms, reduce disability and prevent morbidity. Our aim is palliation. However, when the pattern of metastatic disease results in rapidly progressive organ failure, such as metastatic liver disease or lymphangitis carcinomatosa, its reversal by treatment almost certainly prolongs life in such circumstances.

INCIDENCE AND PREVALENCE

The incidence of breast cancer in the UK is 25 000 new cases per year, but the prevalence of the condition in the population is estimated at 105 000 (Cancer Research Campaign, 1990). It is informative to contrast these figures with

Cancer Surveys Volume 18: *Breast Cancer*
© 1993 Imperial Cancer Research Fund. 0-87969-394-0/93. $5.00 + .00

those for the other two most common cancers, lung and colorectal. The incidence of lung cancer is 40 000 per year, but with its high mortality, the prevalence is only 26 000. For colorectal cancer, the figures are 27 000 and 56 000, respectively. These figures illustrate the chronicity of breast cancer resulting in a high prevalence of more than four times its annual incidence. These statistics show that, of all cancers, carcinoma of the breast almost certainly makes the greatest demands on health care resources.

SELECTION OF TREATMENT

Table 1 lists the wide variety of treatments available for advanced breast cancer. In this highly heterogeneous disease, much skill is needed in the optimal selection of treatment for individual patients. Clinical research has to some extent provided useful guidelines. For localized lesions, radiotherapy can be particularly effective, especially for painful bone metastases. Surgical excision supplemented by radiotherapy may suffice for superficial soft tissue lesions. However, for the palliation of more widespread disease, systemic anti-cancer agents, endocrine therapy or cytotoxic chemotherapy must be considered. Selection of treatment is guided by attention to three factors: extent, pattern and aggressiveness of the disease; steroid receptor levels; and menstrual status.

For patients with rapidly progressing visceral lesions, death is likely to ensue quickly unless the progress of the disease can be reversed. The principal examples are lymphangitis carcinomatosa causing severe breathlessness or hepatic metastases with markedly deranged liver biochemistry. This type of disease is rarely responsive to hormonal treatment, chemotherapy being necessary if there is to be a chance of the disease remitting. For less aggressive disease, it can be helpful to consider the oestrogen and progesterone receptor status of the tumour. With low levels of these receptors, a response to endocrine treatment is unlikely and chemotherapy should be considered. For patients with steroid receptor positive tumours, menstrual status can assist in the selection of treatment. The established treatment for premenopausal patients with receptor positive tumours is ovarian ablation, although the use of gonadotrophin releasing hormone agonists or tamoxifen is a reasonable alternative. For postmenopausal patients, the preferred treatment is tamoxifen. On progression of disease after response to primary hormone treatment, other forms of endocrine treatment may be considered before chemotherapy is needed.

ENDOCRINE TREATMENT

The rationale for endocrine therapy has been to reduce the oestrogenic stimulus to tumour growth. This may be achieved by removing sites of oestrogen production, removing the source of or inhibiting gonadotrophins,

TABLE 1. Treatments available for advanced breast cancer

Radiotherapy
Surgery
Endocrine therapy
  ovarian ablation
  anti-oestrogens
  aromatase inhibitors
  progestogens
  gonadotrophin releasing hormone agonists
Cytotoxic chemotherapy
Corticosteroids
Bisphosphonates
Isotope therapy
Immunotherapy
Symptom control

blocking oestrogenic action, antagonizing oestrogens with androgens or progestogens or inhibiting oestrogen synthesis.

Removal of the source of oestrogen production is by ovarian ablation either surgically or by pelvic irradiation; bilateral adrenalectomy is now obsolete. Removing the source of gonadotrophins by hypophysectomy is also no longer performed as medical approaches to gonadotrophin inhibition have been developed including the use of gonadotrophin releasing hormone agonists, danazol and progestogens.

Tamoxifen has been the principal agent used to block binding of oestrogen to its receptor. Its activity in advanced breast cancer is enhanced by the concomitant use of prednisolone (Rubens *et al*, 1988). It has also been found that tamoxifen has another potentially important anti-tumour action of inducing the production of the inhibitory transforming growth factor beta (Butta *et al*, 1992). Immunohistochemistry shows that the induction of this growth factor in the stroma of human breast cancer occurs in both oestrogen receptor negative and positive tumours. The mechanisms of acquired resistance to tamoxifen are being clarified and attributed to mutations in the oestrogen receptor (Jiang and Jordan, 1992; Fuqua *et al*, 1993). Because tamoxifen has oestrogen agonist effects on certain tissues, such as the bone and endometrium and on lipid metabolism, new less oestrogenic compounds such as droloxifene (Bruning, 1992) and toremifene (Vogel *et al*, 1993) have been developed and are undergoing clinical trial. A further intriguing potential for these agents is their ability to reverse P-glycoprotein mediated multidrug resistance to cytotoxic drugs (Wiebe *et al*, 1992).

Of particular interest in recent years in the development of endocrine therapy has been the production of agents to inhibit oestrogen synthesis. The first such agent, aminoglutethimide, was originally introduced because it inhibited the desmolase enzyme responsible for converting cholesterol to pregnenolone in the adrenal cortex, so interfering with the production of all adrenocortical hormones. Subsequently, it became clear that the principal action of the drug is to inhibit the aromatase enzyme, which converts C19 androgens to C18 oestrogens, a more specific effect achieved by concentrations that do not inhibit desmolase. Moreover, inhibition of aromatase also prevents the peripheral synthesis of oestrogens from androgens in adipose tissue, the liver and breast cancer (Santen *et al*, 1978). These findings have stimulated the search for more specific aromatase inhibitors, both steroidal and non-steroidal, and these agents are likely to become increasingly important endocrine treatments for breast cancer. It has also been suggested that the effectiveness of this approach could be enhanced by the concomitant use of agents that inhibit oestrone sulphatase to prevent the hydrolysis of oestrone sulphate to oestrone (Duncan *et al*, 1993).

CHEMOTHERAPY

The principal cytotoxic agents used for the treatment of breast cancer are doxorubicin, cyclophosphamide, methotrexate, 5-fluorouracil, mitomycin C and mitoxantrone. They are frequently used in combinations that may also include prednisolone. No clearly superior combination has emerged, and it is uncertain whether any are significantly more effective than doxorubicin alone, widely recognized as the most active single drug. Ideally, the contribution of any drug in a combination should be confirmed by a clinical trial in order to use the available treatments optimally. This has only rarely been done, and such trials have demonstrated the lack of value of vincristine in combinations (Steiner *et al*, 1983). Few important new drugs have become established in recent years for use in breast cancer, although taxol is showing considerable promise (Holmes *et al*, 1991) and epirubicin may have advantages over doxorubicin (Launchbury and Habboubi, 1993). Considerable progress has been made in the reduction of the toxic effects of chemotherapy, particularly with the use of more effective anti-emetics. There are no good predictors of response to chemotherapy, although crude measures of tumour bulk and performance status do give some information; a large tumour burden and poor performance status correlate with low response rates (Fischer *et al*, 1982).

Dose-response relationships have been demonstrated for cytotoxic drugs (Carmo-Pereira *et al*, 1987; Engelsman *et al*, 1991). Testing the concept of dose intensification has been facilitated by the use of haematopoietic growth factors and autologous bone marrow transplantation (Eddy, 1992). However, there is no evidence so far to suggest that this enhances either the palliation or curability of advanced breast cancer. This stage of the disease has acted as a test-bed of this approach for potential application in the curative treatment of high risk early disease.

COST EFFECTIVENESS OF TREATMENT

Whether or not a patient judges treatment for advanced breast cancer to be worthwhile will depend on any benefits, such as symptom relief or reduction

TABLE 2. Typical eligibility restrictions in protocols of chemotherapy for advanced breast cancer that often result in patients in clinical trials not being representative of those seen in routine practice

1. Age (eg <70 years)
2. Performance status (eg ≤2 on UICC criteria)
3. Lesions must be measurable
4. Defined limits for haematological tests
5. Defined limits for biochemical tests
6. Exclusion of concomitant illnesses
7. Unacceptability of certain prior treatments
8. Exclusion of certan metastatic lesions
9. Requirement of "informed consent"

UICC = International Union Against Cancer

in disability, outweighing any adverse effects including toxicity and psychosocial disruption from hospital visits. The balance between beneficial and harmful effects can be particularly fine when using cytotoxic chemotherapy for the palliative treatment of cancer. Judgments on cost effectiveness are difficult to make as the relevant factors are not easily compared with each other nor are they readily amenable to quantitative measurement. Clinical trials have usually relied on strict criteria of objective response to determine the efficacy of treatment (Hayward *et al*, 1977), but in recent years, more weight is being given to the evaluation of symptom relief and quality of life (Selby and Robertson, 1987). A particular problem in placing too much reliance on clinical trials to provide useful information in planning treatment for individual patients is that they often have highly restrictive entry criteria and so may not represent the generality of patients with advanced cancer (Table 2).

To develop criteria for good clinical practice, trial results need to be supplemented by information from collective clinical experience (Rubens *et al*, 1992). The appropriateness of such guidelines must be scrutinized carefully. One approach is medical audit, which is defined as the systematic critical analysis of medical activity. Should this process disclose that intended outcomes are not being achieved, changes in the previously determined criteria would be necessary and these again would have to be subjected to audit in due course. Preliminary experience of this approach in advanced breast cancer suggests that objective criteria of response correlate well with the acquisition of benefits in terms of symptom relief and reduction in disability (Rubens, 1993a). However, with the use of successive lines of chemotherapy, effectiveness wanes and benefits from third and fourth line regimens may be negligible.

Audit is by definition a retrospective process and is conducted by medical and nursing personnel perusing case records. To be confident that audit provides subjectively important information, the method needs corroboration by prospective data gathered directly from patients. Techniques for this are well established, and the use of instruments such as the Rotterdam Symptom Checklist (De Haes *et al*, 1990) is being increasingly incorporated into both the design of clinical trials and routine oncological practice. In a recent report, two different schedules of doxorubicin that gave equal dose intensity per unit of time were compared. Although no differences were found between the regimens in terms of objective response, time to progressive disease or physical toxicity, significant advantages were demonstrated in the improvement of psychological status when using a regimen given every 3 weeks, rather than one requiring weekly injections (Richards *et al,* 1992). This illustrates how the omission of quality of life evaluation from clinical trials in advanced cancer might lead to erroneous conclusions being drawn about the relative efficacies of regimens by ignoring aspects of outcome of major importance to patients.

Conduct of clinical practice along these lines with the systematic gathering of global outcome measures is to be encouraged. The extensive data obtained should be used to create databases for multivariate analysis of predictive factors and the automation of audit. The development of such systems can be expected to enhance both decision making and our confidence in selecting treatment for individual patients as well as discarding treatment predicted to be of no value.

EFFECTS OF PRIOR ADJUVANT TREATMENT

Most patients with early breast cancer now receive adjuvant systemic therapy as part of primary treatment, and this leads to a significant improvement in survival (Early Breast Cancer Trialists' Collaborative Group, 1992). However, evidence is accumulating that this results in a lowering of the responsiveness of the disease to systemic treatment after relapse. Response rates for endocrine treatment are lower after either adjuvant tamoxifen (Fornander *et al,* 1987; Rubens, 1993b) or chemotherapy (Houston *et al,* 1993), the latter also being associated with a reduced response of advanced disease to chemotherapy (Bonneterre and Mercier, 1993; Houston *et al,* 1993) and the overall utility of treatment (Rubens, 1993b). Although the impaired responsiveness of the advanced disease does not outweigh the benefits of adjuvant treatment, it does diminish our ability to palliate metastatic disease by systemic anti-tumour treatment. This has important implications for the selection of treatment and also emphasizes the importance of using prior adjuvant treatment as a covariate in the analysis of clinical trials in advanced disease. The mechanism of the lowered response after adjuvant treatment is probably partly from the selection of primary resistant disease, although the induction of acquired resistance may also be important.

BONE METASTASES

The skeleton is the most common distant site to which breast cancer spreads. Bone metastases affect 8% of all patients who develop breast cancer, but this rises to 70% in those with advanced disease (Coleman and Rubens, 1987). Secondaries in bone cause much of the morbidity and disability caused by this disease. Complications include pain, pathological fractures, hypercalcaemia, myelosuppression, spinal cord compression and nerve root lesions. Skeletal damage results from bone resorption caused by the stimulation of osteoclasts by tumour derived cytokines (Mundy *et al*, 1985). Procathepsin D, prostaglandin E and parathyroid hormone related protein released by tumour cells stimulate osteoclasts directly. Interleukin 1, interleukin 6, tumour necrosis factor, epidermal growth factor, transforming growth factor alpha and granulocyte–macrophage colony stimulating factor act through intermediary osteoblasts or immune cells, which in turn release osteoclast stimulating factors.

This knowledge has led to the development of agents that inhibit osteoclastic activity (Coleman and Purohit, 1993). Most important are the bisphosphonates in which oxygen in the P-O-P backbone of pyrophosphoric acid is replaced by carbon, which protects these agents from phosphatase digestion. The bisphosphonates bind to hydroxyapatite, thereby protecting it from osteoclastic resorption. Ingested bisphosphonates are also directly toxic to osteoclasts and also inhibit the differentiation of their precursor cells. The efficacy of bisphosphonates in metastatic bone disease was first demonstrated by the reversal of hypercalcaemia, a complication for which these agents are now the treatment of first choice. Subsequent work showed that even in the absence of direct anti-tumour treatment, they could lead to the recalcification of lytic bone metastases. Current work is directed at the formulation of preparations for oral administration and trials are under way to assess the contribution of bisphosphonates to systemic anti-tumour treatment and their potential role in the prevention of bone metastases.

Another new approach to the treatment of metastatic bone disease is the administration of bone seeking isotopes (Clarke, 1991). Strontium-87 is a pure β emitter and, like calcium, is a bone seeking element. Samarium-153 also has β emission for therapeutic use and additional α emission allows imaging to be done. It is targeted to the skeleton by complexing it to a tetraphosphonate. These agents can be highly effective for relieving bone pain, particularly in the late stages of disease when high doses of opioid analgesics are required and external beam radiotherapy is no longer practicable.

APPROPRIATE USE OF INVESTIGATIONS

The use of laboratory and radiological investigations that do not influence either the management or outcome of patients is always undesirable, but particularly so in patients with advanced cancer. Tests should have a clear purpose, such as those necessary to give cytotoxic chemotherapy safely, those needed to diagnose intercurrent problems and those appropriate to monitor response to treatment. Assessing response to treatment in advanced breast cancer can often simply be achieved by clinical examination supplemented by plain radiography of marker lesions. Sometimes ultrasonography and computed tomography may be useful. Magnetic resonance imaging is only occasionally needed but is of especial value when spinal cord compression is suspected.

A particular problem in monitoring disease progress on treatment is the evaluation of bone metastases. Assessing response to treatment at these sites is difficult compared with disease in soft tissues. Response is usually judged by the recalcification of previously lytic disease seen on plain radiographs according to criteria of the International Union Against Cancer (UICC) (Hayward *et al*, 1977). However, this method does not observe tumour regression directly, but rather a delayed consequential healing. This results in reported response frequencies being lower in the skeleton compared with soft tissue disease (Coleman and Rubens, 1987). This is almost certainly a reflection of the insensitivity of the assessment method rather than a true difference in response rates.

The isotope scan is the most sensitive method for screening for bone metastases. It images function rather than structure and reflects osteoblastic activity. For this reason, it is not of value for the early assessment of response to treatment, because increased osteoblastic activity associated with progression of bone disease is indistinguishable from that due to bone healing (Coleman *et al*, 1988a).

Because of these limitations of imaging techniques, efforts have been made to identify other parameters of response in bone. Biochemical factors studied have included the bone isoenzyme of alkaline phosphatase (ALP-BI), the osteoblast product, osteocalcin, and urinary calcium excretion. The increased osteoblastic activity associated with an ultimate radiological response according to UICC criteria is characterized by an elevation of the serum osteocalcin and ALP-BI 1 month after starting treatment, when there is also a drop in the urinary calcium excretion (Coleman *et al*, 1988b). The combination of a rise in ALP-BI and osteocalcin and a fall in urinary calcium excretion gives a diagnostic efficiency of 89% for discriminating between response and progression. Preliminary observations on the urinary excretion of the crosslinking aminoacids of collagen, pyridinoline and deoxypyridinoline have shown a significant decrease in patients with bone metastases 4 weeks after starting treatment with the osteoclast inhibiting agent pamidronate (Coleman *et al*, 1992).

The importance of these results lies in the aim of the treatment of bone metastases being palliative rather than curative. Early information at 1 month indicative of either response or progressive disease is particularly helpful in determining whether or not treatment should be continued. This cannot be achieved if reliance is placed solely upon imaging tests.

SUMMARY

Treatment for advanced breast cancer is not yet curative but aims to palliate the disease to make life as symptom free and as active for as long as possible with the minimum of adverse effects of treatment. The high prevalence and often long time course of the disease leads breast cancer to make major demands on health care resources. Radiotherapy is valuable for localized lesions, but more widespread disease relies on systemic treatment. Tamoxifen is the main agent for endocrine therapy, although aromatase inhibitors and progestogens are also important. Improvements in cytotoxic chemotherapy have come as much from methods to reduce toxicity as from new agents. Intensive chemotherapy with bone marrow support has not found a routine place in advanced breast cancer, but experience gained may have more application in the adjuvant treatment of high risk operable disease. Incorporation of quality of life measures is being increasingly recognized as essential for the proper evaluation of response to treatment. Although postoperative adjuvant systemic therapy now has an established place for early breast cancer, subsequent relapse responds less well to either endocrine or cytotoxic agents. Bone metastases are a major problem in advanced breast cancer, most of the damage being mediated by the stimulation of osteoclasts by tumour derived cytokines. Important advances in treatment have come from the use of bisphosphonates and β emitting isotopes. Monitoring of bone metastases is enhanced by using biochemical parameters of response in addition to imaging techniques.

References

Bonneterre J and Mercier M (1993) Response to chemotherapy after relapse in patients with or without previous adjuvant chemotherapy for breast cancer. *Cancer Treatment Reviews* **19 (Supplement B)** 21–30

Bruning PF (1992) Droloxifene, a new anti-oestrogen in postmenopausal advanced breast cancer: preliminary results of a double-blind dose finding phase II trial. *European Journal of Cancer* **28A(8/9)** 1401–1407

Butta A, MacLennan K, Flanders KC *et al* (1992) Induction of transforming growth factor beta$_1$ in human breast cancer in vivo following tamoxifen treatment. *Cancer Research* **52** 4261–4264

Cancer Research Campaign (1990) *Incidence—UK Fact Sheet* 11

Carmo-Pereira J, Oliveira Costa F, Henriques E *et al* (1987) A comparison of two doses of adriamycin in the primary chemotherapy of disseminated breast carcinoma. *British Journal of Cancer* **56** 471–473

Clarke SEM (1991) Isotope therapy for bone metastases, In: Rubens RD and Fogelman I (eds). *Bone Metastases, Diagnosis and Treatment*, pp 187–205, Springer-Verlag, London

Coleman RE and Purohit OP (1993) Osteoclast inhibition for the treatment of bone metastases. *Cancer Treatment Reviews* **19** 79–103

Coleman RE and Rubens RD (1987) The clinical course of bone metastases in breast cancer. *British Journal of Cancer* **55** 61–66

Coleman RE, Houston S, James I *et al* (1992) Preliminary results of the use of urinary excretion of pyridinium crosslinks for monitoring metastatic bone disease. *British Journal of Cancer* **65** 766–768

Coleman RE, Mashiter G, Whitaker KB, Moss DW, Rubens RD and Fogelman I (1988a) Bone scan flare predicts successful systemic therapy for bone metastases. *Journal of Nuclear Medicine* **29** 1354–1359

Coleman RE, Whitaker KB, Moss DW, Mashiter G, Fogelman I and Rubens RD (1988b) Biochemical prediction of response of bone metastases to treatment. *British Journal of Cancer* **58** 205–210

de Haes JCJM, van Knippenberg FCE and Neijt JP (1990) Measuring psychological and physical distress in cancer patients: structure and application of the Rotterdam Symptom Check-list. *British Journal of Cancer* **62** 1034–1038

Duncan L, Purohit A, Howarth M, Potter BVL and Reed MJ (1993) Inhibition of estrone sul-fatase activity by estrone-3-methylthiophosphonate: a potential therapeutic agent in breast cancer. *Cancer Research* **53** 298–303

Early Breast Cancer Trialists' Collaborative Group (1992) The systemic treatment of early breast cancer by hormonal, cytotoxic, or immune therapy. *Lancet* **339** 1–15 and 71–85

Eddy DM (1992) High dose chemotherapy with autologous bone marrow transplantation for the treatment of metastatic breast cancer. *Journal of Clinical Oncology* **10** 657–670

Engelsman E, Klijn JCM, Rubens RD *et al* (1991) "Classical" CMF versus a three weekly in-travenous CMF schedule in postmenopausal patients with advanced breast cancer. *European Journal of Cancer* **27** 966–970

Fischer J, Rose CJ and Rubens RD (1982) Duration of complete response to chemotherapy in advanced breast cancer. *European Journal of Clinical Oncology* **18** 747–754

Fornander T, Rutqvist LE and Glas U (1987) Response to tamoxifen and fluoxemesterone in a group of breast cancer patients with disease recurrence after cessation of adjuvant tamoxifen. *Cancer Treatment Reports* **71** 685–688

Fuqua SAW, Chamness GC and McGuire WL (1993) Estrogen receptor mutations in breast cancer. *Journal of Cellular Biochemistry* **51** 135–149

Hayward JL, Carbone PP, Heuson JC, Kumaoka S, Segaloff A and Rubens RD (1977) Assess-ment of response to therapy in advanced breast cancer. *European Journal of Clinical On-cology* **13** 89–94

Holmes FA, Walters RS, Theriault RL *et al* (1991) Phase II trial of taxol, an active drug in the treatment of metastatic breast cancer. *Journal of the National Cancer Institute* **83** 1797–1805

Houston SJ, Richards MA, Bentley AE, Smith P and Rubens RD (1993) The influence of ad-juvant chemotherapy on outcome after relapse for patients with breast cancer. *European Journal of Cancer* **29A** 1513–1518

Jiang S-Y and Jordan VC (1992) A molecular strategy to control tamoxifen resistant breast can-cer. *Cancer Surveys* **14** 55–70

Launchbury AP and Habboubi N (1993) Epirubicin and doxorubicin: a comparison of their characteristics, therapeutic activity and toxicity. *Cancer Treatment Reviews* **19** 197–228

Mundy GR, Ibbotson KJ and D'Souza SM (1985) Tumor products and the hypercalcemia of malignancy. *Journal of Clinical Investigation* **76** 391–394

Richards MA, Hopwood P, Ramirez AJ *et al* (1992) Doxorubicin in advanced breast cancer: in-fluence of schedule on response, survival and quality of life. *European Journal of Cancer* **28A** 1023–1028

Rubens RD (1993a) Approaches to palliation and its evaluation. *Cancer Treatment Reviews* **19 (Supplement)** 67–71

Rubens RD (1993b) Effects of adjuvant systemic therapy on response to treatment after relapse. *Cancer Treatment Reviews* **19 (Supplement B)** 3–10

Rubens RD, Tinson CL, Coleman RE *et al* (1988) Prednisolone improves the response to pri-mary endocrine treatment for advanced breast cancer. *British Journal of Cancer* **58** 626–630

Rubens RD, Towlson KE, Ramirez AJ *et al* (1992) Appropriate chemotherapy for palliating ad-vanced cancer. *British Medical Journal* **304** 35–40

Santen RJ, Santner SJ, Davis B *et al* (1978) Aminoglutethimide inhibits extraglandular estrogen production in postmenopausal women with breast carcinoma. *Journal of Clinical Endocrin-ology and Metabolism* **47** 1257–1265

Selby PJ and Robertson B (1987) Measurement of quality of life in patients with cancer. *Cancer Surveys* **6** 521–543

Steiner R, Stewart JF, Cantwell BMJ, Minton MJ, Knight RK and Rubens RD (1983) Adria-mycin alone or in combination with vincristine in the treatment of advanced breast cancer.

European Journal of Cancer and Clinical Oncology **19** 1553–1557

Vogel CL, Shemano I, Schoenfelder J, Gams RA and Green MR (1993) Multicentre phase II efficacy trial of toremifene in tamoxifen refractory patients with advanced breast cancer. *Journal of Clinical Oncology* **11** 345–350

Wiebe V, Koester S, Lindberg M *et al* (1992) Toremifene and its metabolites enhance doxorubicin accumulation in estrogen receptor negative multidrug resistant human breast cancer cells. *Investigational New Drugs* **10** 63–71

The author is responsible for the accuracy of the references.

Risk Factors and the Prevention of Breast Cancer with Tamoxifen

MONICA MORROW[1] • V CRAIG JORDAN[2]

[1]*Department of Surgery, University of Chicago, Chicago, Illinois 60637;* [2]*Department of Human Oncology, University of Wisconsin Comprehensive Cancer Center, Madison, Wisconsin 53792*

INTRODUCTION

The American Cancer Society estimates that in 1993, 189 000 new cases of breast cancer will be diagnosed in the USA and 44 000 women will die from the disease (Boring *et al*, 1992). These figures make it clear that although screening mammography and the increased use of breast conserving surgery and adjuvant chemotherapy have improved the quality of life and prolonged survival for women with breast cancer, additional therapeutic strategies are needed to combat the disease. In the mid 1980s, a pilot trial was started at the Royal Marsden Hospital to evaluate the use of tamoxifen in high risk women to prevent breast cancer (Powles *et al*, 1989a,b, 1990). However, nationwide recruitment to the trial was stopped after 2000 women had entered amid debate about animal toxicological data and safety issues. The Department of Health has now approved the recruitment of volunteers to complete the trial in the UK. In 1992, the National Surgical Adjuvant Breast and Bowel Project (NSABP) launched a trial to test tamoxifen as a preventive agent in women at increased risk for the development of breast cancer. These trials have generated considerable debate regarding what risk-benefit ratio is appropriate for an intervention to be undertaken in healthy subjects, the majority of whom will never develop breast cancer. This chapter discusses the rationale and design of the current trials, the known toxicities of tamoxifen and additional potential benefits of the drug beyond the prevention of breast cancer and critically reviews the patient population selected for inclusion in the prevention studies.

ADVANTAGES OF TAMOXIFEN

The salient pharmacology and rationale for the use of tamoxifen as an agent to prevent breast cancer have been reviewed extensively (Furr and Jordan, 1984; Jordan and Murphy, 1990; Morrow and Jordan, 1992; Jordan and Morrow, 1993). Tamoxifen effectively inhibits mammary carcinogenesis in laboratory animals (Jordan, 1976, 1983; Jordan et al, 1979, 1990, 1991b; Gottardis and Jordan, 1987). Overall, the animal studies demonstrate two principles: firstly, that the anti-oestrogen must be administered as soon as possible after the carcinogenic insult, and secondly, a long duration of therapy is more effective than short term treatment.

In addition, a large body of clinical evidence from adjuvant studies also suggests that the drug is effective as a potential preventive agent. In the Stockholm trial (Fornander et al, 1989), after local therapy, 1846 postmenopausal women under age 71 were randomized to treatment with tamoxifen at a dose of 40 mg daily for 2 or 5 years or no endocrine therapy. After a median follow-up of 7 years, a 40% reduction in the incidence of contralateral breast cancers was observed in the tamoxifen treated women when compared with control subjects. No differences in contralateral cancer incidence were observed between women treated for 2 or 5 years with tamoxifen (Rutqvist et al, 1991). Risk reduction was greatest during the first 1–2 years of therapy, but benefit persisted for more than 10 years after treatment was stopped. Tamoxifen at a dose of 20 mg daily has also been shown to decrease breast cancer risk. In NSABP Protocol B14 (Fisher et al, 1989), 2892 pre- and postmenopausal women with node negative breast cancer were treated with tamoxifen or placebo for at least 5 years. With a mean follow-up of 59 months, a 50% reduction in contralateral breast cancer was seen in the tamoxifen treated women. In the overview analysis (Early Breast Cancer Trialists' Collaborative Study, 1992), a review of all the randomized clinical trials of tamoxifen therapy demonstrated a 39% decrease in the risk of a second primary breast cancer for women taking tamoxifen.

In addition, there are emerging data that tamoxifen has a protective effect on bone density and blood cholesterol. The relevant studies on bone and lipids are summarized in Tables 1 and 2, respectively. These additional benefits to women have been very important in encouraging clinical investigation. Tamoxifen's demonstrated effectiveness as an anti-tumour agent, as well as its potential impact on osteoporosis and demonstrated ability to reduce fatal

TABLE 1. Bone mineral content in radius and spine of tamoxifen treated and control postmenopausal breast cancer patients (adapted from Ursin *et al*, 1993)

Design differences	Duration of tamoxifen (years)	Control (n)	Tamoxifen	
Radius				
g/cm^2 at time of study				
Fornander *et al* (1990)				
Proximal	2	1.04 (28)	0.99 (26)	−0.08 (NS)
Distal		0.74 (28)	0.70 (26)	−0.08 (NS)
Proximal	5	1.05 (28)	1.06 (21)	+0.01 (NS)
Distal		0.74 (28)	0.78 (21)	+0.04 (NS)
Love *et al* (1988)	2+	0.63 (27)	0.63 (33)	+0.02 (NS)
%/year change in bone mineral density				
Love *et al* (1992)	2	1.29 (68)	0.88 (66)	+0.4 (NS)
Spine				
g/cm^2 at time of study				
Wright *et al* (1990)	not given	1.21 (9)	1.29 (11)	+0.08 (NS)
Love *et al* (1988)	2+	1.21 (27)	1.22 (33)	+0.11 (NS)
%/year change in body mass index				
Love *et al* (1992a)	2	−1.0 (67)	+0.6 (66)	+1.6 (p<0.001)
Turken *et al* (1989)	1	−2.7 (10)	−2.4 (10)	+5.1 (p<0.003)
Ryan *et al* (1991)	1	control	+4.3 (7)	

NS = not significant

myocardial infarction (McDonald and Stewart, 1991), makes it an ideal agent for prevention trials. Nevertheless, a number of toxicological issues need to be placed in perspective as potential risks to women.

TOXICITY OF TAMOXIFEN

Tamoxifen has been used successfully for the treatment of breast carcinoma for 20 years, allowing the accumulation of a large body of knowledge regarding the toxicity of the drug. In women with both node positive and node negative breast cancer, the administration of tamoxifen results in improvements in both disease free and overall survival (Early Breast Cancer Trialists' Collaborative Group, 1992). For the woman with breast cancer, there is no doubt that the benefits of tamoxifen therapy outweigh the risks. However, in the setting of a prevention study, where many of the participants will never develop breast

TABLE 2. Changes in circulating lipids during tamoxifen therapy in pre- and postmenopausal women

Study	Patients	Tamoxifen (mg daily)	Duration (months)	HDLC	LDLC	Ratio HDL/total	Total cholesterol	Triglycerides
Postmenopausal								
Rossner and Wallgren (1984)	23	40	>2	↕	→	←	→	←
Bruning et al (1988)	46	30	2–6	↕	→	←	→	←
Bertelli et al (1988)	55	20	>3	↕	→	←	↕	←
Bagdade et al (1990)	8	20	3	←	→	←	↑	←
Love et al (1991b)	70	20	24	↕	→	←	→	←
Ingram (1990)	13	not given	3–6	↕	→	←	↕	←
Cuzick et al (1992)	14	20	72			→		↑
Premenopausal								
Bruning et al (1988)	8	30	2	↕	→	←	→	↕
Callefi et al (1988)	10	10	3	↕	↕	↕	↕	↕
Cuzick et al (1992)	1	20	not given	→	↕	→	→	↑

HDLC = high density liproprotein cholesterol
LDLC = low density lipoprotein cholesterol

TABLE 3. Reports of documented number of endometrial tumours observed in patients receiving different daily doses of tamoxifen for different durations for the treatment of breast cancers

Study	No. of tumours	Duration (years) of tamoxifen treatment	Dose (mg daily)
Anderson et al (1991)	7	1	30
Atlante et al (1990)	4	2–4	30–60
Fornander et al (1989)	13	2–5	40
Hardell (1988)	11	1–9	40
Killackey et al (1980)	13	0.5–1.3	20
Magriples et al (1993)	15	0.25–10	40
Malfetano (1990)	7	1.5–4	20
Mathew et al (1990)	5	4–8	20
Neven et al (1990)	1	3	20
Sunderland and Osborne (1991)	4	1	20

carcinoma, a careful examination of tamoxifen toxicities is warranted. Side effects that represent an acceptable risk for a woman with cancer may have different implications for the healthy woman. It is essential to evaluate the real situation regarding the potential increase in uterine cancers, liver tumours, eye problems and thrombosis as this is of major significance to prospective volunteers.

Uterine Cancer

There are an increasing number of reports that link tamoxifen therapy for breast cancer with the development of endometrial carcinoma (Table 3). However, analysis of the 70 reported cases demonstrates that 65% of women developing uterine carcinoma received a higher dose, 30–60 mg daily, than the 20 mg daily used in prevention trials. Furthermore, of the women who received 20 mg daily, only 8 of the 20 received the drug for more than 2 years (Table 4). This suggests that patients had pre-existing disease of various stages and grades and the use of tamoxifen caused increases in uterine size (Anteby et al, 1992) or spotting that led to tumour detection.

The oestrogenicity of tamoxifen could lead to an increased detection rate of early stage endometrial carcinoma. This hypothesis has been advanced to explain the increased detection of early stage endometrial carcinoma in oestrogen users (Horwitz and Feinstein, 1986; Kelsey et al, 1982). The incidence of occult endometrial cancer found at autopsy is five times the incidence of clinical disease (Horwitz and Feinstein, 1986; Horwitz et al, 1981). An increase in bleeding due to oestrogen therapy could result in an increased rate of detection of subclinical tumours, resulting in the apparent increased incidence of endometrial carcinoma in users of oestrogen. There is, however, no

TABLE 4. Daily dose and duration of therapy for the 70 cases of confirmed endometrial cancer that occurred in breast cancer patients during or after tamoxifen therapy

	Daily dose (mg)			
	20	**30**	**40**	**60**
All cases	20	8	41	1
Patients with <2 years' therapy	12	8	7	0

Patients receiving less than 2 years of tamoxifen therapy before endometrial cancer was detected are listed on the bottom line

clinical database for those given 20 mg tamoxifen daily to support or refute this assumption. Indeed, it is not possible to make any general statement about tumour grade or stage at diagnosis as these data are not available for 35 of the 70 women treated with tamoxifen.

Liver Cancer

Oestrogens are known to induce hepatocellular carcinomas in rats (Wanless and Medline, 1982). Similarly, tamoxifen and other triphenylethylene analogues (Dragan et al, 1991; Meschter et al, 1991; White et al, 1993; Williams et al, 1993) cause hepatocellular carcinoma in rats. These observations raised concerns about the safety of long term tamoxifen therapy in women (Williams et al, 1992). Since tamoxifen has oestrogenic properties, it can be classified as a promoter of rat liver carcinogenesis (Meschter et al, 1991); however, there is evidence that anti-oestrogens can cause adduct formation to rat liver DNA (Han and Leihr, 1992; White et al, 1993; Williams et al, 1992, 1993). Anti-oestrogens could therefore be considered to be initiators of carcinogenesis. Nevertheless, the clinical relevance of these laboratory studies remains unclear. Only two documented cases of human hepatocellular carcinomas have been published, and both patients were treated with 40 mg of tamoxifen daily (Fornander et al, 1989). Surprisingly, there are no reports of any cases of hepatocellular carcinoma in patients being treated with 20 mg of tamoxifen daily. The incidence of hepatocellular carcinoma is 5 in 100 000, so with such widespread use of tamoxifen, there is no doubt that cases will occur in women taking the drug. Whether this incidence of hepatocellular carcinoma will be significantly higher than the normal incidence will be difficult to ascertain unless rigorous pathological and epidemiological studies are initiated.

Ocular Toxicity

The available data on ocular toxicity are summarized in Table 5. Several studies have failed to demonstrate an association between tamoxifen therapy

TABLE 5. Ocular toxicity in tamoxifen treated patients

Study	No. studied	Mean age	Daily dose (mg)	Mean duration of therapy	No. with ocular toxicity
Pavlidis et al (1992)	63	58	20	25 months	4
Ashford et al (1988)	1	42	20	11 months	1
Griffiths (1987)	1	42	20	3 weeks	1
Vinding and Nelson (1983)	17	67.5	20–30	16 months	2
Pugesgaard and von Eyeben (1986)	1	57	30–40	6 months	1
Gerner (1989)	1	44	30–40	26 months	1
Bentley et al (1992)	1	72	40	1 month	1
Kaiser-Kupfer and Lippman (1978)	4	59	240–320	20.5 months	4

and retinopathy. Beck and Mills (1979) found no evidence of the corneal and retinal changes of tamoxifen toxicity in 19 women taking 20–40 mg of tamoxifen daily for a mean of 15 months (range 3–48 months). A prospective study of 79 women receiving conventional dose tamoxifen also failed to find evidence of ocular toxicity (Longstaff et al, 1989). In a large group of breast cancer patients receiving adjuvant therapy, symptomatic ocular toxicity occurred in only 0.2% of 2375 women receiving tamoxifen alone or in combination with chemotherapy (ICI Pharmaceuticals Group, 1990). Non-specific visual complaints were reported by 5.2% of 1486 women receiving cytotoxic chemotherapy, 3.5% of 1449 women treated with tamoxifen plus cytotoxic therapy, 0.8% of 926 women receiving tamoxifen alone and 0.7% of 941 women on placebo. From these data, it is apparent that if tamoxifen at doses of 20 mg causes ocular toxicity, it is an extremely rare occurrence. The pathogenesis of the retinopathy is uncertain, although a single autopsy case suggests that axonal degeneration is the underlying lesion (Kaiser-Kupfer et al, 1981). No clear relationship between total tamoxifen dose or duration of treatment is evident in the reported cases. A careful ophthalmological evaluation of a large number of women treated with tamoxifen and a matched control group is needed to evaluate the role of tamoxifen alone as a cause of ocular toxicity.

Thromboembolic Disorders

The possibility of an association between tamoxifen and thrombosis was raised by several case reports (Navasaari et al, 1978; Jacquot et al, 1981; Dahan et al, 1985). A significant decrease in anti-thrombin III levels has been observed in women taking tamoxifen (Jordan et al, 1987; Bertelli et al, 1988; Love et al, 1992b) and may account for this observation. However, the occurrence of thrombosis in women with metastatic breast cancer has limited relevance to

TABLE 6. Exclusion criteria for breast cancer prevention trial

Prior diagnosis of
  invasive breast carcinoma
  ductal carcinoma in situ
  invasive carcinoma at other site (excluding basal or squamous cell cancers
    of skin) within 10 years
Age less than 35
Life expectancy less than 10 years
Current use of oestrogen-progesterone replacement, oral
  contraceptives or androgens
Current use of *warfarin*
History of deep venous thrombosis or pulmonary embolus
History of macular degeneration of the retina

the prevention trial since advanced cancer is often associated with hyper-coagulability. In the adjuvant role, the incidence of thrombosis in women treated with tamoxifen alone is low. Fornander *et al* (1991) reviewed the incidence of thrombotic events in 931 women taking adjuvant tamoxifen at a dose of 40 mg daily and 915 control women at a median follow-up of 54 months. Altogether, 432 of the women treated with tamoxifen also received chemotherapy or radiotherapy. A slight increase in the number of hospital admissions for thrombotic events was seen in the tamoxifen group (relative risk 1.2), but this did not reach statistical significance. The addition of chemotherapy or radiotherapy to tamoxifen did not alter this risk. However, a retrospective review of Eastern Cooperative Oncology Group (ECOG) trials demonstrated that the combination of tamoxifen and cyclophosphamide, methotrexate, fluorouracil and prednisone was associated with an increased incidence of arterial thrombosis (Healey *et al*, 1987). Although the sample size of the adjuvant studies may be insufficient to exclude a very small increase in the incidence of thrombosis, hypercoagulability does not appear to be a major problem when tamoxifen is used in an adjuvant role. The exclusion of women with a significant history of thrombosis from the prevention trial will minimize further the risk of thromboembolic disorders.

DESIGN OF THE NSABP TRIAL

The NSABP Prevention Trial will recruit 16 000 women over a 2 year period, and they will be randomized to treatment with tamoxifen 20 mg daily or placebo for a minimum of 5 years. Women with a prior diagnosis of invasive breast carcinoma or ductal carcinoma in situ are excluded from the trial. Other exclusion criteria are summarized in Table 6. In the absence of defined exclusion criteria, all women over the age of 60 are eligible for entry to the study. Women between the ages of 35 and 59 must have a 5 year probability of developing invasive breast cancer which is equal to that of a 60 year old women. Breast cancer risk is determined on the basis of age of participant parity, age at first completed pregnancy, age at menarche, number of first degree relatives with breast cancer and number of breast biopsies. A model that incorporates these risk factor combinations has been developed by Gail *et al* (1989). This model is one of the few that incorporates multiple risk factors and expresses risk in terms of defined time intervals. In addition, the model was derived from data from the Breast Cancer Detection Demonstration Project in which many of the self selected women were at increased risk of developing breast cancer, suggesting that the risk predictions derived from that population will be applicable to women in the prevention trial.

Study participants will be examined 3 months after beginning drug therapy and then at 6 month intervals. The stated endpoints of the trial are breast cancer incidence, breast cancer mortality, cardiovascular deaths and fractures. All participants will undergo annual mammography, annual pelvic examination and cervical smear and monitoring of complete blood count, blood chemistries and lipid profiles at 6 month intervals. Women over age 50 will have yearly electrocardiograms. Ocular toxicity and osteoporosis will be investigated on the basis of symptoms, and regular quality of life questionnaires will be completed. Compliance will be monitored by tablet counts, but drug levels will not be obtained.

DEFINITION OF A HIGH RISK POPULATION

One of the major issues surrounding the current breast cancer prevention trial is the population of women selected for study. The inclusion of premenopausal women (discussed below) as well as all women over 60 years old has been questioned. The average 60 year old woman has a 3.6% risk of developing breast cancer between the ages of 60 and 70 (Ries *et al*, 1987), and her risk of breast cancer death is one third of the risk of developing the disease. In contrast, the risk of myocardial infarction in the same interval is twice the risk of breast cancer development (Cummings *et al*, 1989). Postmenopausal oestrogen replacement is known to reduce the risk of coronary heart disease (Barrett-Connor and Bush, 1989; Sullivan *et al*, 1988), but participants in the prevention trial cannot use hormone replacement. The evidence suggesting that tamoxifen may lower blood cholesterol and reduce the incidence of fatal myocardial infarction has been reviewed. Although these data suggest some benefit, it is not at all clear that the magnitude of risk reduction equals that seen with oestrogen replacement. In addition, half of the women in the prevention trial will receive a placebo. Thus, concern over a relatively low, but emotionally charged, risk of breast cancer may result in a woman increasing her already significant, but less well publicized, risk of coronary artery disease.

A similar argument could be made regarding the risk of osteoporosis, also a significant cause of morbidity in elderly women.

Several other entry criteria of the study are open to question. Higher levels of risk are required for the entry of younger women into the study. The Gail model (Gail *et al*, 1989) considers only first degree relatives in assessing risk, and thus tends to underestimate the risk seen in women with potential hereditary breast cancer. For example, a 35 year old woman with a mother with bilateral premenopausal breast cancer, a maternal grandmother with premenopausal breast cancer and three maternal aunts with premenopausal breast cancer is not eligible for study entry in the absence of other risk factors, although her pedigree is strongly suggestive of hereditary breast cancer. Although such women are a minority of the population, accounting for only 5–10% of breast cancer cases, they represent an extremely high risk group, often subjected to pressure to undergo prophylactic mastectomy.

Estimates of risk may be artificially elevated in other potential trial participants by the inclusion of any breast biopsy or aspiration of non-cystic masses as a risk factor. The relationship of benign breast disease to breast cancer risk is controversial (Morrow, 1991). The work of Dupont and Page (1985) suggests that 80% of breast biopsies done for clinical breast lesions are non-proliferative and associated with no increased breast cancer risk. Clearly, the review of all biopsy specimens dating back over a woman's lifetime is not feasible, but the consideration of any biopsy as evidence of increased risk does not seem justified.

HIGH RISK PREMENOPAUSAL WOMEN

The rationale, efficacy and safety of tamoxifen administration to premenopausal women have been challenged and have been the subject of some controversy. The present strategy of including premenopausal women in the prevention trial is based on both laboratory principles and clinical experience. Simply stated, the available laboratory data suggest that carcinogenesis involves a long process of promotion, but initiation occurs in early puberty. Mammary tissue in older animals is not receptive to carcinogens (Jordan and Morrow, 1993). In humans, we are unaware of the timing or nature of the carcinogenic insult, but breast tissue appears to be most receptive to known initiators in early puberty. Young girls who were survivors of the atomic bombs were found to have the greatest increase in the incidence of breast cancer later in life (Tokunaga *et al*, 1987). Similar evidence comes from thymic irradiation (Hildreth *et al*, 1989), irradiation during fluoroscopic examination for tuberculosis (Miller *et al*, 1989) and irradiation of girls with Hodgkin's disease (Janjan and Zellmer, 1992). Thus, an early initiating event is followed by a long period of promotion. The major role of oestrogen in the process of carcinogenesis is illustrated by the fact that women with non-functioning ovaries have only 1% of the incidence of breast cancer of normal women, and women who have an early oophorectomy at age 35 (Pike *et al*, 1989) have a breast cancer incidence which is 50% of that seen in the normal population. As in the laboratory experience, early intervention appears to be more effective. As stated previously (Design of the NSABP Trial), only premenopausal women with the highest risk are eligible for recruitment to the NSABP trial, but they provide a critical group to study the predictive risk factors, genetics and potentially the molecular biology of breast cancer. The demonstration of an effective therapy for a woman predicted to have breast cancer will be a major advance.

There are concerns that tamoxifen may be ineffective as a preventive in premenopausal women. Tamoxifen is a competitive inhibitor of oestrogen action at the tumour oestrogen receptor (Jordan and Koerner, 1975), but it is known that in premenopausal women, tamoxifen causes an increase in circulating oestrogen (Jordan *et al*, 1991a) that could potentially reverse its antitumour effects. However, laboratory studies demonstrate that it is difficult to reverse the anti-tumour action of tamoxifen in animal models of human disease (Iino *et al*, 1991), and 5 years or more of tamoxifen is known to have efficacy in oestrogen receptor positive, node negative, premenopausal women (Fisher *et al*, 1989). It is important to note though that the long term follow-up of recent adjuvant studies demonstrates that tamoxifen appears to be a suboptimal adjuvant therapy in node positive, premenopausal women (Kaufman *et al*, 1993) and may be unable to prevent contralateral breast cancers (Cancer Research Campaign Breast Cancer Trials Group, 1992). However, these studies illustrate the laboratory principle that stopping tamoxifen treatment prematurely is not advisable (Jordan, 1983). The recent reports (Cancer Research Campaign Breast Cancer Trials Group, 1992; Kaufman *et al*, 1993) address the value of only 2 years of tamoxifen therapy, whereas the prevention trial is using at least 5 years of tamoxifen therapy. In the Cancer Research Campaign Study, there was an early dramatic effect of tamoxifen that produced a complete suppression of contralateral breast cancer at 3 years (Cuzick and Baum, 1985). However, the drug was stopped at 2 years, and by 9 years, no difference in the incidence of contralateral breast cancer was observed (Cancer Research Campaign Breast Cancer Trials Group, 1992). By contrast, the greatest decrease in contralateral breast cancer in NSABP B14 (Fisher *et al*, 1989) was observed in premenopausal women during therapy. Therefore, tamoxifen may only be beneficial in premenopausal women for as long as it is administered, but then disease is reactivated by oestrogen after the antioestrogen is stopped.

Finally, it is important to consider whether the potential survival benefits to selected women at high risk for breast cancer outweigh the physiological

TABLE 7. Symptomatic side effects reported with tamoxifen therapy (adapted from Fritsch and Wolf, in press)

Complaint	Incidence (%)
Fatigue	5–70
Vasomotor instability (hot flashes)	17–67
Insomnia	0–54
Headache	9–37
Depression	1–33
Altered menses	1–31
Fluid retention	2–25
Nausea	3–21
Anorexia	1–16
Vomiting	1–12
Diarrhoea	8–10
Constipation	2–4
Weight gain	4

risks. Young women taking tamoxifen are at risk for pregnancy, but women planning a family are not candidates for the prevention trial. Indeed, like the related compound clomiphene, tamoxifen has been used as a pro-fertility agent to induce ovulation in subfertile women (Furr and Jordan, 1984). Barrier contraceptives should be used to avoid accidental pregnancy. If pregnancy does occur, women must stop taking tamoxifen because of possible teratogenesis. However, it is important to stress that no specific malformations have been described in the literature that are associated with tamoxifen use.

The effects of tamoxifen on bones and lipids will be monitored in the NSABP's double blind prevention trial so that treated women can be compared to placebo treated women without bias. Regrettably, there are as yet no large studies of effects of tamoxifen on bone mineral density in premenopausal women. Powles and co-workers (1989a) did not show a difference in bone mineral loss in the forearm of premenopausal women compared with post-menopausal women. Similarly, Fentiman et al (1989) found no effect on bone density in premenopausal women receiving tamoxifen for mastalgia. However, only a few dozen women were involved and neither study evaluated patients who had taken tamoxifen for longer than 18 months.

At present, very little information on the effect of tamoxifen on blood lipids is available for premenopausal patients (Table 3), and it is difficult to make general conclusions from so few patients. Nevertheless, low density lipoprotein cholesterol consistently decreases.

QUALITY OF LIFE ISSUES

Tamoxifen is well tolerated as an anti-cancer drug. In NSABP B14 (Fisher et al, 1989), treatment was discontinued due to toxicity in 9.4% of tamoxifen patients and 6.3% of control women. However, minor side effects that may be acceptable to a woman diagnosed with breast cancer may be poorly tolerated in a healthy woman. A variety of symptomatic side effects have been reported in women taking tamoxifen. These have recently been reviewed in detail (Fritsch and Wolf, in press) and are summarized in Table 7. Although the list is extensive, it is important to note that in placebo controlled trials, only vasomotor instability was consistently found to be significantly more frequent in women taking tamoxifen (Love *et al*, 1991a; Fritsch and Wolf, in press). However, the frequency of minor symptoms may be underestimated in treatment studies designed to monitor major life threatening toxicities. As part of the double blind, placebo controlled Wisconsin tamoxifen study, the postmenopausal subjects participating in the trial were queried in detail regarding symptomatic side effects of therapy (Love *et al*, 1991a). Over a 12 month interval, no differences in general quality of life were identified between women taking tamoxifen or placebo. Mild gynecological symptoms, defined as vaginal discharge, irritation or bleeding, appeared to be more frequent in women taking tamoxifen, but these differences were statistically significant only at 6 months and fluctuated over the study period. No other symptoms were found to occur more frequently in tamoxifen treated women.

Information more relevant to tamoxifen as a preventive agent is available from the pilot study of Powles and co-authors (1989a,b, 1990). A total of 435 healthy women at increased risk for breast cancer were randomized to tamoxifen 20 mg daily or placebo as a feasibility study for a larger prevention trial, and approximately half of the participants were premenopausal. Toxicity and compliance were monitored at 6 month intervals. The only significant difference in toxicity noted was an increased incidence of hot flashes in the women taking tamoxifen. At 12 months, an 83% compliance rate was noted for women in the tamoxifen arm of the trial which had decreased to approximately 70% at 2 years. This high rate of compliance in healthy women supports the data from adjuvant studies that tamoxifen is well tolerated.

CONCLUSIONS

From the available information on tamoxifen, a number of conclusions can be drawn, and many additional questions can be asked. The clinical and laboratory evidence suggesting that tamoxifen will be effective in preventing some, although certainly not all, breast cancers is strong. A detailed review of the toxicities of tamoxifen does not give rise to major concerns about the development of endometrial carcinoma, hepatocellular carcinoma or ocular problems. It is difficult to attribute many of the reported cases of endometrial carcinoma occurring during tamoxifen therapy to the drug, since in many cases, tumours were detected after a very short time on tamoxifen treatment.

Ocular toxicity requires further evaluation in a large group of women whose baseline visual acuity is established before beginning therapy. It is extremely difficult, in selected small groups of women chosen from an unknown number of women taking tamoxifen, to draw any sound conclusions regarding retinal problems.

On the other hand, although concerns regarding the major toxicities mentioned above may be overstated, it is likely that symptomatic side effects, particularly those related to the anti-oestrogenic effects of tamoxifen in the premenopausal woman, may be more frequent than appreciated in data from trials designed to collect information on major, life threatening toxicities. Further information on menstrual irregularities and other gynecological effects in premenopausal women is needed to evaluate the acceptability of tamoxifen as an intervention in large numbers of women.

Important questions regarding lipids and bones remain unanswered in both pre- and postmenopausal women. Premenopausal women taking tamoxifen for breast cancer treatment are an excellent source with which to answer these questions in a timely fashion. In postmenopausal women, a comparison between tamoxifen and oestrogen replacement therapy will become critical if tamoxifen is to be considered for routine use in normal postmenopausal women.

Although it is evident that all the potential concerns regarding the use of tamoxifen for breast cancer prevention have not been completely addressed, the available data suggest that tamoxifen is both a safe and an efficacious means of preventing breast cancer. Without a carefully monitored, prospective study such as is currently in place, answers to the question of breast cancer prevention will not be obtained.

SUMMARY

Oestrogen is intimately involved in the growth and development of breast cancer. Tamoxifen, a non-steroidal anti-oestrogen, not only is an effective adjuvant therapy for node positive and node negative disease, but also has several attractive pharmacological features that have enhanced interest in testing it as a preventive drug for breast cancer in high risk women. Tamoxifen is known to prevent contralateral breast cancer, but it also has significant oestrogenicity for reducing circulating cholestrol and preventing bone loss in the lumbar spine of postmenopausal women. Several clinical trials have been initiated around the world; however, there has been increasing concern about the safety of tamoxifen. Nevertheless, current reports indicate that there is little risk of developing endometrial and liver cancer, although further clinical studies must be planned. Concerns about retinal and thromboembolic problems remain anecdotal, and again additional research is essential. The prevention trials with tamoxifen are necessary to establish the worth and feasibility of a pharmacological intervention. If tamoxifen is found to be of value to prevent breast cancer in a broad population, then the future ability to predict breast cancer through molecular markers will provide the physician for the first time with a therapeutic option to treat the targeted patient.

References

Anderson M, Storm HH and Mouridsen HT (1991) Incidence of new primary cancers after adjuvant tamoxifen therapy and radiotherapy for early breast cancer. *Journal of the National Cancer Institute* **83** 1013–1017

Anteby E, Yagel S, Zacut D, Palti Z and Hochner-Celnikier D (1992) False sonographic appearance of endometrial neoplasia in postmenopausal women treated with tamoxifen. *Lancet* **1** 433–434

Ashford A, Donev I, Tiwati R and Garrett T (1988) Reversible ocular toxicity related to tamoxifen therapy. *Cancer* **61** 33–35

Atlante G, Pozzi M, Vincenzoni C and Vocaturo G (1990) Four case reports presenting new acquisitions on the association between breast and endometrial carcinoma. *Gynecological Oncology* **37** 378–380

Bagdade JD, Wolter J and Subbaiah PV (1990) Effects of tamoxifen treatment on plasma lipids and lipoprotein lipid composition. *Journal of Clinical Endocrinology and Metabolism* **70** 1132–1135

Barrett-Connor E and Bush T (1980) Estrogen replacement and coronary heart disease. *Cardiovascular Clinicians* **19** 159–172

Beck M and Mills P (1979) Ocular assessment of patients treated with tamoxifen. *Cancer Treatment Reports* **63** 1833–1834

Bentley C, Davies G and Aclimandos W (1992) Tamoxifen retinopathy: a rare but serious complication. *British Medical Journal* **304** 495–6

Bertelli G, Pronzato P, Ameroso D *et al* (1988) Adjuvant tamoxifen in primary breast cancer: influence on plasma lipid S and antithrombin III levels. *Breast Cancer Research and Treatment* **12** 307–310

Boring C, Squires T and Tong T (1992) Cancer statistics 1992. *CA-A Cancer Journal for Clinicians* **42** 19–38

Bruning PF, Bonfrer JMG, Hart AAM *et al* (1988) Tamoxifen, serum lipoproteins and cardiovascular risk. *British Journal of Cancer* **58** 497–499

Caleffi M, Fentimen IS, Clark GM *et al* (1988) Effect of tamoxifen on oestrogen binding, lipid and lipoprotein concentrations and blood clotting parameters in premenopausal women with breast pain. *Journal of Endocrinology* **119** 335–340

Cancer Research Campaign Breast Cancer Trials Group (1992) The effect of adjuvant tamoxifen: the latest results from the Cancer Research Campaign Adjunct Breast Trial. *European Journal of Cancer* **28A** 904–907

Cummings S, Black D and Rubin S (1989) Lifetime risks of hip, Colles or vertebral fracture and coronary heart disease among white postmenopausal women. *Archives of Internal Medicine* **149** 2445–2448

Cuzick J and Baum M (1985) Tamoxifen and contralateral breast cancer. *Lancet* **ii** 282

Cuzick J, Allen D, Baum M *et al* (1992) Long-term effects of tamoxifen. *European Journal of Cancer* **29A** 15–21

Dahan R, Espie M, Mignot L, Houlbert D and Chanu B (1985) Tamoxifen and arterial thrombosis. *Lancet* **1** 638

Dragan YP, Xu YMD and Pitot HC (1991) Tumor promotion as a target for estrogen/antiestrogen effects in rat hepatocellular carcinogenesis. *Preventive Medicine* **20** 15–26

Dupont W and Page D (1985) Risk factors for breast cancer in women with proliferative breast disease. *New England Journal of Medicine* **312** 146–151

Early Breast Cancer Trialists Collaborative Group (1992) Systemic treatment of early breast cancer by hormonal, cytotoxic or immune therapy. *Lancet* **339** 1–15

Fentiman IS, Caleffi M, Rodin A, Murby B and Fogelman I (1989) Bone mineral content of women receiving tamoxifen for mastalgia. *British Journal of Cancer* **60** 262–264

Fisher B, Costantino J, Redmond C *et al* (1989) A randomized clinical trial evaluating tamoxifen in the treatment of patients with node-negative breast cancer who have estrogen receptor positive tumors. *New England Journal of Medicine* **32** 479–484

Fornander T, Rutqvist L, Cedermark B *et al* (1989) Adjuvant tamoxifen in early breast cancer: occurrence of new primary cancers. *Lancet* **ii** 117–120

Fornander T, Rutqvist LE, Sjoberg HE, Blomqvist L, Mattsson A and Glas U (1990) Long-term adjuvant tamoxifen in early breast cancer: effect on bone mineral density in post-menopausal women. *Journal of Clinical Oncology* **8** 1019–1024

Fornander T, Rutquist L, Cedermark B *et al* (1991) Adjuvant tamoxifen in early stage breast cancer: effects on intercurrent morbidity and mortality. *Journal of Clinical Oncology* **9** 1740–1748

Fritsch M and Wolf D Symptomatic side effects of tamoxifen therapy, In: Jordan VC (ed). *Long-Term Tamoxifen Therapy*, University of Wisconsin Press, Madison (in press)

Furr BJA and Jordan VC (1984) Pharmacology and clinical uses of tamoxifen. *Pharmacology and Therapeutics* **25** 127–205

Gail MH, Brinton LA, Byar DP *et al* (1989) Projecting individualized probabilities of developing breast cancer for white females who are being examined annually. *Journal of the National Cancer Institute* **81** 1879–1884

Gerner E (1989) Ocular toxicity of tamoxifen. *Annals of Ophthalmology* **21** 420–423

Gottardis MM and Jordan VC (1987) The antitumor actions of keoxifene and tamoxifen in the N-nitrosomethylurea induced rat mammary carcinoma model. *Cancer Research* **47** 4020–4024

Griffiths M (1987) Tamoxifen retinopathy at low dosage. *American Journal of Ophthalmology* **104** 185–186

Han X and Leihr JG (1992) Induction of covalent DNA adducts in rodents by tamoxifen. *Cancer Research* **52** 1360–1363

Hardell L (1988) Tamoxifen as risk factor for carcinoma of corpus uteri. *Lancet* **ii** 563

Healey B, Tormey D and Gray R (1987) Arterial and venous thrombotic events in ECOG adjuvant breast cancer trials. *Proceedings of the American Society of Clinical Oncology* **6** 54

Hildreth NG, Shore R and Dvaretski P (1989) The risk of breast cancer after irradiation of the thymus in infancy. *New England Journal of Medicine* **321** 1281–1284

Horwitz RI and Feinstein AR (1986) Estrogens and endometrial cancer. *American Journal of Medicine* **81** 503–507

Horwitz RI, Feinstein AR, Horwitz SM and Robboy SJ (1981) Necropsy diagnosis of endometrial cancer and detection bias in case control studies. *Lancet* **ii** 66–68

ICI Pharmaceuticals Group (1990) Data presented at the Food and Drug Administration Oncology Drugs Advisory Committee Meeting, Bethesda MD, 29 June

Iino Y, Wolf DM, Langan-Fahey SA *et al* (1991) Reversible control of oestradiol-stimulated growth of MCF-7 tumours by tamoxifen in the athymic mouse. *British Journal of Cancer* **64** 1019–1024

Ingram D (1990) Tamoxifen use, oestrogen binding and serum lipids in postmenopausal women with breast cancer. *Australian and New Zealand Journal of Surgery* **60** 673–675

Jacquot C, Craterol R, Bariety J *et al* (1981) DES versus tamoxifen in advanced breast cancer. *New England Journal of Medicine* **304** 1041–1043

Janjan N and Zellmer D (1992) Calculated risk of breast cancer following mantle irradiation determined by measured dose. *Cancer Detection and Prevention* **16** 273–282

Jordan VC (1976) Effect of tamoxifen (ICI 46 474) on initiation and growth of DMBA-induced rat mammary carcinoma. *European Journal of Cancer* **12** 419–423

Jordan VC (1983) Laboratory studies to develop general principles for the adjuvant treatment of breast cancer with antiestrogens: problems and potential for future clinical applications. *Breast Cancer Research and Treatment* **3** (**Supplement**) 73–86

Jordan VC and Koerner S (1975) Tamoxifen (ICI 46 474) and the human carcinoma 8S oestrogen receptor. *European Journal of Cancer* **11** 205–206

Jordan VC and Morrow M (1993) An evaluation of strategies to reduce the incidence of breast cancer. *Stem Cell* **11** 252–262

Jordan VC and Murphy CS (1990) Endocrine pharmacology of antiestrogens as antitumor agents. *Endocrine Review* **11** 578–593

Jordan VC, Dix CJ and Allen KE (1979) The effectiveness of long term treatment in a laboratory model for adjunct hormone therapy of breast cancer, In: Salmon SE and Jones SE (eds). *Adjuvant Therapy of Cancer II*, pp 19–21, Grune and Stratton, New York

Jordan VC, Fritz NF and Tormey DC (1987) Long-term adjuvant therapy with tamoxifen: effect on sex hormone binding globulin and antithrombin III. *Cancer Research* **47** 4517–4519

Jordan VC, Lababidi MK and Mirecki SM (1990) The antioestrogeneic and antitumour properties of prolonged tamoxifen therapy in C3H/OUJ mice. *European Journal of Cancer* **26** 718–722

Jordan VC, Fritz NF, Thompson M, Langan-Fahey S and Tormey DC (1991a) Alteration of endocrine parameters in premenopausal women with breast cancer during long-term adjuvant tamoxifen nontherapy. *Journal of the National Cancer Institute* **83** 1488–1491

Jordan VC, Lababidi MK and Langan-Fahey SM (1991b) Suppression of mouse mammary tumorigenesis by long-term tamoxifen therapy. *Journal of the National Cancer Institute* **83** 492–495

Kaiser-Kupfer M and Lippman M (1978) Tamoxifen retinopathy. *Cancer Treatment Reports* **62** 315–320

Kaiser-Kupfer M, Kupfer C and Rodriques M (1981) Tamoxifen retinopathy: a clinicopathologic report. *Ophthalmology* **88** 89–93

Kaufman M, Jonat W, Albel U *et al* (1993) Adjuvant randomized trials of doxorubicin/cyclophosphamide versus doxorubicin/cyclophosphamide/tamoxifen and CMF chemotherapy versus tamoxifen in women with node-positive breast cancer. *Journal of Clinical Oncology* **11** 445–460

Kelsey JL, LiVolse VA, Holford TR *et al* (1982) A case-control study of cancer of the endometrium. *American Journal of Epidemiology* **116** 333–342

Killackey MA, Hakes TB and Pierce VK (1980) Endometrial adenocarcinoma in breast cancer patients receiving antiestrogens. *Cancer Treatment Reports* **69** 237–238

Longstaff S, Sigurdsson H, O'Keefe M, Ogston S and Preece P (1989) A controlled study of the ocular effects of tamoxifen in conventional dosage in the treatment of breast carcinoma. *European Journal of Cancer and Clinical Oncology* **25** 1805–1808

Love RR, Mazess RB, Tormey DC, Barden HS, Newcomb PA and Jordan VC (1988) Bone mineral density in women with breast cancer treated with adjuvant tamoxifen for at least two years. *Breast Cancer Research and Treatment* **12** 297–301

Love R, Cameron L, Connell B and Leventhal H (1991a) Symptoms associated with tamoxifen treatment in postmenopausal women. *Archives of Internal Medicine* **151** 1842–1847

Love RR, Wiebe D, Newcomb P *et al* (1991b) Effect of tamoxifen on cardiovascular risk factors in postmenopausal women. *Annals of Internal Medicine* **115** 860–864

Love RR, Mazess RB, Barden HS *et al* (1992a) Effect of tamoxifen on bone mineral density in postmenopausal women with breast cancer. *New England Journal of Medicine* **326** 852–856

Love R, Surawicz T and Williams E (1992b) Antithrombin III level, fibrinogen level, and platelet count changes with adjuvant tamoxifen therapy. *Archives of Internal Medicine* **152** 317–320

Magriples U, Naftolin F, Schwarz PE and Carcangiu ML (1993) High grade endometrial carcinoma in tamoxifen-treated breast cancer patients. *Journal of Clinical Oncology* **11** 485–490

Malfetano JH (1990) Tamoxifen-associated endometrial carcinoma in postmenopausal breast cancer patients. *Gynecologic Oncology* **39** 82–84

Mathew A, Chabon AB, Kabakow B, Drucker M and Hirschman RJ (1990) Endometrial carcinoma in five patients with breast cancer on tamoxifen therapy. *New York State Journal of Medicine* **90** 207–208

McDonald CC and Stewart HJ (1991) Fatal myocardial infarction in the Scottish adjuvant tamoxifen trial. *British Medical Journal* **303** 435–437

Meschter C, Kendall M, Rose DP *et al* (1991) Carcinogenicity of tamoxifen. *The Toxicologist* **11** 695

Miller AB, Howe GR, Sherman GS *et al* (1989) Mortality from breast cancer irradiation during fluoroscopic examinations in patients being treated for tuberculosis. *New England Journal of Medicine* **321** 1285–1289

Morrow M (1991) Pre-cancerous breast lesions: implications for breast cancer prevention trials. *International Journal of Radiation Oncology, Biology, Physics* **23** 1071–1078

Morrow M and Jordan VC (1992) Prospects for the prevention of breast cancer, In: Harris JR (ed). *Breast Diseases Update*, pp 1–12, Lippincott Health Care, Philadelphia

Navasaari K, Heikkinen M and Taskinen P (1978) Tamoxifen and thrombosis. *Lancet* **ii** 946–947

Neven P, DeMuylder Y, VanBelle Y, Vanderick G and DeMuylder E (1990) Hysteroscopic follow-up during tamoxifen treatment. *European Journal of Obstetrics, Gynecology and Reproductive Biology* **35** 235–238

Pavlidis NA, Petris C, Briassoulis E *et al* (1992) Clear evidence that long-term low-dose tamoxifen treatment can induce ocular toxicity. *Cancer* **69** 2961–2964

Pike MC, Ross RK, Lobo RA, Key TJ, Potts M and Henderson BE (1989) LHRH agonists and the prevention of breast and ovarian cancer. *British Journal of Cancer* **60** 142–148

Powles TJ, Hardy JR, Ashley SE *et al* (1989a) A pilot trial to evaluate the acute toxicity and feasibility of tamoxifen prevention in breast cancer. *British Journal of Cancer* **60** 126–131

Powles TJ, Hardy JR, Ashley SE *et al* (1989b) Chemoprevention of breast cancer. *Breast Cancer Research and Treatment* **14** 23–31

Powles TJ, Tillyer CR, Jones AL *et al* (1990) Prevention of breast cancer with tamoxifen—an update on the Royal Marsden Hospital pilot program. *European Journal of Cancer* **26** 680–684

Pugesgaard T and von Eyeben F (1986) Bilateral optic neuritis evolved during tamoxifen treatment. *Cancer* **58** 383–386

Ries LAB, Hankey BF and Edwards BK (eds) (1987) *Cancer Statistics Review 1983-1987*. National Cancer Institute Division of Cancer Prevention and Control Program, NIH Publication No 90-2789, Bethesda MD

Rossner S and Wallgren A (1984) Serum lipoproteins and proteins after breast cancer surgery and effects of tamoxifen. *Atherosclerosis* **52** 334–346

Rutqvist L, Cedermark, B, Glas VU *et al* (1991) Contralateral primary tumors in breast cancer patients in a randomized trial of adjuvant tamoxifen therapy. *Journal of the National Cancer Institutte* **83** 1299–1306

Ryan WG, Wolter J and Bagdade J (1991) Apparent beneficial effects of tamoxifen on bone mineral content in patients with breast cancer: preliminary study. *Osteoporosis International* **2** 39–41

Sullivan JM, Vander Zwaag R, Lemp GF *et al* (1988) Postmenopausal estrogen use and coronary atherosclerosis. *Annals of Internal Medicine* **108** 358–363

Sunderland MC and Osborne CK (1991) Tamoxifen in premenopausal patients with metastatic breast cancer: a review. *Journal of Clinical Oncology* **9** 1283–1297

Tokunaga M, Land CE, Yamamoto T *et al* (1987) Incidence of female breast cancer among atomic bomb survivors: Hiroshima and Nagasaki 1950-1980. *Radiation Research* **112** 243–272

Turken S, Siris E, Seldin D, Flaster E, Hyman G and Lindsay R (1989) Effects of tamoxifen on spinal bone density in women with breast cancer. *Journal of the National Cancer Institute* **81** 1086–1088

Ursin G, Spicer D and Pike M (1993) Tamoxifen and prevention. *Lancet* **341** 693–694

Vinding T and Nielsen N (1983) Retinopathy caused by treatment with tamoxifen in low dose. *Acta Ophthalmology* **61** 45–50

Wanless IR and Medline A (1982) Role of estrogens as promoters of hepatic neoplasia. *Laboratory Investigation* **46** 313–320

White INH, deMalteis F, Davis A *et al* (1993) Genotoxic potential of tamoxifen and analogs in female Fisher F344/n rats, DBA/2 and C57 BL/6 mice and in human HCL-5 cells. *Carcinogenesis* **14** 315–317

Williams GM, Iatropoulos MJ and Hard GC (1992) Long-term prophylactic use of tamoxifen: Is it safe? *European Journal of Cancer Prevention* **1** 386–387

Williams GM, Iatropoulos HJ, Djordjevic MV and Kaltenberg OP (1993) The triphenylethylene drug tamoxifen is a strong liver carcinogen in the rat. *Carcinogenesis* **14** 315–317

Wright CDP, Evans WD, Mansel RE *et al* (1990) Effect of long-term tamoxifen therapy on bone mass. *Bone* **11** 221

The authors are responsible for the accuracy of the references.

Biographical Notes

Jiri Bartek, MD, PhD, graduated from Palacky University, Olomouc, Czechoslovakia, in 1979 and received his PhD at the Institute of Molecular Genetics in Prague. He was awarded two ICRF visiting fellowships (in 1983 and 1988–1989) and fellowships at the German Cancer Centre in Heidelberg and CRC laboratories in Dundee. He headed the department of tumour biology at the Institute of Haematology in Prague and is now senior scientist at the Danish Cancer Society's division for cancer biology in Copenhagen. His work is focused on cell and molecular biology of tumour suppressors and aberrations of the cell cycle control in cancer cells.

Jirina Bartkova, MD, PhD, graduated from Palacky University, Olomouc, Czechoslovakia, in 1979 and trained in tumour pathology and cell biology at the Charles University in Prague. She was awarded an ICRF visiting fellowship in 1988. She joined the Danish Cancer Society in Copenhagen in 1993 as an assistant senior researcher in the department of cell cycle and cancer. Her research interests are the cell biology of epithelial cells and the molecular pathology of breast, colon and testicular cancer.

Els MJJ Berns obtained her BSc in biology in 1978 and her MSc in biology in 1981 at the University of Utrecht. In 1986 she received her PhD in biochemistry at Erasmus University in Rotterdam. After a 2 year postdoctoral research fellowship at Baylor College of Medicine, Houston, Texas, she joined the division of endocrine oncology at the Dr Daniel den Hoed Cancer Centre, Rotterdam, in 1988. Her main research interests are genetic alterations in endocrine independent solid tumours.

Sharon Brookes joined the ICRF in 1981 after graduating with honours from Bristol University. She worked first in the viral carcinogenesis laboratory and subsequently the molecular oncology laboratory, where she is now a senior scientific officer.

Joy Burchell is on the permanent staff of the ICRF, working in the epithelial cell biology laboratory. She has done pioneering work on the molecular and immunological analysis of the *MUC1* gene and the aberrant glycosylation of its product.

Robert Callahan graduated from Grove City College, Grove City, Pennsylvania, in 1965. He obtained a PhD in molecular biology and bacterial genetics under Elias Balbinder at Syracuse University in 1970, then became a Damon Runyon cancer research fellow in the National Institute of Child Health and Human Development, National Institutes of Health, until 1972 and subsequently a staff research fellow there until 1973. During this period he studied T7 bacteriophage and the in vitro translation of human adenovirus proteins. In 1973 he joined the National Cancer Institute (NCI). His interests during the next 7 years were the role of genetically transmitted and infectious retroviruses in the aetiology of cancer. In 1982 he joined the laboratory of tumour immunology and biology (NCI) as chief of the oncogenetics section. Over the past 13 years his major research interests have focused on the molecular pathology of breast cancer.

Clive Dickson is a principal scientist and head of the viral carcinogenesis laboratory at ICRF. He received his PhD training in the ICRF environmental carcinogenesis unit and spent 3 years as a postdoctoral fellow at the University of California in Berkeley before returning to ICRF in 1976. He was appointed to the permanent staff in 1979. He has a longstanding interest in mammary tumorigenesis, which encompasses the identification and characterization of *INT2/FGF3* and the amplification of the 11q13 region in human cancers.

231

Douglas Easton graduated in mathematics from Cambridge University and obtained a PhD in genetic epidemiology at the University of London. He now works at the Institute of Cancer Research in London. His major interests are the genetic epidemiology of cancer and other common diseases and the development of statistical methods for application to various problems in epidemiology and genetics.

Rosalind A Eeles is a medical graduate of Cambridge University and St Thomas's Hospital, London. Following her higher medical training she trained in radiotherapy and oncology at the Royal Marsden Hospital, London and Sutton. Her current research interests are genetic predisposition to cancer, in particular breast and prostate cancer. She has a particular interest in germline mutations in the *TP52* gene and together with Dr Mike Stratton has set up predictive *TP53* testing at the Royal Marsden Hospital. She is currently a clinical research fellow in molecular genetics and oncology in the CRC section of molecular carcinogenesis and academic unit of radiotherapy, Royal Marsden Hospital, Sutton.

Vera Fantl obtained her BSc from Westfield College, London, and worked at King's College Hospital before joining the ICRF in 1977 as a scientific officer in the clinical endocrinology laboratory. She was awarded a PhD degree from London University in 1987 and transferred to the viral carcinogenesis laboratory, where she is now a chief scientific officer.

Ian Fentiman graduated in medicine from the University of London in 1968. He trained in general surgery and became an FRCS in 1974. In 1975 he started work with Joyce Taylor-Papadimitriou and Sir Michael Stoker in the tumour cell laboratory at ICRF, receiving his MD from the University of London in 1978. He is now consultant surgeon at Guy's Hospital and is the deputy director of the ICRF clinical oncology unit. His research interests include treatment and prevention of breast cancer.

John A Foekens obtained his BSc in chemistry in 1974 and his MSc in biochemistry in 1977 from the University of Leiden. He received his PhD from Erasmus University, Rotterdam, in 1982. In 1985, following a 2 year postdoctoral research fellowship in Canada at the Cancer Control Agency of British Columbia, he was appointed head of the laboratory of tumour endocrinology at the Dr Danial den Hoed Cancer Centre in Rotterdam. His major research interests involve the study of prognostic factors in endocrine related cancers and the mechanism of action of hormones and growth factors in in vitro and in vivo model systems.

Deborah Ford received an MSc in statistics from the University of Southampton. In 1990 she joined the section of epidemiology at the Institute of Cancer Research, where the majority of her work has been in cancer genetics.

Rosalind Graham graduated from Leicester University in 1987 with a BSc in biological sciences. She obtained a PhD from Manchester University in 1992 and subsequently joined the epithelial cell biology laboratory at ICRF. Her research has focused on the development of preclinical mouse models for evaluation of *MUC1* based immunogens in tumour rejection and in stimulating an immune response.

Walter Gregory is senior lecturer in medical statistics at Guy's Hospital in the ICRF breast cancer unit. He graduated with a BSc in mathematics and philosophy from Nottingham University in 1977 and recently obtained a PhD at University College London. His main research interests have been in mathematical models relating duration of response in cancer patients following treatment to the underlying kinetics and biology of the disease.

Jeffrey T Holt, MD, is a graduate of Kalamazoo College and the University of Michigan School of Medicine. He trained in pathology at the University of Rochester and in 1983 became a research associate in the laboratory of Dr Arthur Nienhuis in the clinical haematology branch of the National Heart, Lung, and Blood Institute. During this time Dr Holt's work concentrated on the utilization of antisense RNA to study gene expression. In 1987 he was appointed assistant professor in the departments of cell biology and pathology at the Vanderbilt University School of

Medicine and was promoted to associate professor in 1991. His current research interests concern transcriptional regulation in neoplasia and in the identification of differentially expressed genes in cancer.

Roy A Jensen, MD, is an assistant professor in pathology and cell biology at Vanderbilt University School of Medicine. He received his MD at Vanderbilt and subsequently did his residency and fellowship in anatomical pathology at that institution. In 1988 he accepted a position as a biotechnology training fellow in the laboratory of Dr Stuart Aaronson at the National Cancer Institute. His current research interests concern the molecular and cellular biology of breast neoplasia and the identification of the growth control mechanisms in breast epithelial cells.

V Craig Jordan obtained BSc, PhD and DSc degrees from the University of Leeds department of pharmacology. From 1972 to 1974 he was a visiting scientist at the Worcester Foundation for Experimental Biology in Massachusetts before returning to Leeds as lecturer in pharmacology. Following his appointment as head of the endocrine unit for the Ludwig Institute for Cancer Research in Bern, Switzerland, he moved to the University of Wisconsin, Madison, where he is currently professor of human oncology and pharmacology and director of the breast cancer program for the Comprehensive Cancer Center.

Jan GM Klijn graduated in medicine at the University of Amsterdam in 1972 and trained in internal medicine and endocrinology at the academic hospital Dijkzigt of Erasmus University in Rotterdam, where he received his PhD in 1987. Since 1981 he has been head of the division of endocrine oncology, consisting of a clinical section and a laboratory of tumour endocrinology, at the Rotterdam Cancer Institute (Dr Danial den Hoed Kliniek). His main research interest is endocrine manipulation of cancer. He established a group working on preclinical and clinical applications of new endocrine treatment modalities and on cell biological prognostic factors. He has performed preclinical studies on LHRH analogues, somatostatin analogues and antiprogestins.

David P Lane graduated in microbiology from University College London, taking his PhD there in 1976 in the faculty of medicine. After a year as postdoctoral research fellow at ICRF, he lectured in zoology at Imperial College, London. From 1978 to 1980 he was Robertson research fellow, CRI fellow, at Cold Spring Harbor Laboratories, New York. He returned to Imperial College as lecturer from 1981 to 1985, moving to ICRF Clare Hall laboratories in 1985. In 1990 he was appointed professor of molecular oncology at the University of Dundee, where he is also director of the Cancer Research Campaign cell transformation research group.

Monica Morrow obtained BS and MD degrees from Penn State University and Jefferson Medical College, Philadelphia. She trained as a surgeon at the University of Vermont and completed a surgical oncology fellowship at the Memorial Sloan-Kettering Cancer Center, New York, in 1983. Following a faculty appointment at State University of New York, Down State Medical Center, New York, she moved to the University of Chicago, where she is currently associate professor of surgery and director of the multidisciplinary breast cancer programme.

David L Page, MD, received his medical training at Johns Hopkins University and subsequently received residency training at Vanderbilt University, Massachusetts General Hospital, the National Institutes of Health and Johns Hopkins University. He is currently director of anatomical pathology at Vanderbilt University Medical Center. Since the early 1970s he has had an interest in histological indicators of increased breast cancer risk. In 1979 he was a visiting professor at the University of Edinburgh, where he began a long and fruitful collaboration with Dr Thomas J Anderson. This collaboration resulted in the publication of *Diagnostic Histopathology of the Breast*, a widely used textbook in breast pathology.

Gordon Peters was an undergraduate at Aberdeen University and a postgraduate student at Edinburgh University before doing postdoctoral research at the University of Wisconsin. He became a research fellow at the ICRF in 1977 and was appointed to the permanent staff in 1983. He is currently a principal scientist and head of the molecular oncology laboratory, where the main focus of research has turned from *INT2/FGF3* to the mapping of human chromosome 11q13 and the biology of the D type cyclins.

Julian Peto is Cancer Research Campaign professor of epidemiology at the Institute of Cancer Research. In addition to cancer genetics his research interests include the aetiology of breast cancer, papillomaviruses and cervical cancer, industrial epidemiology and clinical trials.

R D Rubens is professor of clinical oncology at the United Medical and Dental Schools of Guy's and St Thomas's Hospitals, London. He is a consultant physician and honorary director of the ICRF unit at Guy's Hospital. His particular interest is in the treatment of breast cancer and he is the current chairman of the breast cancer cooperative group of the European Organization for Research and Treatment of Cancer.

David S Salomon is chief of the tumour growth factor section of the laboratory of tumour immunology and biology at the National Cancer Institute, National Institutes of Health. His major interest is the role of growth factors in the pathogenesis of breast and colon cancer. He obtained his PhD in developmental biology and biochemistry at the department of biological sciences, State University of New York, Albany, and was subsequently a postdoctoral fellow at the Roche Institute of Molecular Biology, where he studied the role of hormones and growth factors in pre- and postimplantation development in the mouse. In 1975 he moved to the National Institute of Dental Research at NIH in Dr George Martin's laboratory as a staff fellow, where he studied the interaction between different growth factors and the extracellular matrix. He went to the NCI in 1982.

Rosalind Smith obtained her BSc from Leeds University and is currently a chief scientific officer in the ICRF viral carcinogenesis laboratory, where she has worked since 1980. She was previously in the translation laboratory at ICRF.

Martha Stampfer trained in biology at Harvard University and received her PhD in cell biology from the Massachusetts Institute of Technology in 1972 under David Baltimore and Harvey Lodish. She did her postdoctoral training at the University of California, San Francisco, under the late Gordon Tomkins. In 1976 she joined the staff of the Lawrence Berkeley laboratory, where she began studies on development and characterization of a human mammary epithelial cell system.

Joyce Taylor-Papadimitriou is a principal scientist and head of the epithelial cell biology laboratory at ICRF central laboratories in Lincoln's Inn Fields, where her research is focused on various aspects of the cell and molecular biology of breast cancer. She graduated as a biochemist from Cambridge University and took her PhD in Toronto before spending some time at the Medical Research Council in Mill Hill, London, where she worked in virology and on the mechanism of action of interferon. She worked for several years in Greece as head of the virology department of the Theagenion Cancer Institute, where she pursued her interest in interferon. She began her research in breast cancer when she came to the ICRF in 1974.

Paul Yaswen trained in biology at Tufts University and received his PhD in cell and molecular biology from Brown University under Nelson Fausto. He did his postdoctoral training at the Dana-Farber Cancer Institute and Lawrence Berkeley laboratory. He became a staff scientist at Lawrence Berkeley laboratory in 1990 and is currently studying molecular aspects of mammary epithelial cell differentiation.

Index

235

LIST OF PREVIOUS ISSUES

VOLUME 1 1982

No. 1: Inheritance of Susceptibility to Cancer in Man
Guest Editor: W F Bodmer

No. 2: Maturation and Differentiation in Leukaemias
Guest Editor: M F Greaves

No. 3: Experimental Approaches to Drug Targeting
Guest Editors: A J S Davies and M J Crumpton

No. 4: Cancers Induced by Therapy
Guest Editor: I Penn

VOLUME 2 1983

No. 1: Embryonic & Germ Cell Tumours in Man and Animals
Guest Editor: R L Gardner

No. 2: Retinoids and Cancer
Guest Editor: M B Sporn

No. 3: Precancer
Guest Editor: J J DeCosse

No. 4: Tumour Promotion and Human Cancer
Guest Editors: T J Slaga and R Montesano

VOLUME 3 1984

No. 1: Viruses in Human and Animal Cancers
Guest Editors: J Wyke and R Weiss

No. 2: Gene Regulation in the Expression of Malignancy
Guest Editor: L Sachs

No. 3: Consistent Chromosomal Aberrations and Oncogenes in Human Tumours
Guest Editor: J D Rowley

No. 4: Clinical Management of Solid Tumours in Childhood
Guest Editor: T J McElwain

VOLUME 4 1985

No. 1: Tumour Antigens in Experimental and Human Systems
Guest Editor: L W Law

No. 2: Recent Advances in the Treatment and Research in Lymphoma and Hodgkin's Disease
Guest Editor: R Hoppe

No. 3: Carcinogenesis and DNA Repair
Guest Editor: T Lindahl

No. 4: Growth Factors and Malignancy
Guest Editors: A B Roberts and M B Sporn

VOLUME 5 1986

No. 1: Drug Resistance
Guest Editors: G Stark and H Calvert

No. 2: Biochemical Mechanisms of Oncogene Activity: Proteins Encoded by Oncogenes
Guest Editors: H E Varmus and J M Bishop

No. 3: Hormones and Cancer: 90 Years after Beatson
Guest Editor: R D Bulbrook

No. 4: Experimental, Epidemiological and Clinical Aspects of Liver Carcinogenesis
Guest Editor: E Farber

VOLUME 6 1987

No. 1: Naturally Occurring Tumours in Animals as a Model for Human Disease
Guest Editors: D Onions and W Jarrett

No. 2: New Approaches to Tumour Localization
Guest Editor: K Britton

No. 3: Psychological Aspects of Cancer
Guest Editor: S Greer

No. 4: Diet and Cancer
Guest Editors: C Campbell and L Kinlen

VOLUME 7 1988

No. 1: Pain and Cancer
Guest Editor: G W Hanks

No. 2: Somatic Cell Genetics and Cancer
Guest Editor: L M Franks

No. 3: Prospects for Primary and Secondary Prevention of Cervix Cancer
Guest Editors: G Knox and C Woodman

No. 4: Tumour Progression and Metastasis
Guest Editor: I Hart

VOLUME 8 1989

No. 1: Colorectal Cancer
Guest Editor: J Northover

No. 2: Nitrate, Nitrite and Nitroso Compounds in Human Cancer
Guest Editors: D Forman and D E G Shuker

No. 3: A Critical Assessment of Cancer Chemotherapy
Guest Editor: A H Calvert

No. 4: Biological Response Modifiers
Guest Editors: F R Balkwill and W Fiers

VOLUME 9 1990

No. 1: Haemopoietic Growth Factors: Their Role in the Treatment of Cancer
Guest Editor: M Dexter

No. 2: Germ Cell Tumours of the Testis: A Clinico-Pathological Perspective
Guest Editors: P Andrews and T Oliver

No. 3: Genetics and Cancer— Part I
Guest Editors: W Cavenee, B Ponder and E Solomon

No. 4: Genetics and Cancer— Part II
Guest Editors: W Cavenee, B Ponder and E Solomon

VOLUME 10 1991

Cancer, HIV and AIDS
Guest Editors: V Beral, H W Jaffe and R A Weiss

VOLUME 11 1991

Prostate Cancer: Cell and Molecular Mechanisms in Diagnosis and Treatment
Guest Editor: J T Isaacs

VOLUME 12 1992

Tumour Suppressor Genes, the Cell Cycle
and Cancer
Guest Editor: A J Levine

VOLUME 13 1992

A New Look at Tumour Immunology
Guest Editors: A J McMichael and W F Bodmer

VOLUME 14 1992

Growth Regulation by Nuclear Hormone Receptors
Guest Editor: M G Parker

VOLUME 15 1992

Oncogenes in the Development of Leukaemia
Guest Editor: O N Witte

VOLUME 16 1993

The Molecular Pathology of Cancer
Guest Editors: N R Lemoine and N A Wright

VOLUME 17 1993

Pharmacokinetics and Cancer Chemotherapy
Guest Editors: P Workman and M A Graham